Resilient Grandparent Caregivers

The study of grandparents raising grandchildren, now almost two decades old, has tended to have a negative bias, emphasizing the difficulties such people face and the negative impact that grandparent caregiving has on them physically, socially, and emotionally. This edited book seeks to reverse this trend by taking a positive approach to understanding grandparent caregivers, focusing on their resilience and resourcefulness. This method reflects a strengths-based approach and the importance of benefit-finding and positive coping. Chapters feature information from both qualitative and quantitative studies and are written by a diverse range of professionals, such as counselors, psychologists, geriatric social workers, and nurse practitioners, to provide multidisciplinary perspectives for practitioners working with grandparent caregivers. Part I discusses the positive qualities that custodial grandparents possess—resilience, resourcefulness, and benefit finding. The second part considers the sociocultural aspects of resilience and resourcefulness in grandparent caregivers. Finally, Part III presents strengths-based interventions for working with custodial grandparents. Practitioners will find this to be a valuable resource in their work and the field as a whole, stimulating positive changes in attitudes toward and practices with grandparent caregivers.

Bert Hayslip, Jr., PhD, is a professor in the Department of Psychology at the University of North Texas.

Gregory C. Smith, PhD, is a professor and the director of the Human Development Center at Kent State University.

Resilient Grandparent Caregivers

A Strengths-Based Perspective

Edited by
Bert Hayslip, Jr. and Gregory C. Smith

Routledge
Taylor & Francis Group
NEW YORK AND LONDON

First published 2013
by Routledge
711 Third Avenue, New York, NY 10017

Simultaneously published in the UK
by Routledge
27 Church Road, Hove, East Sussex BN3 2FA

Routledge is an imprint of the Taylor & Francis Group, an informa business

Library of Congress Cataloging in Publication Data
Resilient grandparent caregivers : a strengths-based perspective / [edited by]
Bert Hayslip, Jr. and Gregory C. Smith.
p. cm.
Includes bibliographical references and index.
1. Grandparents as parents–United States. 2. Caregivers–United States.
3. Intergenerational relations–United States. 4. Custody of children–United States.
I. Hayslip, Bert. II. Smith, Gregory C., 1951–
HQ759.9.R475 2013
306.874'50973–dc23

2012023105

ISBN: 978-0-415-89754-9 (hbk)
ISBN: 978-0-415-89755-6 (pbk)
ISBN: 978-0-203-80390-5 (ebk)

Typeset in Minion
by Graphicraft Limited, Hong Kong

To my wonderful granddaughter, Kemble Kate Hayslip

To Dorothy and Carl Smith, whose love and support as parents and grandparents have contributed in so many ways to this volume

Contents

About the Editors

Dr. Bert Hayslip, Jr. received his doctorate in Experimental Developmental Psychology from the University of Akron in 1975. After teaching at Hood College in Frederick, MD for three years, he joined the faculty at the University of North Texas, where he is now Regents Professor of Psychology. Dr. Hayslip is a Fellow of the American Psychological Association, the Gerontological Society of America, and The Association for Gerontology in Higher Education, and has held research grants from the National Institute on Aging, The Hilgenfeld Foundation, and the National Endowment for the Humanities. He is currently Associate Editor of *Experimental Aging Research*, Editor of *The International Journal of Aging and Human Development*, and is Associate Editor of *Developmental Psychology*. His published research deals with cognitive processes in aging, interventions to enhance cognitive functioning in later life, personality-ability interrelationships in aged persons, grandparents who raise their grandchildren, grief and bereavement, hospice care, death anxiety, and mental health and aging. He is coauthor of *Hospice Care* (Sage, 1992), *Psychology and Aging: An Annotated Bibliography* (Greenwood, 1995), *Grandparents Raising Grandchildren: Theoretical, Empirical, and Clinical Perspectives* (Springer, 2000), *Adult Development and Aging* (Krieger, 2011), *Working with Custodial Grandparents* (Springer, 2003), *Cultural Changes in Attitudes toward Death, Dying, and Bereavement* (Springer, 2005), *Diversity among Custodial Grandparents* (Springer, 2006), and *Parenting the Custodial Grandchild: Implications for Clinical Practice* (Springer, 2008). He recently completed a focus group study of rural and urban grandparent caregivers detailing their needs and concerns, funded by the North Central Texas Area Agency on Aging. He recently received as a Co-PI a grant from the National Institute of Nursing Research to examine the impact of several clinical interventions on grandparent caregiver and grandchild well-being.

Dr. Gregory C. Smith earned his doctorate in Human Development (Specialization in Psychology of Adult Development and Aging) from the University of Rochester, a master's in Psychology from Villanova University, and a bachelor's in Psychology from the State University of New York. Since 2001, he has been Professor of Human Development, Family Studies, & Gerontology and Director of the Human Development Center at Kent State University. He is also on the

Graduate Faculty in the Department of Psychology. He came to KSU after five years as Research Associate in the Ringel Institute of Gerontology (Nelson A. Rockefeller College of Public Affairs and Policy, University at Albany) and 11 years as a tenured faculty member in the Department of Human Development (University of Maryland, College Park). His applied experiences include internships in rehabilitation psychology and gerontological counseling, and serving as Special Administrative Assistant in a multi-level care gerontology center. He is a Fellow of the Gerontological Society of America, a member of the Board of Trustees for the Ohio Association of Gerontology & Education, and Associate Editor of the *International Journal of Aging and Human Development*, and a peer reviewer on various NIH study sections. His primary research focus is on caregiving issues within aging families, and he has been the PI and C0-PI of studies funded by the National Institute on Aging, the National Institute of Mental Health, and the National Institute of Nursing Research. He recently received as a Co-PI a grant from the National Institute of Nursing Research to examine the impact of several clinical interventions on grandparent caregiver and grandchild well-being.

Contributors

Araceli Alvarez-Nunez, MSW, Pacific Clinics, Santa Fe Springs, CA

Sandra J. Bailey, PhD, CFLE, Department of Health and Human Development, Montana State University, Boseman, MT

Kimberly Bundy-Fazioli, LCSW, PhD, School of Social Work, Colorado State University, Fort Collins, CO

Peter E. Campos, PhD, Project Healthy Grandparents, Georgia State University, Atlanta, GA

Gloria F. Carr, PhD Loewenberg School of Nursing, University of Memphis, Memphis, TN

Katherine D. Castillo, MA, Department of Psychology, Sam Houston State University, Huntsville, TX

Nathan S. Consedine, PhD, Department of Psychological Medicine, The University of Auckland, School of Medicine, Auckland, New Zealand

Francine Conway, PhD, Derner Institute of Advanced Psychological Studies, Adelphi University, Garden City, NY

Linda L. Dannison, PhD, Department of Family and Consumer Sciences, Western Michigan University, Kalamazoo, MI

Shanna R. Davis, MS, Department of Psychology, University of North Texas, Denton, TX

Megan L. Dolbin-MacNab, PhD, LMFT, Department of Human Development, Virginia Polytechnic Institute and State University, Blacksburg, VA

Minde Erickson, MS, Department of Health and Human Development Montana State University, Boseman, MT

Patricia Ernandez, MSW, Kaiser Permanente, Tri-Central Hospice/Palliative Care, Harbor City, CA

Christopher R. Ferrante, MA, Department of Psychology, Pacific University, Portland, Oregon

Lisa A. Ferretti, LMSW, State University of New York, Center for Excellence in Aging Services, School of Social Welfare, Albany, NY

Jack W. Finney, PhD, Department of Psychology, Virginia Polytechnic Institute and State University, Blacksburg, VA

Christine A. Fruhauf, PhD, Department of Human Development & Family Studies Colorado State University, Fort Collins, CO

Catherine Goodman, DSW, School of Social Work, California State University-Long Beach, Long Beach, CA

Heather Greenwood, MA, University of Hawaii at Manoa Cooperative Extension, University of Manoa, Manoa, HI

Bert Hayslip Jr., PhD, Department of Psychology, University of North Texas, Denton, TX

Craig E. Henderson, PhD, Department of Psychology, Sam Houston State University, Huntsville, TX

Sarah A. Himmelheber, MSW, School of Social Work, University of Georgia, Atlanta, GA

Linda C. James, Family Resource Centers of Crestwood Children's Center, Hillside Family of Agencies, Rochester, NY

Melodye James, MA, Department of Human Development & Family Studies Colorado State University, Fort Collins, CO

Susan J. Kelley, PhD, Byrdine F. Lewis School of Nursing and Health Professions, Georgia State University, Atlanta, GA

Jwakym Kim, MSW, State University of New York, Center for Excellence in Aging Services, School of Social Welfare, Albany, NY

Stacey R. Kolomer, PhD, School of Social Work, University of Georgia, Atlanta, GA

Rebecca Koltz, PhD, Department of Health and Human Development, Montana State University, Bozeman, MT

Bethany L. Letiecq, PhD, Department of Health and Human Development, Montana State University, Boseman, MT

Robert J. Maiden, PhD, Department of Psychology, Alfred University, Alfred, NY

Philip McCallion, PhD State University of New York, Center for Excellence in Aging Services, School of Social Welfare, Albany, NY

Cara V. Murray, MSW, Children's Healthcare of Atlanta, Atlanta, GA

Carol M. Musil, PhD, RN, FAAN, FGSA, Frances Payne Bolton School of Nursing, Case Western Reserve University, Cleveland, OH

Craig S. Neumann, PhD, Department of Psychology, University of North Texas, Denton, TX

Lindsey W. North, MA, Department of Psychology, Sam Houston State University, Huntsville, TX

Karen A. Roberto, PhD, Center for Gerontology and Institute for Society, Culture, and the Environment, Virginia Polytechnic Institute and State University, Blacksburg, VA

Dolores Scorzo, MSG, SCAN Health Plan, Long Beach, CA

Andrea B. Smith, PhD, College of Education, Western Michigan University, Kalamazoo, MI

Gregory C. Smith, PhD, College of Health, Education, and Human Services, Kent State University, Kent, OH

Deborah M. Whitley, PhD, School of Social Work, Georgia State University, Atlanta, GA

Loriena A. Yancura, PhD, Department of Family and Consumer Science, University of Hawaii at Manoa, Manoa, HI

Jaclene A. Zauszniewski, PhD, RN-BC, FAAN, Frances Payne Bolton School of Nursing, Case Western Reserve University, Cleveland, OH

Craig Zuckerman, PhD Department of Counselor Education, St. Bonaventure University, St. Bonaventure, NY

Foreword

"Joey is my cruise." Adrian, Joey's grandmother, concluded her remarks at the National Press Club smiling as she explained she felt isolated from many of her peer group as they set out on cruises to exotic locations. Instead she spends her days raising her 12-year-old grandson and caregiving for her husband and mother. She said she cruises everyday to the doctors, to school and elsewhere and she wouldn't have it any other way. Joey is her masterpiece.

Grandfamilies, families in which grandparents and other relatives are raising children, face complex, multiple challenges. They come together suddenly, often without warning, such as the case of the grandmother I once met in Kansas City. With her last child grown and out of the house, she redecorated, turning her condo into the dream home she'd always wanted. White carpets and crystal figurines in the living room, it was a perfect place for a single woman. Then the knock came in the middle of the night. The authorities walked in with her two young grandchildren. The figurines were boxed up and put in the closet and white carpet didn't last long. Dreams deferred.

These grandparents make tremendous sacrifices to care for another generation and yet I've never met a grandparent who said they wouldn't take their grandchild in when faced with raising the child or turning the child over to the state. As another grandparent said "Other people don't realize how hard it is, or how gratifying it is." Grandparents know a child ages out of a system but never ages out of a family.

When Generations United stepped to the forefront in 1996 and joined national children, youth and aging organizations to raise a positive profile of grandfamilies and advocate for supportive policies, the landscape was much bleaker than today. Media portrayals painted the families as broken, perpetuating intergenerational cycles of poverty (the apple doesn't fall far from the tree) and raising the children only because of the benefits they would receive to do so. One article was particularly infuriating, calling the caregivers "country club grandparents" because they would get a "child only" grant of $116 each month to care for a child. $116? Since I don't golf, I asked a friend what $116 would get you at a country club. She said not much—no green fees, caddie or dinner and cocktails afterwards. Yet that relatively tiny amount was supposed to be enough to feed a child, clothe a child and put a roof over a child's head.

The media coverage in recent years has more accurately told the tale. A front-page story in the *Wall Street Journal* hit an entirely different note. With the caption, "Grandfamilies come under pressure," the article explored the impact of the economy on these families, acknowledging they play a critical role in caring for our country's children. Ironically, while these families struggle to stretch their limited incomes, they are saving the government significant amounts of money. In fact, over ten years ago Generations United crunched an important number. We conservatively estimated that if even half of the children raised by grandparents outside the formal foster care system were to enter that system, it would cost our country more than 6.5 billion dollars a year.

We've come a long way, but have miles to go. With this book, Bert Hayslip and Gregory Smith are giving a welcome boost to persuasive arguments by demonstrating how grandfamilies use their resiliency and resourcefulness to overcome challenges. The authors of each chapter have explored existing research and evaluation and programmatic examples. From that exploration, they have developed a valuable platform focused on the strengths of the caregivers, children and youth who are members of "grand" families. Essentially their message to policy makers is this: grandfamilies not only deserve our respect, they deserve our support. They understand that fragmented policies and services can wear down even the most stalwart grandparents and advocates. And they recommend that rather than ignore grandfamilies' needs as well as strengths, we should conduct more research and promote wider implementation of grandfamily-friendly policies and evidence-based programs. That way, grandfamilies will have the wherewithal to do what they do best: raise healthy children who contribute to our economic and societal strength.

This book on resilient grandparent caregivers conveys the importance of weaving a continuum of supports for grandfamilies. As with all families, they have multiple generations and unique problems and strengths. One family may only need occasional respite, while another needs help accessing health care and yet another needs a home big enough to house a larger family. Relative caregivers can be amazingly resourceful. Take Kirk Franklin's aunt for example. Born in Fort Worth, Texas, to a teenage mother, Franklin never knew his father and was adopted at the age of three by the only mother he ever really knew—his great-aunt Gertrude. At an early age, she took special interest in assisting Franklin to develop his interest in music. She and her young nephew would collect cans and newspapers to recycle. They used that money to fund his piano lessons beginning at age four. Her commitment to helping him find his passion has resulted in Franklin receiving numerous awards including the two Grammy's he received at the 54th Annual Grammy Awards for Best Gospel Song and Best Gospel Album. There's no doubt that great-aunt Gertrude was on his mind as he accepted these awards. "She taught me everything. She taught me how to respect people and respect myself, and that's something I'll never forget."

Is Kirk Franklin an exception? How do the children raised in grandfamilies fare? The authors have explored this nascent area of study, and others of us continue to collect stories that help shine a light on the successful products of grandfamilies. It bolsters the children and inspires their caregivers to know their sacrifices will yield positive results in the end. Another of those stories is that of President Barrack Obama. When accepting the nomination of his party he said, "My grandmother . . . she's the one who taught me about hard work. She's the one who put off buying a new car or a new dress for herself so that I could have a better life. She poured everything she had into me. And although she can no longer travel, I know that she's watching tonight and that tonight is her night, as well."

In 1948, the United Nations declared: "The family is the natural and fundamental group unit of society and is entitled to protection by society and the State." It would be easy for grandparents to give up. Given the difficulties they face it would be understandable. The fact they don't give up is a sign of real strength, real ability to cope and a testament to the power of love.

Another testament to that power occurred back at the National Press Club. After his grandmother finished speaking, Joey took the stage. He answered questions about his family and told a story about a recent Sunday morning when he fed the dog and cat and brought his grandmother coffee and the paper in bed telling her she could have an easy day. When asked why he did such a thoughtful thing he said, "She works a lot for me and does a lot for the family. I'll pay her back one day, so I might as well do it now." Grandfamilies are resilient, resourceful, strong and indeed, grand.

Donna M. Butts, Executive Director, Generations United
February 11, 2012

Preface

Gerontologists often emphasize the salience of loss and more generally maladaptive coping in understanding the aging process. Indeed, the study of grandparents raising grandchildren, while almost two decades old, largely reflects this negative bias in documenting the difficulties such persons face and more often than not, focusing on the negative impact that grandparent caregiving has on them physically, socially, and emotionally. *Resilient Grandparent Caregivers: A Strengths-Based Perspective* takes a positive approach to understanding grandparent caregivers in emphasizing their resilience and resourcefulness to reflect a strengths-based approach to caregiving as well as the importance of benefit finding and positive coping that characterizes many grandparent caregivers. The multidisciplinary chapters that define this book are organized into (1) those emphasizing the positive qualities that custodial grandparents possess, i.e., resilience, resourcefulness, and benefit finding, viewing resilience as a personal attribute or characteristic, as well as an ongoing process of adaptation to change, (2) those seeking to understand such qualities in the larger context of grandparents' relationships with others, and (3) intervention-based work taking a strengths-based approach with grandparent caregivers. Both qualitative and quantitative approaches are included as are projects that are descriptive and intervention-oriented. Each chapter is written/co-written by a practitioner (e.g., geriatric social worker, nurse practitioner, counselor, psychologist, geriatrician) to ensure that its focus is an applied one—to stress not only the understanding of resilience—its dispositional, process-oriented, and interpersonal aspects —among grandparent caregivers, but also stressing the understanding and implementation of interventions whose purpose it is to maintain or enhance resilience among grandparent caregivers.

The first section of *Resilient Grandparent Caregivers: A Strengths-Based Perspective* addresses questions regarding the nature of resilience as a personal attribute or characteristic as well as a process. It explores related constructs, e.g., those of resourcefulness and benefit finding, as well as their relationships to a variety of indicators of well-being in grandparent caregivers. Its focus is on understanding resilience in grandparent caregivers: its antecedents and its consequences. It allows us to more clearly see the advantages of being a resilient caregiver, in contrast to a deficit-oriented approach which has characterized much of the work with grandparent caregivers to date. Questions that are addressed in this section relate to for example, how does resilience manifest itself in grandparent caregivers? Do they think about their roles in a positive manner? Is this beneficial to them and their grandchildren? What is it about grandparent caregiving that enhances their well-being, happiness, mental or physical health, or cognitive functioning? Do grandparents who are better problem solvers or who are more spiritual function more adaptively in the context of the demands of their role? What are the ways that resilient grandparents think about their roles and the impact of these roles on them? How does successful parenting impact the well-being of grandparent caregivers and grandchildren? How do resilient grandparents adjust to their new roles as parents? What self-care skills do resilient grandparent caregivers employ?

Part II of *Resilient Grandparent Caregivers* addresses resilience in the context of relationships with others. It examines resilience in terms of the support that grandparents receive from others as well as the support that they might provide to one another. Questions that this section addresses relate to: How is resilience expressed in terms of relationships with others among grandparent caregivers? How does the support grandparent caregivers can provide to one another both reflect and contribute to resilience? How can the transmission of cultural values be an expression of resilience?

Part III of *Resilient Grandparent Caregivers* addresses the question of how we might enhance resilience and benefit finding among grandparent caregivers. It therefore directly speaks to interventions with grandparent caregivers to enhance resilience. How might such interventions be designed with grandparent caregivers in mind? What social policies work for or against such efforts? How can grandparent caregivers be empowered to enhance their resilience? How can increasing knowledge about community resources enhance this sense of empowerment? How can we educate grandparent caregivers to better attend to their health? How can mental health practitioners work to enhance resilience of grandparents and grandchildren? How might a strengths-based approach to working with custodial grandparents be designed? What might its effects be?

Clearly, our intention and hope is that this book will ultimately stimulate practice and policy, and to an extent, research pertaining to grandparent caregivers that emphasizes what they are doing *right*—how they are coping positively and indeed growing from the experience of raising a grandchild, rather than focusing on the negative impact that caregiving has on them and stressing the difficulties they are facing in caring for a grandchild. We hope that it will be a valuable resource for those professionals and practitioners who work with grandparents raising grandchildren: educators, counselors, social service providers, and social workers.

Bert Hayslip Jr.
Gregory C. Smith

Part I

Resilience and Resourcefulness Among Grandparent Caregivers

1 The Role of Negative and Positive Caregiving Appraisals in Key Outcomes for Custodial Grandmothers and Grandchildren[1]

Gregory C. Smith and Megan L. Dolbin-MacNab

Abstract

To conceptualize how custodial grandmothers' positive and negative appraisals of their caregiving responsibilities impact their psychological well-being, parenting behavior, and the adjustment of their grandchildren, we present a model integrating the Family Stress Model (Conger, Reuter, & Conger, 2000) and the two-factor model of caregiving appraisals and adjustment (Lawton, Moss, Kleban, Glicksman, & Rovine, 1991). In addition, we draw on data from a sample of custodial grandmothers to examine the extent to which the proposed integrated model has empirical support. Study findings lend support to our integrated model, and suggest that how grandmothers appraise their caregiving situations influences their psychological well-being and, in turn, their parenting. Dysfunctional parenting was associated with greater grandchild total difficulties and prosocial behavior. Implications for practitioners are addressed.

Introduction

As the number of families in which grandparents are raising their grandchildren continues to grow (Kreider & Ellis, 2011), there has been increased interest in the adjustment of the grandchildren (e.g., Billing, Ehrle, & Kortenkamp, 2002; Dolbin-MacNab & Keiley, 2009; Smith & Palmieri, 2007; Solomon & Marx, 1995). These children often struggle with a variety of internalizing and externalizing problems including depression, anxiety, reactive attachment disorder, aggression, hyperactivity, inattention, and impulsivity (Grant, Gordon, & Cohen, 1997). Evidence further suggests that custodial grandchildren experience these problems at higher rates than normative samples (Smith & Palmieri, 2007). With increased recognition of the difficulties facing custodial grandchildren, attempts have been made to gain insight into factors that influence grandchildren's well-being. Two sets of factors that may be particularly relevant to the adjustment of custodial grandchildren are grandparents' parenting behaviors and grandparents' psychological adjustment (Hayslip, Shore, Henderson, & Lambert, 1998; Sands & Goldberg-Glen, 2000; Smith & Hancock, 2010; Smith, Palmieri, Hancock, & Richardson, 2008; Smith & Richardson, 2008; Young & Dawson, 2003).

Unfortunately, to date, much of the literature on custodial grandfamilies has emphasized stressors and negative outcomes. While there is little question that grandparents experience a variety of stressors (Hayslip & Kaminski, 2005) that lead to psychological distress and other negative outcomes (see, for example, Hughes, Waite, LaPierre, & Luo, 2007; Minkler & Fuller-Thomson, 1999; Minkler, Fuller-Thomson, Miller, & Driver, 1997), there are also positive aspects of the caregiving arrangement for both grandparents (Hayslip & Kaminski, 2005; Hughes et al., 2007) and their grandchildren (Dolbin-MacNab & Keiley, 2009; Dolbin-MacNab, Rodgers, & Traylor, 2009). For example, grandchildren often report that being raised by their grandparents has given them more opportunities and put them on a better trajectory for the rest of their lives (Dolbin-MacNab & Keiley, 2009; Dolbin-MacNab et al., 2009). Similarly, grandparents' love for and commitment to their grandchildren can lend value and satisfaction to the caregiving role, as does grandparents' knowledge that they are contributing to a better life for their grandchildren (Hayslip & Kaminski, 2005). Thus, raising grandchildren can be a mixed valence experience for grandparents that includes both positive and negative emotions and outcomes.

Given that the experience of raising grandchildren is not entirely negative or positive, it becomes important to learn more about those grandparents and grandchildren who are resilient in the face of multiple stressors. One prominent definition refers to resilience as the "capacity to maintain, or regain, psychological well-being in the face of challenge" (Ryff, Friedman, Morozink, & Tsenkova, in press, pp. 3–4). The resilience literature suggests that there are a large number of individual attributes, relationships, and external support systems that are protective and promote individual resilience (Garmezy, 1985; Ong, Bergeman, & Boker, 2009; Smith & Hayslip, in press). These resilience factors reflect not only the absence of negative characteristics and stressors, but also the presence of positive influences (Ryff et al., in press). One potential resilience factor, which is the focus of this chapter, is appraisals, or whether grandparents interpret their caregiving situation positively or negatively (Lawton, Moss, Kleban, Glicksman, & Rovine, 1991). Of particular interest is grandparents' positive appraisals and how they influence their psychological well-being, their parenting behavior, and ultimately, their grandchildren's adjustment.

A Proposed Model of Family Stress and Resilience

To examine how custodial grandmothers' appraisals of their caregiving responsibilities impact their psychological well-being, parenting behavior, and the adjustment of their grandchildren, in this chapter, we present a model integrating the Family Stress Model (FSM; Conger, Reuter, & Conger, 2000) and the two-factor model of caregiving appraisals and adjustment (TFM; Lawton et al., 1991). In addition to providing an overview of this integrated model, we also use data from a sample of custodial grandmothers to examine the extent to which the model has empirical support. Our integrated model improves on previous theorizing and research in that it provides a dynamic explanation for grandparents' psychological well-being while, at the same time, capturing the interdependent nature of the grandparent-grandchild relationship. Identifying the mechanisms by which grandparents impact their custodial grandchildren is essential for practitioners interested in identifying ways to promote resilience for grandparents and grandchildren alike.

In our integrated model (see Figure 1.1), the FSM (Conger et al., 2000) helps to explain how grandparent well-being influences grandchildren's adjustment. According to the FSM, stressors result in caregivers experiencing psychological difficulties such as depression or anxiety. Psychological distress then leads to caregivers displaying less effective parenting behaviors toward their children. This dysfunctional parenting behavior, in turn, results in increased child difficulties. Previous studies with grandparents raising grandchildren have established that grandparents' psychological distress is associated with elevated levels of grandchild behavior problems (Hayslip et al., 1998; Young & Dawson, 2003; Sands & Goldberg-Glen, 2000). Additional research based on the FSM with custodial grandparents has demonstrated that the linkage between grandparents' psychological distress and grandchildren's maladjustment is indirect

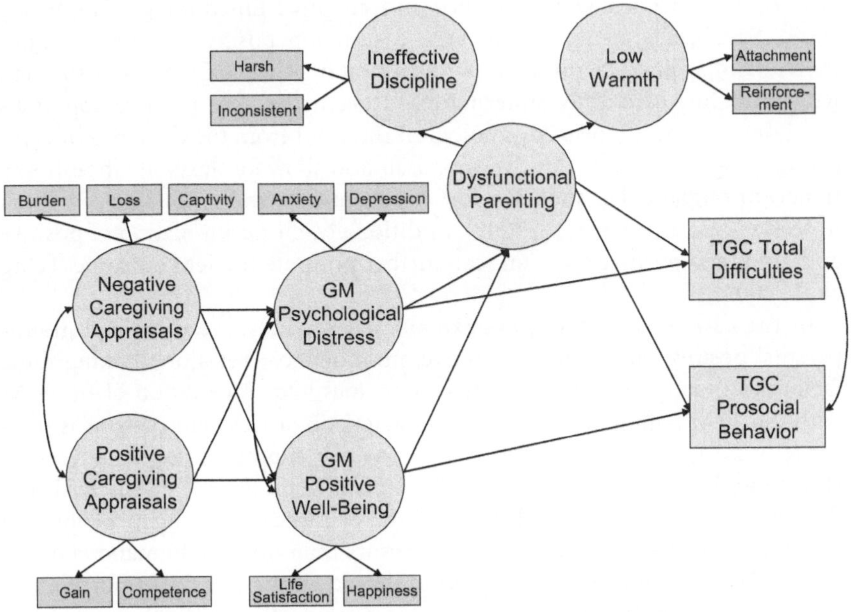

Figure 1.1 The hypothesized structural and measurement model

through grandparents' ineffective parenting behaviors (Smith et al., 2008; Smith & Hancock, 2010). Based on these studies, it appears that the FSM is a useful means for conceptualizing familial influences on grandchild adjustment—those grandchildren raised by grandparents with higher levels of psychological distress are likely to experience dysfunctional parenting and, in turn, greater emotional and behavioral problems.

While the FSM (Conger et al., 2000) helps conceptualize the intersection between grandparent psychological distress and grandchild adjustment, it does not explain resilience within these families. That is, the FSM fails to consider how positive outcomes can still occur for grandparents and grandchildren, despite their experience of considerable stressors and high levels of risk. By integrating the TFM (Lawton et al., 1991) into the FSM, a more complete conceptualization of the processes influencing custodial grandparent and grandchild resilience can emerge. The TFM holds that providing care is a mixed valence experience—it can be a positive experience, but caregiving may also be a stressor that creates additional demands and a sense of burden for grandparents (Lawton et al., 1991). Given this mixed valence nature of caregiving, the TFM would suggest that raising grandchildren is associated with appraisals and outcomes that can be either positive or negative in nature. Positive appraisals are said to be related to positive emotionality within caregivers, while negative appraisals are associated with negative emotionality and the demands and responsibilities of caregiving (Lawton et al., 1991).

Central to the focus of this chapter, although positive and negative appraisals are normative reactions to the demands of caregiving, positive appraisals have been associated with resilience and adaptive functioning (Ong et al., 2009). Specifically, being able to view a situation positively helps to buffer individuals against disruptions, stressors, and other difficulties associated with providing care. This buffering effect occurs because positive appraisals are thought to be a type of psychological time-out from the demands of caregiving (Ong et al., 2009). Positive appraisals also allow for flexibility in response to new or ongoing demands, support coping efforts, and encourage caregivers to seek resources (Ong et al., 2009). Additionally, the accumulation of positive appraisals and positive emotions can further promote resilient outcomes (Ong et al., 2009).

In the case of custodial grandparents, few studies have examined grandparents' positive appraisals or positive emotionality—let alone linking these factors to grandparent or grandchild outcomes. Our integration of the FSM with the TFM highlights that a key characteristic of "resilient persons is their capacity for generative experiences and positive appraisals despite adversity" (Bonanno, 2004; Bonanno, Westphal, & Mancini, in press, p. 10). Thus, resilience does not mean a complete absence of stress. Moreover, resilient people are not necessarily better at coping with stressors than others (Bonnano et al., in press). Our integration is meaningful in that it emphasizes the importance of considering the role of positive appraisals in promoting grandparent psychological well-being which, in turn, should enhance their parenting behavior and their grandchildren's positive adjustment.

To examine the extent to which there is empirical support for our integration of the FSM and the TFM, we used data from a sample of custodial grandmothers and the statistical technique of structural equation modeling (SEM; for more information about this approach see Byrne, 2006) to test our model (see Figure 1.1 for the measurement and structural models we examined). According to the basic tenets of the FSM, we hypothesized that the impact of custodial grandmothers' appraisals and psychological well-being on grandchild adjustment would be primarily indirect through their parenting behavior. In turn, and following the TFM, we hypothesized that model constructs of a similar valence (i.e., either positive or negative) would be more strongly related to each other than to model constructs of the opposite valence. More specifically, we hypothesized that negative appraisals of the caregiving situation would have a greater impact on grandmothers' psychological distress than on their positive psychological well-being. In contrast, we expected positive appraisals of the caregiving situation to have a greater impact on grandmothers' positive well-being than on grandmothers' psychological distress.

Study Overview

To test our integrative model empirically, we drew on data collected from 733 custodial grandmothers ($M = 56$ years, $SD = 8.1$) who had provided full-time care to a grandchild in the absence of the grandchild's parents for at least three months ($M = 6.4$ years of caregiving, $SD = 4.0$, Range = 3 months to 16 years). For this study, a target grandchild (TG) was also selected as the focus of investigation. In cases where there were multiple grandchildren, the TG was selected using the most recent birthday technique. The TG were 391 girls and 342 boys ($M = 9.8$ years, SD = 3.7, Range = 4 to 17 years). The majority (65.8%) of grandmothers were providing care to a TG born to a daughter. Most grandmothers reported multiple reasons for their raising the TG, with the majority of reasons concerning a crisis or tragedy within the parent generation. Some of these crises or tragedies included parental substance abuse (55.4%) or parental incarceration (42.6%). Other key demographic information regarding the grandmothers who participated in the study is provided in Table 1.1.

Grandmothers were recruited across the 48 contiguous states through a combination of convenience and population-based methods. Specifically, quota sampling was used to obtain a sample that was half Black and half White. Grandmothers were excluded if they were providing care due to the death of their own child. Further details regarding the recruitment of this sample can be found in Smith et al. (2008).

Measuring Model Constructs

The grandmothers completed a series of self-report questionnaires administered in a telephone interview conducted by professionally trained interviewers at a public research university in Ohio. Each of the indicators in our model (see the squares in Figure 1.1) was measured during the telephone interview.

Table 1.1 Descriptive Demographic Statistics of Grandmothers and Target Grandchildren (N = 733)

Variable	*n*	%
Marital Status		
Married	352	48.0
Divorced	159	21.7
Widowed	102	13.9
Single, Never Married	66	9.0
Separated	49	6.7
Living with Partner (Not Married)	5	0.7
Education		
Less than 5 years	5	0.7
5–8 years	19	2.6
Some High School	99	13.5
High School Graduate	205	28.0
Some College	260	35.5
College Graduate	95	13.0
Graduate/Professional Training	50	6.8
Residential Locale		
Urban	350	47.7
Rural	238	32.5
Suburban	141	19.2
Other	4	0.5
Work Status		
Not Working	202	27.6
Retired	144	19.6
Working Full or Part-Time	329	44.9
Full-Time Homemaker	41	5.6
Seeking Employment	17	2.3
Income		
Under $10,000	123	16.8
$10,000–$15,000	109	14.9
$16,000–$20,000	85	11.6
$21,000–$25,000	90	12.3
$26,000–$35,000	112	15.3
$36,000–$50,000	99	13.5
$51,000–$75,000	59	8.0
$76,000–$100,000	19	2.6
$101,000–$125,000	4	0.7
More than $125,000	5	0.7
Missing[a]	28	3.8
Target Grandchild Age		
4–7 years	235	32.1
8–10 years	194	26.5
11–14 years	206	28.1
15–17 years	98	13.4
Formal Legal Arrangements		
Formal Custody	271	37.0
Foster Parent Status	16	2.2
Adoption	90	12.3
Guardianship	215	29.3
Currently Seeking Legal Custody	69	9.4
None	72	9.8

Table 1.1 (cont'd)

Variable	*n*	%
Relationship of Target Grandchild's Parent to Grandmother		
Son	227	31.0
Step-Son	7	1.0
Daughter	482	65.8
Step-Daughter	16	2.2
Missing Data	1	0.1
Reasons for Care[a]		
Child abandonment	205	28.0
Physical or emotional abuse	201	27.4
Removed from parental custody	225	30.7
Parents' mental health problems	218	29.7
Parents' teen pregnancy	133	18.1
Parental substance abuse	406	55.4
Parents' incarceration	312	42.6
Parents' HIV-AIDS	11	1.5
Other (not AIDS) health problems	114	15.6
One of the parents deceased	47	6.4

[a]Missing data were less than 10 percent and mean substitution was used for imputation in the data analyses.
[b]Respondents were asked to report any and all reasons for assuming care of the target grandchild that applied to their situation.

All of the indicators were measured with self-report instruments that have established reliability and validity.

Grandchild Outcomes

To test our integrated model, we needed to examine grandchildren's behavioral and emotional problems, as well as their prosocial behavior. Grandchildren's total difficulties and prosocial behavior were measured with scales from the parent-informant version of the Strengths and Difficulties Questionnaire (SDQ; Goodman, 2001). A grandchild's score for the total difficulty scale ($\alpha = .88$) was derived by summing all items from the hyperactivity-inattention, conduct problems, emotional symptoms, and peer problems subscales. Grandchildren's prosocial behavior was assessed with the five items from the SDQ prosocial subscale ($\alpha = .71$). For all items on the SDQ, grandmothers indicted whether a given behavior ranged from "not true" (0) to "certainly true" (2) for her grandchild. Higher scores for grandchildren's overall level of difficulty indicate greater amounts of psychological difficulties in the grandchild. Similarly, higher scores on the prosocial behavior questions indicate greater levels of prosocial behavior.

Dysfunctional Parenting

In our integrated model, dysfunctional parenting is thought to predict grandchildren's outcomes. Measures of low warmth and ineffective discipline were used in our model as indicators of dysfunctional parenting. Low warmth was assessed with items from the Reinforces Parent subscale ($\alpha = .69$) and the Attachment subscale ($\alpha = .60$) of the Parenting Stress Index (Abidin, 1995). The Reinforces Parent subscale examines the extent to which a caregiver projects negative responses onto a target child. The Attachment subscale assesses the caregiver's emotional closeness to the child and the real or perceived inability to observe and understand the child's needs and feelings. Grandmothers' indicated their degree of agreement (ranging from 1 = strongly agree to 5 = strongly disagree) with each item, and higher summed scores suggest a more problematic parent—child relationship.

Scales measuring grandmothers' use of harsh and inconsistent discipline, respectively, served as indicators of ineffective discipline. Six items were adapted from the Parenting Practices Interview (PPI), which was derived from the Oregon Social Learning Center's discipline questionnaire (Webster-Stratton, Reid, & Hammond, 2001). Grandmothers indicated how often (ranging from 1 = never to 5 = very often) they engaged in a variety of parenting behaviors (e.g., raise your voice, scold, or yell; threaten to punish your grandchild but not really punish him/her) in response to their grandchild misbehaving. The summed scores for harsh ($\alpha = .66$) and inconsistent ($\alpha = .54$) discipline were calculated so that higher scores indicate greater use of the parenting practices.

Grandmother Psychological Distress

Our integrated model suggests that when grandmothers are psychologically distressed, they are more likely to engage in dysfunctional parenting, which results in more negative grandchild outcomes. In testing this model, we viewed depression and anxiety as two key indicators of grandmothers' psychological health (see Figure 1.1). Depression was assessed with the Center for Epidemiologic Studies Depression Scale (CES-D, Radloff, 1977). For each item, participants endorsed the response that best described how often they had felt a particular way in the past week. Response options ranged from 0 (rarely or none of the time—less than 1 day) to 3 (most or all of the time—5 to 7 days). Higher scores indicated greater depression symptoms ($\alpha = .90$). Anxiety was assessed by the three item anxiety scale from the Mental Health Inventory II (Stewart, Ware, Sherbourne & Wells, 1992). Grandmothers rated how often (ranging from 1 = all of the time to 6 = none of the time) during the past month they had been very nervous, tense, or restless. For this scale, higher scores indicated greater anxiety ($\alpha = .84$).

Grandmother Positive Well-Being

Just as grandmothers' psychological distress was hypothesized to influence their parenting, we also hypothesized that parenting behavior would be influenced by grandmothers' positive well-being. Positive well-being involved two indicators—life satisfaction and happiness. Life satisfaction was measured with the Satisfaction with Life Scale (Diener, Emmons, Larsen, & Griffin, 1985). For this scale, participants rated each item from 1 (strongly disagree) to 7 (strongly agree) and higher scores indicated greater life satisfaction ($\alpha = .82$). Happiness was measured by a single item ("On average, what percent of the time do you feel happy?") that was rated from 0 to 100%.

Caregiving Appraisals

The final component of the integrated model that needed to be measured was negative and positive caregiving appraisals. In the model (see Figure 1.1), these appraisals are hypothesized to influence grandmothers' positive well-being and psychological distress. Three indicators were used to measure negative caregiving appraisals—developmental burden, role captivity, and loss of self. Developmental Burden ($\alpha = .75$) was measured by an adaptation of a scale developed by Novak and Guest (1989), with grandmothers indicating their agreement with each item (e.g., "You feel that you are missing out on the best years of your life"). Response options were on a scale from 1 (strongly disagree) to 5 (strongly agree). Role Captivity ($\alpha = .75$) was measured with the Role Captivity Scale (Pearlin, Mullan, Semple, & Skaff, 1990). Grandmothers noted how often (ranging from 1 = never to 4 = very often) they endorsed each item (e.g., "You felt trapped by caring for your grandchild"). Finally, Loss of Self ($\alpha = .75$) was measured by two items from the Loss of Self Scale (Pearlin et al., 1990), with grandmothers noting how often (ranging from 1 = never to 4 = very often) they experienced each item (e.g., "Felt that you've lost a sense of who you are"). For each of these indicators of negative caregiving appraisals, higher scores suggested greater burden, role captivity, and loss of self.

Positive caregiving appraisals were measured with two indicators, perceived gain and competence. Perceived Gain ($\alpha = .67$) was measured by four items (e.g. "As a caregiver, you feel as though you've grown as a person"). Competence measured by two items (e.g., "As a caregiver, you've learned to cope with a very difficult situation"). For both indicators, responses were given on a scale from 1 (never) to 4 (very often). Higher scores on these indicators of positive caregiving appraisals indicated greater perceived gain and competence.

Statistically Testing the Integrated Model

To statistically examine the extent to which there was empirical support for our integrated model, we analyzed the data via structural equation modeling (EQS 6.0; for more information about this approach see Byrne, 2006). A maximum likelihood solution with the Satorra-Bentler correction for non-normality was applied (Curran, West, & Finch, 1996). Both the measurement and structural features of the proposed model were examined. In testing our model, rather than conceptualizing dysfunctional parenting as a first-order latent construct assessed by several indicators, we modeled this construct as a higher-order factor encompassing two first-order factors labeled ineffective discipline and low warmth (see Figure 1.1). This approach was confirmed in our prior research with custodial grandparents (Smith et al., 2008) and is consistent with the widespread view that ineffective discipline and low warmth are distinct, yet highly correlated, constructs that comprise the most influential parenting mechanisms affecting the development of adjustment problems in children (see, for example, Locke & Prinz, 2002; Rubin & Burgess, 2002).

The overall fit of our integrated model to the data gathered in the study was good: Comparative Fit Index = .96 (good fitting models are close to 1.00); Root Mean Square Error of Approximation = .05 (good fitting models are ≤ .05); Standardized Root Mean Square Residual = .04 (values < .08 indicate good model fit). Having good overall fit suggests that our integrated model has some empirical support.

Table 1.2 presents the results of the measurement model, or the standardized and unstandardized factor loadings of each indicator (e.g., anxiety and depression) on each of the model's latent constructs (e.g., grandmother

Table 1.2 Estimated Standardized and Unstandardized Factor Loadings (N = 733)

Latent Factors and Indicators	*Factor Loadings*	
	Standardized	*Unstandardized*
Dysfunctional Parenting (*Second Order*)		
Ineffective Discipline†	*.70*	*1.00*
Harsh	.62	1.00
Inconsistent	.63	.99
Low Warmth†	*.83*	*2.43*
Attachment	.82	1.00
Reinforcement	.83	1.01
GM Psychological Distress		
Anxiety	.75	1.00
Depression	.87	10.59
GM Positive Well-Being		
Life Satisfaction	.74	1.00
Happiness	.77	2.30
Negative Caregiving Appraisals		
Burden	.70	1.00
Role Loss	.84	.43
Role Captivity	.78	.59
Positive Caregiving Appraisals		
Gain	.67	3.98
Competence	.85	1.00

Note: All factor loadings were statistically significant ($p < .05$). One indicator per factor had its loading fixed at 1.00 to establish the factor scale.
†Values in this row represent loadings on the second order Dysfunctional Parenting factor.

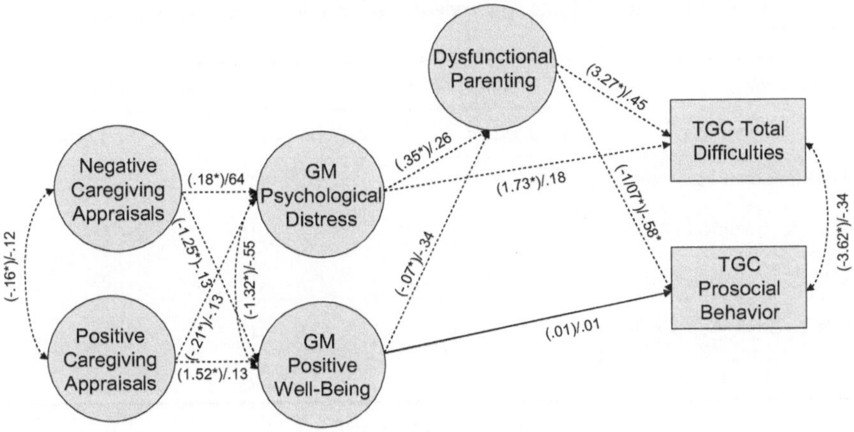

Figure 1.2 Results for the structural model
Note: Pathways in dot line are statistically significant; $p > .05$, unstandardized coefficients in parentheses.

psychological distress). All indicators loaded onto their respective latent constructs at statistically significant levels and there were no indicators that cross loaded onto other constructs.

Figure 1.2 shows the results for the structural model, or the relationships among the various latent constructs (or circles) in the model. In this model, the estimated standardized and unstandardized (in parentheses) path coefficients for each of the model's hypothesized pathways were statistically significant except for the path hypothesized from grandmother positive well-being to the target grandchild's prosocial behavior. Together, findings from this analysis suggest that there was statistical support for the model, as it was conceptualized.

Finally, Table 1.3 presents the total effects (i.e., both direct and indirect effects) of the model constructs on the outcomes of grandchild total difficulties and prosocial behavior. As anticipated, all antecedent constructs in the model had statistically significant total effects on both grandchild total difficulties and grandchild prosocial behavior.

Summary and Discussion of Study Findings

To test our integration of the FSM (Conger et al., 2000) and the TFM (Lawton et al., 1991), we examined data from a national survey of grandmothers raising grandchildren. The findings from this study, which are described in detail below, lend empirical support to our integrated model and offer valuable insight into the role of grandmothers' negative and positive caregiving appraisals in influencing key outcomes for both grandmothers and their grandchildren. In particular, our findings highlight how positive appraisals, grandmothers'

Table 1.3 Total Effects of Model Antecedents on Grandchildren's Mental Health (N = 733)

Antecedents	*Total Difficulties*		*Prosocial Behavior*	
	Standardized	*Unstandardized*	*Standardized*	*Unstandardized*
Dysfunctional Parenting	.45	3.27	−.58	−1.07
GM Psychological Distress	.30	2.88	−.15	−.38
GM Positive Well-Being	−.16	−.23	.19	.07
GM Negative Appraisals	.29	.81	−.22	−.16
GM Positive Appraisals	−.06	−.95	.04	.18

Note: All reported total effect were statistically significant; $p > .05$.

psychological well-being, and effective parenting behavior can result in resilient outcomes for grandparents and grandchildren alike.

As would be predicted from the FSM (Conger et al., 2000), our findings show that dysfunctional parenting had the greatest total effect on grandchildren's total difficulties, as well as on their prosocial behavior. Thus, higher levels of dysfunctional parenting were associated with more grandchild emotional and behavioral problems and less prosocial behavior. Given the varied stressors associated with parenting grandchildren (Dolbin-MacNab, 2006; Gibson, 2005) and the negative impact of poor parenting on grandchildren's well-being, our findings highlight the importance of practitioners indentifying those grandparents who might benefit from parent training and other interventions to support their efforts in parenting their grandchildren.

Consistent with the FSM (Conger et al., 2000), our findings further show that custodial grandmothers' psychological well-being has a direct effect on the quality of their parenting, and an indirect effect on grandchildren's total difficulties and prosocial behavior. As would also be expected from the TFM (Lawton et al., 1991), grandmothers' psychological distress was associated with higher levels of dysfunctional parenting, and was indirectly related to greater grandchild emotional and behavioral difficulties and less prosocial behavior. Conversely, grandmother positive well-being was related to less dysfunctional parenting directly, and indirectly related to fewer grandchild difficulties and greater prosocial behavior. From a resilience perspective, these findings emphasize that positive grandmother psychological well-being is key to promoting more functional parenting and better grandchild outcomes.

Our examination of the role of positive and negative caregiving appraisals within the context of the proposed model suggests that the effects of grandmothers' positive and negative caregiving appraisals on grandchildren's well-being were indirect, via their total effects on the grandmothers' psychological distress, positive well-being, and dysfunctional parenting. The finding that both positive and negative appraisals are relevant to grandmother outcomes lends additional support to the application of the TFM (Lawton et al., 1991) to custodial grandfamilies. Our findings further reveal that how custodial grandmothers appraise the caregiving situation has significant implications for their mental health, as well as the adjustment of their grandchildren.

Although our findings suggest that both positive and negative appraisals were important to grandparent well-being, they appeared to operate by different mechanisms. Grandmothers' negative appraisals were related more strongly to their psychological distress than to their positive well-being. In contrast, and unexpectedly, grandmothers' positive caregiving appraisals were similarly related to their psychological distress and to their positive well-being. The TFM argues that negative appraisals of a caregiving situation will increase negative affect (and negative outcomes, such as depression and anxiety) to a greater extent than reducing positive affect or outcomes (Lawton et al., 1991). It also suggests that positive appraisals should be associated with positive well-being and positive outcomes, but not as strongly related to negative affect and outcomes such as psychological distress (Lawton et al., 1991). Our unexpected findings related to grandmothers' appraisals may suggest that, for many grandmothers, negative appraisals tend to dominate their lives. In contrast, those grandmothers with strong positive caregiving appraisals may be coping with their caregiving responsibilities unusually well.

In examining the link between grandmothers' appraisals and grandchildren's outcomes, we found that both negative and positive appraisals had significant total effects on grandchildren's total difficulties and prosocial behavior. However, the magnitude of the effects of grandmothers' positive appraisals on these particular outcomes was not as great as it was for negative appraisals. This finding, which only partially supports the TFM (Lawton et al., 1991), could be because custodial grandmothers are experiencing so many stressors (e.g., legal, financial, social, etc.) that their negative appraisals are realistic and, therefore, are a more salient part of their caregiving experience. In addition, there may be some bidirectional processes at work. Some studies have suggested that, when grandchildren have severe emotional and behavioral problems, grandparents may experience higher levels of depression, anxiety, and psychological distress (e.g., Hayslip et al., 1998; Young & Dawson, 2003; Sands & Goldberg-Glen, 2000). As such, perhaps grandparents' negative appraisals are a reflection of the parenting challenges and stress they experience on a daily basis.

While our findings provide valuable insight into factors that influence grandmother and grandchild well-being, several study limitations should be noted. First, the data were self-reported by grandmothers and might be biased in some systematic way. In addition, the study was cross-sectional in nature, and does not permit causal inferences despite the use of SEM. While the current sample was reasonably diverse, it only included White and African-American grandmothers. To better represent the larger population of grandparents raising grandchildren, more information would be needed about grandfathers and Latino grandparent-headed families, for instance. Finally, despite the value of the current model for understanding factors that influence grandmother and grandchild outcomes, further model development and refinement is needed. It is possible that other, more sensitive indicators of the constructs could be used. Also, there may be key constructs that should be in the model, but were not included here. For example, perhaps social support or family resources have an influence on grandparents' positive and negative appraisals. Similarly, characteristics of the grandchildren, such as affect regulation, could influence their emotional and behavior problems, as well as their prosocial behavior.

Practice Implications

For clinicians who are interested in promoting the resilience of grandparents and their custodial grandchildren, the findings from this study have a number of important practice implications. These practice implications highlight the possibility (and necessity) of intervening with grandfamilies in multiple arenas—from parent training to interventions designed to promote grandmother psychological well-being. To encourage resilient outcomes for grandparents and their grandchildren, we recommend that practitioners adopt a multifaceted approach that targets the needs of both grandparents and their grandchildren.

Implications for Parenting Interventions

Given our finding that the influence of grandmothers' psychological distress on grandchildren's adjustment is largely indirect through their parenting practices, it is sensible to conclude that the adjustment of many custodial grandchildren may be enhanced by making parent training programs available to their grandparents. Parent training programs follow the premise that dysfunctional parenting practices contribute to the development, progression, and maintenance of disruptive behaviors across childhood. Thus, these programs are aimed at changing caregivers' behaviors, perceptions, communication, and understanding how to effect desired changes in child behavior (Lundahl, Risser, & Lovejoy, 2006).

Several forms of parent training exist. They differ in theoretical orientation, amount of intervention, qualifications of the trainers, mode of delivery (e.g., individual, group, self-directed), specific therapeutic components (e.g., parenting skills, stress management, marital therapy), and those (e.g., parent only or the parent and the child) who receive treatment (Kazdin, 2005). Recent meta-analyses have shown, however, that programs based on behavioral principles yield the greatest benefits (Garland, Hawley, Brookman-Frazee, & Hurlburt, 2008). Key features of Behavioral Parent Training (BPT) are that (a) caregivers participate in the skills training (focused on cognitive, affective, and behavioral changes in the caregiver); (b) caregivers are encouraged to increase their positive interactions with the child through positive play, increased rewards for good behavior, ignoring unwanted behavior, and improved communication with clear requests and consequences; and (c) sessions include review of homework, video presentations of more or less effective ways of parenting, short lectures and discussions to elicit parenting principles, interactive exercises, modeling and role plays parenting behaviors to be changed, charting and monitoring of parenting and children's behaviors, assignment of homework, and training on effective discipline through timeouts or removal of privileges (Kumpfer & Alvarado, 2003). Within the context of resilience, it is evident from the above description that BPT tends to focus more on positive parent-child interactions and good behaviors than on the negative aspects of children's behavior and problematic interactions with their caregivers. This focus on positives has also been supported by research showing that parenting practices involving warmth and effective discipline have the protective effect of lessening the mental health problems of children previously exposed to major stressors (Sandler et al., 2003).

Presently, the effectiveness of BPT with custodial grandfamilies remains unknown, despite its apparent relevance to promoting resilience for grandparents and grandchildren alike. Nonetheless, to effectively deliver parenting interventions, including BPT, practitioners should consider training sessions held at convenient times and locations. Peer-led workshops or peer support opportunities may also be an effective means for engaging grandparents in examining their parenting attitudes and skills. Practitioners should be careful, however, as they may encounter grandparents who do not see any problems with their parenting and may be unwilling to consider making changes to their parenting beliefs and behavior (Dolbin-MacNab, 2006). Practitioners can still work within these grandparents' existing parenting frameworks to slowly introduce new ideas about child-rearing, while still respecting the grandparents' past experience and wisdom.

Strategies to Promote Grandparent Psychological Well-Being

The results of this study demonstrated that grandmother psychological well-being was associated with better parenting practices and, in turn, better grandchild outcomes. As such, practitioners should realize that there are multiple pathways through which a custodial grandmother's psychological distress could result in disrupted parenting. Depressive symptoms, for instance, may interfere with parenting via (a) sadness or flat affect that impairs grandparents' emotional expression and regulation; (b) hopelessness and low self-worth that diminishes parenting self-efficacy, (c) a heightened self-focus that detracts from parent-child interactions; (d) irritability resulting in decreased warmth and sensitivity and increased criticism; and (e) fatigue leading to inconsistent responding, lack of guidance and limit setting, and withdrawal (Conley et al., 2004). Various parenting processes may be similarly disrupted by the presence of anxiety in custodial grandmothers, with symptoms ranging from everyday worries to extreme levels of nervousness, physiological arousal, and inhibited behavior or avoidance that are characteristic of clinical disorders. For example, caregivers preoccupied by their own worries or anxiety tend to (a) respond less warmly and positively to children; (b) give children less independence; (c) express greater criticism; and (d) form less secure attachments (Conley et al., 2004).

As suggested by our model (see Figure 1.1), it may be that it is custodial grandparents' psychological overload rather than a lack of parenting skill or knowledge that underlies their poor parenting practices. Evidence that therapeutic change in a caregivers' psychological distress can result in improved parenting and positive outcomes for children in the absence of parent training also comes from recent studies on the remission of maternal depression. For example, Foster and colleagues (2008) found that remission of maternal depression was associated with changes in children's (ages 7–17) perceptions of their mother's warmth/acceptance, which in turn partially mediated the relation between maternal depression remission and youth internalizing symptoms. It has also been widely acknowledged that, even without severe distress or psychopathology, parenting behavior can become disrupted within the context normal daily hassles (Elgar, Mills, McGrath, Waschbusch, & Brownridge, 2007).

In light of the above considerations, practitioners interested in promoting resilience among grandfamilies should offer activities and develop interventions that encourage positive grandparent psychological well-being. For example, those grandparents who are highly distressed should be encouraged to seek mental health support via therapy or a well-designed and executed support group (Strom & Strom, 2000). Practitioners can also promote grandparents' psychological well-being by teaching grandparents skills that they can use to manage their depression and anxiety (e.g., coping skills, seeking social support, and mindfulness meditation).

Besides addressing psychological distress via mental health treatment or skills training, practitioners can also engage in a number of other activities designed to promote or reinforce positive grandparent well-being. This approach is consistent with the dual-factor model of mental health and other positive psychology approaches, which suggest that interventions should not just decrease negative symptoms, but should also improve subjective well-being (Ryff et al., in press; Seligman, 2008; Wang, Zhang & Wang, 2011). In the case of custodial grandparents, grandparents may benefit from celebrations designed to acknowledge the efforts and sacrifices they are making to raise their grandchildren. Other strategies for promoting grandparent well-being could include offering respite care, addressing service needs, and assisting with self-care.

Addressing Grandparent Appraisals

The findings of this study and the TFM (Lawton et al., 1991) suggest that positive and negative appraisals may operate independently in terms of their influence on grandparent well-being and grandchild outcomes. As such, interventions should target grandparents' negative *and* positive appraisals. Interventions should also acknowledge their coexistence (versus their exclusivity; Gable & Reis, 2010). By targeting positive and negative appraisals, practitioners can offer multiple means by which interventions can promote grandparent resilience. Practitioners should also realize that positive and negative appraisals occur simultaneously and are not mutually exclusive.

In the current study, grandmothers' negative appraisals had larger total effects on their psychological well-being and the adjustment of their grandchildren than did their positive appraisals. Therefore, practitioners may want to focus their intervention efforts on reducing grandparents' negative appraisals. This can be accomplished by assisting grandparents in removing some of the challenges or stressors they are experiencing through greater access to support services or other resources. Another strategy for reducing grandparents' negative appraisals would be enhancing their ability to access and make use of existing resources. To accomplish this, practitioners could assist grandparents completing paperwork, gathering documentation, making calls, and locating available services.

Practitioners can also combat negative appraisals by adopting a solution- or resource-focused stance (e.g., de Shazer & Dolan, 2007). This stance focuses on encouraging grandparents to identify their problem-solving successes and exceptions to their difficulties. Other, similar approaches that focus on exceptions, alternative narratives, or positives exist as well [e.g., narrative therapy (Freedman & Combs, 1996); Well-Being Therapy (Fava & Ruini, 2003)]. Any of these clinical stances can be used to challenge grandparents' negative appraisals about their caregiving situation, and assist grandparents in creating more neutral or positive appraisals.

Positive appraisals are an important factor determining an individual's resilience to stress (Bonanno et al., in press; Ong et al., 2009). Although the findings from our study did not dramatically support this link, given that positive appraisals have been consistently linked to positive outcomes in many other studies and among numerous other populations, we still encourage practitioners who work with grandfamilies to consider interventions specifically designed to develop and enhance grandparents' positive appraisals. For instance, practitioners could help grandparents make the most of the positive events that occur in their lives (Gable & Reis, 2010). This could include teaching grandparents to savor positive events, count blessings, and share positive events in their lives with supportive others (Bryant, 1989; Emmons & McColough, 2003; Gable & Reis, 2010). Along these lines, practitioners could also teach grandparents to focus on the positive reasons that they are raising their grandchildren (Hayslip & Kaminski, 2005) and how their grandchildren are benefitting from the caregiving arrangement (Dolbin-MacNab & Keiley, 2009; Dolbin-MacNab et al., 2009; Gable & Reis, 2010). Similarly, because positive appraisals occur as people progress toward goals that they value (Carver, 1996; Gable & Reis, 2010), practitioners can assist custodial grandparents in identifying their goals and highlighting the ways in which they are making (or have already made) progress toward those goals. This process could also focus on helping grandparents identify ways that they can obtain the resources they need to further reach their goals. Finally, mindfulness-type interventions could be used to teach grandparents to recognize and make the most of positive events and, in turn, build positive appraisals (Ryff et al., in press) and better psychological health.

Promoting Grandchild Adjustment

In addition to the areas already discussed, the findings from this study have implications for promoting positive outcomes in custodial grandchildren. Given the clear linkages between grandparents' parenting behavior, psychological well-being, and grandchildren's adjustment, practitioners should consider adopting a systemic approach (Cox & Paley, 2003) in their work with grandfamilies. A systemic approach emphasizes how grandchildren's behavior may be influencing grandparents' appraisals and well-being. It also examines how problems with boundaries, hierarchy, and power can result in inconsistent or harsh discipline on the part of the grandparent (Bartram, 1994; Minuchin, 1974). Via parenting training or family therapy, practitioners can work with grandparents to create clear, appropriate hierarchies in which they have appropriate power and leadership over their custodial grandchildren (Minuchin, 1974). By adopting a systemic approach, practitioners can also interrupt problematic feedback loops by helping grandparents interpret their grandchildren's behavior in less negative ways and by teaching grandparents to respond differently to their grandchild's behavior. Grandchildren can also be supported in dealing with their grandparents' stress and encouraged to participate in prosocial activities and relationships. In these ways, the system is likely to respond in a more positive, resilient manner.

Note

1 This research was supported by an award to the first author from the NIMH [R01 MH 066851-02]. An earlier version of this chapter was presented at the annual meeting of the American Psychological Association, August 2010, San Diego, CA.

References

Abidin, R. R. (1995). *Parenting stress index: Professional manual* (3rd ed.). Lutz, FL: Psychological Assessment Resources.

Bartram, M. H. (1994). Clarifying subsystem boundaries in grandfamilies. *Contemporary Family Therapy, 18*, 267–277.

Billing, A., Ehrle, J., & Kortenkamp, K. (2002). Children cared for by relatives: What do we know about their well-being? *New Federalism* (Policy Brief B-46). Washington DC: The Urban Institute.

Bonnano, G. A. (2004). Loss, trauma, and human resilience: Have we underestimated the human capacity to thrive after extremely aversive events? *American Psychologist, 59*, 20–28. doi: 10.1037/1942-9681.S.1.101

Bonanno, G. A., Westphal, M., & Mancini, A. D. (in press). Loss, trauma and resilience in adulthood. In B. Hayslip, Jr. & G. C. Smith (Eds.), *Annual review of gerontology and geriatrics: Emerging perspectives on resilience in later life*. New York, NY: Springer.

Bryant, F. B. (1989). A four-factor model of perceived control: Avoiding, coping, obtaining, and savoring. *Journal of Personality, 57*, 773–797.

Byrne, B. M. (2006). *Structural equation modeling with EQS: Basic concepts, applications, and programming*. (2nd ed.). Mahwah, NJ: Lawrence Erlbaum Associates.

Carver, C. C. (1996). Emergent integration in contemporary personality psychology. *Journal of Research in Personality, 30*, 319–334.

Conger, K. J., Rueter, M. A., & Conger, R. D. (2000). The role of economic pressure in the lives of parents and their adolescents: The Family Stress Model. In L. J. Crockett & R. K. Silbereisen (Eds.), *Negotiating adolescence in times of social change* (pp. 201–223). New York, NY: Cambridge University Press.

Conley, C. S., Caldwell, M. S., Flynn, M., Dupre, A. J., & Rudolph, K. D. (2004). Parenting and mental health. In M. Hoghughi & N. Long (Eds.), *Handbook of parenting: Theory and research for practice* (pp. 276–285). Thousand Oaks, CA: Sage.

Cox, M., & Paley, B. (2003). Understanding families as systems. *Current Directions in Psychological Science, 12*(5), 193–196. doi:10.1111/1467-8721.01259

Curran, P. J., West, S. G., & Finch, J. (1996). The robustness of test statistics to non-normality and specification error in confirmatory factor analysis. *Psychological Methods, 1*, 16–29. doi:10.1037//1082-989X.1.1.16

de Shazer, S., & Dolan, Y. (2005). *More than miracles: The state of the art of solution-focused brief therapy*. New York, NY: Routledge.

Diener, E., Emmons, R. A., Larsen, R. J., & Griffin, S. (1985). The satisfaction with life scale. *Journal of Personality Assessment, 49*, 71–75. doi:10.1207/s15327752jpa4901_13

Dolbin-MacNab, M. L. (2006). Just like raising your own? Grandmothers' perceptions of parenting a second time around. *Family Relations, 55*, 564–575. doi:10.1111/j.1741-3729.2006.00426.x

Dolbin-MacNab, M. L., & Keiley, M. K. (2009). Navigating interdependence: How adolescents raised solely by grandparents experience their family relationships. *Family Relations, 58*, 162–175. doi:10.1111/j.1741-3729.2008.00544.x

Dolbin-MacNab, M. L., Rodgers, B. E., & Traylor, R. M. (2009). Bridging the generations: A retrospective examination of adults' relationships with their kinship caregivers. *Journal of Intergenerational Relationships, 7*, 159–176.

Elgar, F. J., Mills, R. S. L., McGrath, P. J., Waschbusch, D. A., & Brownridge, D. A. (2007). Maternal and paternal depressive symptoms and child maladjustment: The mediating role of parental behavior. *Journal of Abnormal Child Psychology, 35*, 943–955.

Emmons, R. A., & McCullough, M. E. (2003). Counting blessings versus burdens: An experimental investigation of gratitude and subjective well-being in daily life. *Journal of Personality and Social Psychology, 84*, 377–389. doi:10.1037//0022-3514.84.2.377

Fava, G. A., & Ruini, C. (2003). Development and characteristics of a well-being enhancing psychotherapeutic strategy: Well-being therapy. *Journal of Behavior Therapy and Experimental Psychiatry, 34*, 45–63. doi:10.1016/S0005-7916(03)00019-3

Foster, C. E. et al. (2008). Remission of maternal depression: Relations to family functioning and youth internalizing and externalizing symptoms. *Journal of Clinical Child & Adolescent Psychology, 37*, 714–724.

Freedman, J., & Combs, G. (1996). *Narrative therapy: The social construction of preferred realities*. New York, NY: W. W. Norton & Company.

Gable, S. L., & Reis, H. T. (2010). Good news! Capitalizing on positive events in an interpersonal context. *Advances in Experimental Social Psychology, 42*, 195–257. doi:10.1037/a00 18344.

Garland, A. F., Hawley, K. M., Brookman-Frazee, L., & Hurlburt, M. S. (2008). Identifying common elements of evidenced-based psychosocial treatments for children's disruptive. *Journal of the American Academy of Child and Adolescent Psychiatry, 5*, 505–514.

Garmezy, N. (1985). Stress-resistant children: The search for protective factors. In J. E. Stevenson (Ed.), *Recent research in developmental psychopathology: Journal of Child Psychology and Psychiatry book supplement* (pp. 213–233). Oxford: Pergamon Press.

Gibson, P. A. (2005). Intergenerational parenting from the perspective of African American grandmothers. *Family Relations, 54*, 280–297. doi:10.1111/j.0197-6664.2005.00022.x

Goodman, R. (2001). Psychometric properties of the Strengths and Difficulties Questionnaire. *Journal of the American Academy of Adolescent Psychiatry, 40*, 1337–1345. doi:10.1097/00004583-200111000-00015

Grant, R., Gordon, S. G., & Cohen, S. T. (1997). An innovative school-based intergenerational model to serve grandparent caregivers. *Journal of Gerontological Social Work, 28*, 47–61. doi:10.1300/J083v28n01_07

Hayslip, B., & Kaminski, P. L. (2005). Grandparents raising their grandchildren. *Marriage and Family Review, 37*, 147–169. doi:10.1300/J002v37n01_10

Hayslip, B., Shore, R. J., Henderson, C. E., & Lambert, P. L. (1998). Custodial grandparenting and the impact of grandchildren with problems on role satisfaction and role meaning. *Journal of Gerontology: Social Sciences, 53B*, S164–S173. doi:10.1093/geronb/53B.3.S164

Hughes, M. E., Waite, L. J., LaPierre, T. A., & Luo, Y. (2007). All in the family: The impact of caring for grandchildren on grandparents' health. *Journal of Gerontology: Social Sciences, 62B*, S108–S119. doi:10.1093/geronb/62.2.S108

Kazdin, A. E. (2005). *Parent management training: Treatment for oppositional, aggressive, and antisocial behavior in children and adolescents.* New York: Oxford University Press.

Kreider, R. M., & Ellis, R. (2011). *Living arrangements of children: 2009* (Current Population Reports, P70-126). Washington, DC: U. S. Census Bureau. Retrieved from http://www.census.gov/prod/2011pubs/p70-126.pdf

Lawton, M. P., Moss, M., Kleban, M. H., Glicksman, A., & Rovine, M. (1991). A two-factor model of caregiving appraisal and psychological well-being. *Journal of Gerontology, 46*, P181–P189.

Locke, L. M., & Prinz, R. J. (2002). Measurement of parental discipline and nurturance. *Clinical Psychology Review, 22*, 895–929.

Lundahl, B., Risser, H. J., & Lovejoy, C. M. (2006). A meta-analysis of parent training: Moderators and follow-up effects. *Clinical Psychology Review, 26*, 86–104.

Minkler, M., & Fuller-Thomson, E. (1999). The health of grandparents raising grandchildren: Results of a national study. *American Journal of Public Health, 89*, 1384–1392. doi: 10.2105/AJPH.89.9.1384

Minkler, M., Fuller-Thomson, E., Miller, D., & Driver, D. (1997). Depression in grandparents raising grandchildren: Results of a national longitudinal study. *Archives of Family Medicine, 6*, 445–452.

Minuchin, S. (1974). *Families and family therapy.* Cambridge, MA: Harvard University Press.

Novak, M., & Guest, C. I. (1989). Application for a multidimensional Caregiver Burden Inventory. *The Gerontologist, 29*, 798–803.

Ong, A. D., Bergeman, C. S., & Boker, S. N. (2009). Resilience comes of age: Defining features in later adulthood. *Journal of Personality, 77*, 1777–1804. doi: 10.1111/j.1467-6494.2009.00600.x

Pearlin, L. I., Mullan, J., Semple, S., & Skaff, M. (1990). Caregiving and the stress process: An overview of concepts and their measures. *The Gerontologist, 30*, 583–594.

Radloff, L. S. (1977). The CES-D Scale: A self-report depression scale for research in the general population. *Applied Psychological Measurement, 1*, 385–401.

Rubin, K. H., & Burgess, K. (2002). Parents of aggressive and withdrawn children. In M. Bornstein (Ed.), *Handbook of Parenting*. (2nd ed.). Vol. 1, 383–418. Hillsdale, NJ: Lawrence Erlbaum Associates.

Ryff, C. D., Friedman, E. M., Morozink, J. A., & Tsenkova, V. (in press). Psychological resilience in adulthood and later life: Implications for health. In B. Hayslip, Jr. & G. C. Smith (Eds.), *Annual review of gerontology and geriatrics: Emerging perspectives on resilience in later life*. New York, NY: Springer.

Sandler, I. N., Ayers, T. S., Wolchik, S. A. et al. (2003). The Family Bereavement Program: Efficacy evaluation of a theory-based prevention program for parentally bereaved children and adolescents. *Journal of Consulting and Clinical Psychology, 71*, 587–600.

Sands, R. G., & Goldberg-Glen, R. S. (2000). Factors associated with stress among grandparents raising their grandchildren. *Family Relations, 49*, 97–105. doi: 10.1111/j.1741-3729.2000.00097.x

Seligman, M. E. P. (2008). Positive health. *Applied Psychology: An International Review, 57*, 3–18. doi: 10.1111/j.1464-0597.2008.00351.x

Solomon, J. C., & Marx, J. (1995). "To grandmother's house we go:" Health and school adjustment of children raised solely by grandparents. *The Gerontologist, 35*(3), 386–394.

Smith, G. C., & Hancock, G. R. (2010). Custodial grandmother-grandfather dyads: Pathways among marital distress, grandparent dysphoria, parenting practice, and grandchild adjustment. *Family Relations, 59*, 45–59. doi: 10.1111/j.1741-3729.2009.00585.

Smith, G. C., & Hayslip, B. (in press). Resilience in adulthood and later life: What does it mean and where are we heading? In B. Hayslip & G. Smith (Eds.), *Annual review of gerontology and geriatrics: Emerging perspectives on resilience in adulthood and later ife*. New York, NY: Springer.

Smith, G. C., & Palmieri, P. A. (2007). Risk of psychological difficulties among children raised by custodial grandparents. *Psychiatric Services, 58*, 1303–1310.

Smith, G. C., Palmieri, P. A., Hancock, G. R., & Richardson, R. A. (2008). Custodial grandparents' psychological distress, dysfunctional parenting, and grandchildren's adjustment. *International Journal of Aging and Human Development, 67*, 327–367.

Smith, G. C., & Richardson, R. A. (2008). Understanding the parenting practices of custodial grandmothers: Overcompensating, underserving, or overwhelmed? In B. Hayslip, Jr. & P. Kaminski (Eds.), *Parenting the custodial grandchild* (pp. 131–147). New York: Springer.

Stewart, A. L., Ware, J. E., Sherbourne, C. D., & Wells, K. B. (1992). Psychological distress/wellbeing and cognitive functioning measures. In A. L. Stewart & J. E. Ware (Eds.), *Measuring functioning and well-being: The medical outcomes study approach* (pp. 102–142). Durham, NC: Duke University Press.

Strom, R. D., & Strom, S. K. (2000). Meeting the challenge of raising grandchildren. *International Journal of Aging and Human Development, 51*(3), 183–198.

Wang, X., Zhang, D., & Wang, J. (2011). Dual-factor model of mental health: Surpass the traditional mental health model. *Psychology, 2*, 767–772.

Webster-Ratton, C., Reid, M. J., & Hammond, M. (2001). Preventing conduct problems, promoting social competence: A parent and teacher training partnership in Head Start. *Journal of Clinical Child Psychology, 30*, 283–302.

Young, M., & Dawson, T. (2003). Perception of child difficulty and levels of depression in caregiving grandmothers. *Journal of Mental Health and Aging, 9*, 111–122.

2 The Relation Between Caregiving Style, Coping, Benefit Finding, Grandchild Symptoms, and Caregiver Adjustment Among Custodial Grandparents

Katherine D. Castillo, Craig E. Henderson, and Lindsey W. North

Abstract

This study examines factors that influence custodial grandparents' adjustment to the role of caregiving. Specifically, we explored grandparents': (a) caregiving styles, (b) coping styles, (c) perceptions of their grandchild's behavior problems, and (d) ascribed benefits as they all relate to caregiver adjustment. Participants for this study included grandparents raising at least one grandchild. Caregiving styles, coping styles, and benefit finding were found to impact caregiver adjustment. Authoritative caregiving and benefit finding were both related to higher satisfaction with caregiving; benefit finding was also related to caregiver reports that caring for their grandchild had less negative impact on their lives. Findings of this study suggest that custodial grandparents would benefit from an intervention that (at least in part) focuses on developing an authoritative caregiving style and learning to recognize the benefits of raising grandchildren. Effective interventions may also need to involve both custodial grandparents and their grandchildren, as grandchild internalizing and externalizing symptoms may prevent grandparents from capitalizing on their strengths in benefit finding and using certain coping styles to promote adjustment.

The Relation Between Caregiving Style, Coping, Benefit Finding, Grandchild Symptoms, and Caregiver Adjustment Among Custodial Grandparents

The number of grandparents in the United States providing care for their grandchildren is rising considerably, with the 2000 U.S. Census reporting that 5.7 million grandparents are living with their grandchildren, an increase of 30% between 1990 and 2000 (U.S. Bureau of the Census, 2001). Grandparents are increasingly becoming the primary caregivers for their grandchildren for a variety of reasons, including parental substance abuse, teen pregnancy, divorce, parental unemployment, parental incarceration, physical or mental illness, abuse, and neglect (Hayslip & Goldberg-Glen, 2000; Minkler & Fuller-Thomson,

1999). While it is certainly the case that such circumstances, along with national problems such as violence and HIV infection, have led to incapacitation and death of young adults, especially those in low-income communities have led to the increased number of grandparents raising grandchildren, the literature as a whole may have overemphasized the negative aspects of grandparent caregiving. It is also true that despite the stressors that may lead to grandparent caregiving, grandparents often report their caregiving experiences can be rewarding and that their decision to assume the parenting role was made to improve the lives of their grandchildren (Hayslip, Shore, Henderson, & Lambert, 1998; Henderson & Stevenson, 2003).

Indeed, many grandparents claim caregiving brings them feelings of satisfaction, accomplishment, and an increased purpose for living (Henderson & Stevenson, 2003; Jendrek, 1993). In two studies conducted by Burton (1992), the majority of grandparents reported high levels of satisfaction in their roles as custodial caregivers and feelings of deep love and commitment to their grandchildren. Grandparents also report that raising their grandchildren helps them feel young and active and provides them with additional companionship (Kropf & Burnette, 2003; Jendrek, 1993). In addition, caregiving often gives grandparents the opportunity to enjoy a closer relationship with their grandchildren (Fuller-Thomson & Minkler, 2000). That said, it cannot be overlooked that the experience of raising grandchildren also presents hardships. Taking on the role of parent a second time involves making major lifestyle changes. These changes can potentially impact the caregiver's life by causing financial strain, social isolation, and reducing leisure time (Fuller-Thomson & Minkler, 2000; Hayslip, Shore, Henderson, & Lambert, 1998). In addition, assuming the role of caregiver may lead to changes in quality of life such as declines in mental and physical health (Casper & Bryson, 1998).

A more balanced perspective on grandparent caregiving is needed in the field; one that examines the challenges of grandparent caregiving in light of the benefits grandparents may receive from assuming this role again, as well as identifying the factors related to better caregiver adjustment. Such factors may be the focus of future interventions designed to promote the optimal functioning of families of grandparent caregivers. In the following sections, we examine factors that may be related to better (and worse) caregiver adjustment: (a) presence of grandchild problems, (b) grandparents' parenting styles, (c) grandparents' coping, and (d) the extent to which grandparents experience benefits from raising their grandchildren. We then report the results of a study examining these factors as predictors of the psychological adjustment of grandparents raising their grandchildren.

The Impact of Grandchild Problems on Grandparent Adjustment

Grandchildren raised by their grandparents commonly exhibit high rates of internalizing symptoms and externalizing problems (Emick & Hayslip, 1999; Hayslip et al., 1998). Several factors contribute to this tendency. One factor is that grandparents are more likely to be called upon for childcare assistance when the child has problems (Hetherington, 1989). Consequently, grandparents who step in to help their children by raising their grandchild often end up raising grandchildren with existing problems.

Children being raised by grandparents may also experience problems as a result of the circumstances that precipitated grandparent care (Fuller-Thomson & Minkler, 2000; Hayslip et al., 1998). Previous research has found that internalizing and externalizing behaviors are associated with factors such as family disruption and family conflict, both of which are situations which commonly lead to grandparents raising grandchildren (Birmaher et al., 1996; Loeber & Stouthamer-Loeber, 1986; McCord, 1982). In addition, situations such as family conflict and abuse (frequent precipitants of grandparents assuming care responsibility) can increase a child's vulnerability to depression and other forms of psychopathology (Birmaher et al., 1996).

When grandchildren have problems, the stress of dealing with these issues contributes to poor grandparent adjustment and higher levels of anxiety and depression compared to custodial grandparents caring for grandchildren with lower levels (Emik & Hayslip, 1999; Fuller-Thomson & Minkler, 2000; Hayslip et al., 1998; Hayslip & Patrick, 2006; Sands & Goldberg-Glen, 2000). In contrast, when grandchildren have fewer problems, grandparents are more satisfied in their roles as custodial grandparents (Hayslip & Patrick, 2006).

Coping Style

Coping can be described as attempts to deal with stressors in order to reduce their negative impact (Snyders & Pulvers, 2001). When faced with stressful situations, individuals cope in a variety of ways. Over time, individuals develop characteristic behavioral responses that are adjusted and repeated when they are helpful in reducing the individual's stress (Carver, Scheier, & Weintraub, 1989; Snyders & Pulvers, 2001). Although people may employ different coping strategies depending on the nature of the situation, researchers have found individuals tend to adopt characteristic coping styles; that is, people have a particular manner in which they typically cope with stress (Carver et al., 1989). Individuals' coping styles can affect the overall impact that stressful situations have on them and effectiveness in decreasing stress.

There are two primary ways in which coping has traditionally been conceptualized by researchers (Littleton, Horsley, John, & Nelson, 2007). One way to study coping is to distinguish between problem-focused and emotion-focused coping (Lazarus & Folkman, 1984). Another way to conceptualize coping, and the method that will be utilized in the current study, is to distinguish between avoidance coping and approach coping (Roth & Cohen, 1986). Avoidance coping involves avoiding the stressor or one's reaction to it, for example, withdrawing from the situation or denying that it exists. Approach coping includes strategies such as problem solving that focus on directly diminishing the impact of the stressor or on one's reaction to the stressor.

Benefit Finding

Researchers have found that focusing on the positive effects of stressful situations, or "benefit finding," is related to more positive outcomes (Helgeson, Reynolds, & Tomich, 2006). A meta-analysis done by Helgeson et al. (2006) included 77 articles examining the relationship of benefit finding to the mental and physical health outcomes of individuals who had experienced a stressful event (e.g., chronic illness, natural disaster, sexual assault, romantic relationship break-up, unexpected caregiving, etc.). The researchers found that benefit finding was associated with less depression and more positive well-being. In addition, the relationship between benefit finding and adjustment was stronger when more time had elapsed since the stressor had occurred. According to the researchers, because growth takes time, people are more likely to identify benefits from the stressful experience when they have had time to adjust to the stressor.

Few studies have examined benefit finding among caregivers. However, the studies that have been conducted have found that benefit finding leads to better adjustment. McCausland and Pakenham (2003) examined the relationship between benefit finding and adjustment among caregivers of individuals with HIV/AIDS. They found that benefit finding was inversely correlated with depression. Personal growth, increased understanding of others, and positive personality change were the most common benefits reported by the caregivers. Using a sample of caregivers of individuals with dementia, Machac-Burleson et al. (2008) found that benefit finding was associated with more satisfaction with caregiving and less depression. The current study will examine whether these relationships are similar among grandparent caregivers (Hayslip et al., 1998).

Caregiving Styles

Baumrind (1971, 1991) identified three basic styles of parenting: (1) authoritative, characterized by high levels of warmth and attentiveness, (2) authoritarian, characterized by low levels of acceptance and high levels of control, (3) and permissive, characterized by high levels of warmth and low levels of control. King (2004) extended this research to apply to individuals' caregiving styles. King (2004) describes authoritative caregivers as being fairly easy going, warm and involved with the recipients of their care, and using reasonable discipline methods. Authoritarian caregivers are described as utilizing verbal hostility, corporal punishment, punitive strategies, and excessive directiveness. Permissive caregivers are characterized as having an inability to follow through with discipline and directives.

King (2004) claims that some caregiving styles are more adaptive than others. Authoritative caregivers appear to adjust better to caregiving than authoritarian or permissive caregivers, reporting less life disruption, burden, and grief while also appraising their caregiving situation in more positive terms. Further, authoritarian and permissive caregivers report more anxiety in relationships and negative appraisal of their caregiving situation. A study done by Machac-Burleson et al. (2008) with a sample of caregivers of family members with dementia also found caregiving style to influence caregiver adjustment. As in King (2004), authoritative caregiving style was associated with better adjustment and more benefit finding. Contrary to King (2004), however, some positive aspects of adjustment were found to be associated with authoritarian and permissive caregiving styles. Although authoritarian caregiving was associated with lower caregiving satisfaction, it was also associated with higher physical quality of life. Permissive caregiving was associated not only with high levels of burden and impact, but also with more benefit finding.

The Current Study

The current study took a strengths approach in examining specific factors—namely, grandparents' caregiving and coping styles, benefit finding, and perceptions of their grandchildren's behavior problems—that combine to influence the adjustment of grandparents raising grandchildren. Adjustment was measured by grandparents' appraisal of their caregiving situation, depression, and quality of life. Based on current literature, several outcomes were expected. As demonstrated in Machac-Burleson et al. (2008), we anticipated that caregiving style, coping style, and benefit finding would be directly related to caregiver adjustment, and caregiving style would be indirectly related to caregiver adjustment through coping style and benefit finding. Further, we anticipated that the relationship between caregiving style and caregiver adjustment will be impacted by grandparents' perceptions of their grandchildren's behavior problems.

Method

Participants and Procedure

The participants for this study consist of 61 grandparents providing full-time care for their grandchildren. All participants are the primary caregivers for one or more of their grandchildren. Participants were identified from community organizations such as schools, churches, day-care centers, and doctor's offices, establishing contacts with a point-person at each organization and maintaining consistent follow-up. Participants were also recruited by attending conferences for grandparents raising grandchildren in Dallas, TX. Attempts to find participants were also made through word of mouth and by distributing flyers at community organizations and businesses in the Huntsville, TX area. After providing informed consent, each participant was asked to complete a packet of study questionnaires. The participants were also provided with informational handouts including lists of community resources from which they may be able to obtain social support and assistance.

Measures

Participants answered a series of questions regarding demographics (e.g., age, education, race) as well as questions intended to give a better understanding of the participant's caregiving situation (e.g. number of years providing care to grandchild, quality of relationship with grandchild, reason for assuming care of grandchild). *Caregiving style* was assessed using the Caregiving Style Scale (CSS; King, 2004). The CSS is based on the Parenting Practices Questionnaire (PPQ; Robinson, Mandleco, Olsen, & Hart, 1995). The items on the CSS measure authoritative caregiving, authoritarian caregiving, and permissive caregiving characteristics. *Coping* was examined by the Brief COPE (Carver, 1997). The measure is made up of 14 two-item scales, which can be classified into two subscales: approach and avoidant coping. *Benefit finding* was examined using an adaptation of Behr's Positive Contributions Scale (PCS; Tomich & Hegelson, 2004). Each of the 21 items follows the stem, "Caring for my grandchild has . . ." The Strengths and Difficulties Questionnaire (SDQ; Goodman, 1997) was used to assess the *grandchildren's internalizing and externalizing behaviors* as perceived by the participants. The 25-item questionnaire is composed of five scales: conduct problems, hyperactivity-inattention, emotional symptoms, peer problems, and prosocial behavior. For the purposes of this study, the conduct problems and emotional symptoms scales were used.

Caregiver adjustment was operationalized using three interrelated constructs: (a) caregiving appraisal, (b) caregiver perceptions of quality of life, and (c) depression. The Caregiving Appraisal Scale (CAS; Lawton, Kleban, Moss, Rovine, & Glickman, 1989) was used to assess the participants' perceived amount of burden, satisfaction regarding their caregiving situation, and the negative impact caregiving has had on the caregiver's life. The Medical Outcomes Study 36 Item Short Form Health Survey (MOS SF-36; Frytak, 2000; Ware & Sherbourne, 1992) was used to assess quality of life. The MOS SF-36 is made up of eight health concepts: physical functioning, role limitations due to physical problems, social functioning, bodily pain, general mental health, role limitations due to emotional problems, vitality, and general health perceptions. To assess depression, the Geriatric Depression Scale-Short Form (GDS-SF; Sheikh & Yesavage, 1986) was used. Items on the GDS-SF have been shown to be significantly related to diagnostic criteria for depression (Sheikh & Yesavage, 1986).

Results

The majority of participants were married (54.8%), African-American (51.6%), females (82.5%). The age of the participants ranged from 42 to 77 ($M = 60.2$, $SD = 8.0$). Parental drug abuse was the most common reason that participants reported for assuming care of their grandchild (23.8%). This was followed in frequency by a category named "other parental incapacity," which involved reasons such as their grandchildren's parent(s) being young, immature, or irresponsible, or that the parent(s) were experiencing psychological, legal, or other overwhelming life problems. Nineteen percent of grandparents reported reasons for assuming care of their grandchild(ren) that were coded in this category. Other common categories included death of parent, parental abuse and/or neglect, parental professional obligations (which include situations such as the parent moving out of state for work or for school), parental health problems, and other miscellaneous reasons (e.g., out of love for the grandchild, because the child asked to be raised by grandparent, etc.). For the most part, the pattern of reasons that emerged from the data followed what has been found in previous research. For example, previous studies have reported drug abuse to be one of the most common reasons that most custodial grandparents assume the duty of raising their grandchildren (Barth, 1991; Casper & Bryson, 1998; Feig, 1990). However, unlike previous research (Casper & Bryson, 1998), only a small percentage of participants reported divorce as being the reason for assuming care.

The relationships between caregiving style, coping style, and benefit finding, and grandparent adjustment were also explored. All three of the caregiving styles were significantly related to one or more of the adjustment variables. The use of an authoritative caregiving style was positively associated with caregiver satisfaction, while the use of an authoritarian caregiving style was negatively associated with caregiver satisfaction. The use of a permissive caregiving was positively associated with depression and negatively associated with quality of life.

Both coping styles and benefit finding were also significantly associated with one or more adjustment variables. Approach coping was positively associated with caregiver burden and negative impact. Avoidant coping was positively associated with depression, caregiver burden, and negative impact, and was negatively associated with caregiver satisfaction and quality of life. Benefit finding was positively associated with both caregiver satisfaction and quality of life. Grandparents' reports of their grandchildren's internalizing and externalizing symptoms were not correlated with any of the adjustment variables.

Predictors of Grandparent Adjustment

Caregiving style was significantly associated with caregiver satisfaction with the use of an authoritative caregiving style associated with higher caregiver satisfaction. Caregivers' quality of life could also be reliably predicted from their caregiving style. The use of a permissive caregiving style was associated with lower quality of life. Additionally, while caregiving style did not significantly predict depression, there was a marginal trend between the use of a permissive caregiving style and more depression.

Overall, there was a significant relationship between coping style and benefit finding and depression, with avoidant coping being associated with more depression. Finally, grandchild symptoms were not related to any measures of adjustment.

Mediators of the Caregiving-Grandparent Adjustment Relationship

In addition to the direct relationships reported above, we also carried out analyses to examine whether coping and benefit finding mediated the relationship between caregiving style and grandparent adjustment (see Figures 2.1 and 2.2). We found that benefit finding explained the relationship between authoritative caregiving style and caregiver satisfaction; that is, when adjusting for the relationship between benefit finding and caregiver satisfaction, the relationship between authoritative caregiving style and caregiver satisfaction statistically decreased.

In addition, avoidant coping explained the relationship between permissive caregiving style and lower quality of life (see Figure 2.2). When adjusting for the relationship between avoidant coping and quality of life, the relationship between permissive caregiving style and quality of life statistically decreased.

The findings from this study suggest that caregiving style, coping style, and benefit finding are important in understanding the experience of grandparents raising their grandchildren. More specifically, the results support the current literature and our expectation that caregiving style is directly related to caregiver adjustment. This suggests that efforts to promote certain types of caregiving styles may not only help strengthen a grandparent caregiver's relationship with their grandchildren, but improve their overall well-being as well. For example, grandparents who adopt an authoritative caregiving style (those who are warm and involved with their grandchildren but set clear limits on their behavior) reported more satisfaction with their caregiving situation. Conversely, grandparents who adopted a permissive caregiving style—characterized by reluctance or inability to follow through with discipline—reported lower quality of life and marginally higher levels of depression. These findings emphasize that the styles by which grandparents care for their grandchildren exert important effects on their adjustment as caregivers.

Further, as expected, coping and benefit finding are also directly related to caregiver adjustment. Grandparents reporting more benefit finding were

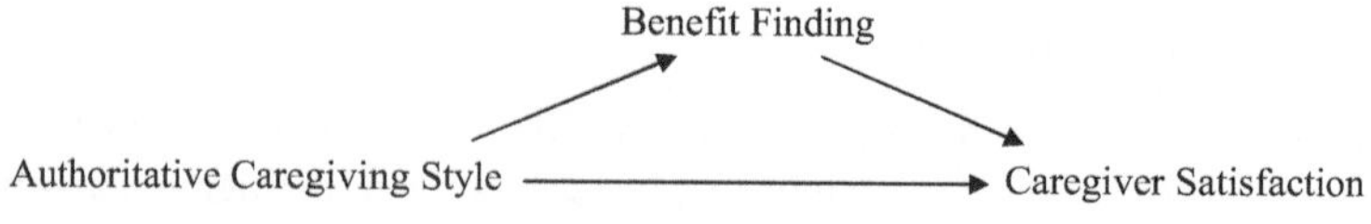

Figure 2.1 Benefit Finding Mediation Model

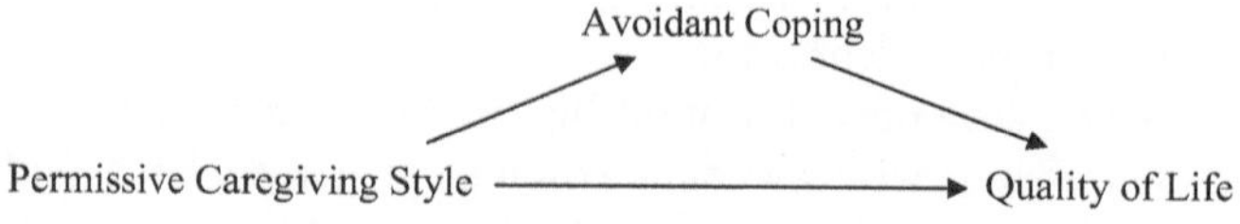

Figure 2.2 Avoidant Coping Mediation Model

more satisfied with caregiving and were less negatively impacted by caring for their grandchild. In addition, grandparents who identified more benefits also reported a marginally higher quality of life. Although Helgeson et al. (2006) recently published a meta-analysis on benefit finding, the literature examining benefit finding specifically in the context of caregiving is limited. However, findings from the current study are consistent with the few studies that have been conducted. These findings on benefit finding also suggest a critical element of interventions aimed at grandparent caregivers is to foster the ability of grandparent caregivers to focus on positive aspects of their caregiving situation. While the evidence is limited, our results indicate helping grandparents to capitalize on the rewards of caregiving may be one pathway to better psychological adjustment and reduce the likelihood of negative psychosocial outcomes.

Additionally, previous research suggests coping style plays an important role in caregiver adjustment. As expected, the study results suggest avoidant coping is associated with negative outcomes. Grandparents who reported using more avoidant coping strategies (e.g., withdrawal, denial) reported higher levels of depression, lower quality of life, and more caregiving burden. Although previous research has found approach coping to be associated with positive outcomes (Ben-Zur, 2005; Penley et al., 2002), similar evidence was not found in the current study.

In fact, contrary to expectations, grandparents who reported using more approach coping (e.g., problem solving, planning) reported perceiving their lives as more burdened and more negatively impacted by their caregiving situation. It is possible that this occurred because grandparents who are in particularly stressful situations may be using a mixture of several coping strategies rather than consistently selecting one manner of coping. Further, they may not be using the approach coping strategies effectively. Thus, effective clinical intervention would help the caregiver to cope with adjustment difficulties by taking an active stance in planning alternative options, brainstorming solutions to adjustment difficulties ahead of time, and learning to recognize when avoidant coping is triggered. While benefit finding appears to be a more important element of adjustment in this sample of custodial grandparents, learning to effectively use active coping strategies (e.g., approach coping) can also play a valuable role in psychological well-being for grandparent caregivers.

Caregiving Style and Coping Strategy

A grandparent's caregiving style and how he or she is coping with the situation may be related to each other. Our findings suggest custodial grandparents who use an authoritative caregiving style are satisfied with their caregiving situation largely because they see more benefits in raising their grandchildren. Currently, little is known about benefit finding in caregivers. However, these findings suggest benefit finding may be more likely to promote satisfaction for authoritative caregivers. It makes sense that grandparents who are easy-going, warm, attentive, and involved with their grandchildren would be more apt to recognize the benefits of caregiving, an ability that leads to satisfaction. In turn, services aimed at helping grandparents to see the positive aspects of caregiving may encourage more involvement and attentiveness to their grandchildren's needs, including more consistent discipline. This authoritative caregiving style then enhances the relationship and overall satisfaction. In contrast, using a permissive caregiving style is related to lower quality of life for custodial grandparents because those who report permissive caregiving are also using more avoidant coping techniques. Avoidant coping tends to be used when an individual feels there is nothing he or she can do about a stressful situation (Lazarus & Folkman, 1984). It stands to reason that permissive grandparents lacking disciplinary follow-through may feel that they have no control over the situation and respond with avoidance.

Therefore, it seems lower quality of life results when custodial grandparents feel ill-equipped to cope with the demands of caregiving. They may be overwhelmed by the needs of their grandchildren or lack the necessary coping strategies to deal with the disciplinary problems they encounter. Equipping grandparents with tools for caregiving, such as communication and rule-setting skills or behavioral management plans, *in addition* to teaching them proactive coping strategies may be most effective. Whatever the case, it seems clear that any intervention aimed at promoting active coping strategies and a warm, consistently rewarding relationship between grandparents and their grandchildren will likely result in more beneficial outcomes.

Limitations, Strengths, and Future Directions

The significance of our findings must be considered in light of the study limitations. First, the population proved to be a difficult population to access, reflected in a small sample size. Furthermore, cross-sectional study design was used, consisting of self-report questionnaires. As such, the strong associations may at least partially emerge because the same individual is reporting on each of the constructs we examined. The findings would be richer if grandchildren also reported on their grandparents' caregiving style and adjustment.

However, despite these limitations, the relationships between the constructs examined in the current study have not been investigated in custodial grandparents. To our knowledge, this is the first study examining benefit finding in custodial grandparents, and along with King (2004), it is one of the first studies investigating caregiving style. A second strength of the study is that an ethnically balanced sample was obtained, which suggests greater generalizability of these findings to a broader spectrum of grandparents.

Future studies using a longitudinal design should be conducted. A longitudinal study would allow researchers to determine the temporal order of caregiving, coping, and benefit finding. For example, it is possible that people first adopt a caregiving style, which then influences their perspective as caregivers, making them more likely to focus on the positive aspects of caregiving.

Alternatively, it is possible that grandparents who frequently engage in benefit finding tend to adopt certain caregiving styles more than others. Longitudinal studies would also allow researchers to examine grandparents' change in adjustment over time. For example, the meta-analysis done by Helgeson et al. (2006) examining benefit finding in individuals who had experienced a stressful event found the relationship between benefit finding and adjustment to be stronger when more time had elapsed since the stressor had occurred. It is also important for future studies to obtain the perspective of the grandchild, examining how well he or she has adjusted to being raised by their grandparent.

Conclusion

In summary, the findings of the current study suggest when examining custodial grandparent adjustment, not only do grandchild symptoms need to be considered, but so do grandparents' caregiving style, coping style, and benefit finding. These constructs influence each other and therefore need to be examined and understood together. The current study adds to a limited body of research on an underserved population. These findings can help shape interventions aimed at assisting grandparents in adjusting to their caregiving situation by capitalizing on individual strengths in coping and caregiving style. Specifically, it is suggested that these types of interventions promote the use of authoritative caregiving strategies, provide psychoeducation, and emphasize the importance of recognizing the many benefits that come with being a custodial grandparent.

References

Barth, R. (1991). Educational implications of prenatally drug-exposed children. *Social Work in Education, 13*, 130–136.

Baumrind, D. (1971). Current patterns of parental authority. *Developmental Psychology*, 4, (2), 1–103.

Baumrind, D. (1991). Parenting styles and adolescent development. In J. Brooks-Gunn, R. Lerner & A. C. Petersen (Eds.), *Encyclopedia of adolescence, II*. New York: Garland.

Ben-Zur, H. (2005). Coping, distress, and life events in a community sample. *International Journal of Stress Management, 12*, 188–196.

Birhamer, B., Ryan, N. D., Williamson, D. E., Brent, D. A., Kaufman, J., Dahl, R. E., et al. (1996). *Journal of the American Academy of Child and Adolescent Psychiatry, 35*, 1427–1439.

Burton, L. M. (1992). Black grandparents rearing children of drug-addicted parents: Stressors, outcomes, and social service needs. *The Gerontologist, 32*, 744–751.

Carver, C. S. (1997). You want to measure coping but your protocol's too long: Consider the Brief COPE. *International Journal of Behavioral Medicine, 4*, 92–100.

Carver, C. S., Scheier, M. F., & Weintraub, J. K. (1989). Assessing coping strategies: A theoretically cased approach. *Journal of Personality and Social Psychology, 56*, 267–283.

Casper, L., & Bryson, K. (1998). *Co-resident grandparents and their grandchildren: Grandparent-maintained families* (Population Division technical working paper, 26). Washington, DC: U.S. Bureau of the Census.

Emick, M., & Hayslip, B. (1999). Custodial grandparenting: Stresses, coping skills, and relationships with grandchildren. *International Journal of Aging and Human Development, 48*, 35–62.

Frytak, J. R. (2000). Assessment of quality of life in older adults. In R. L. Kane & R. A. Kane (Eds.), *Assessing older persons: Measures, meaning, and practical applications* (pp. 200–236). New York: Oxford University Press.

Fuller-Thomson, E., & Minkler, M. (2000). The mental and physical health of grandmothers who are raising their grandchildren. *Journal of Mental Health and Aging, 6*, 311–323.

Goodman, R. (1997). The strengths and difficulties questionnaire: A research note. *Journal of Child Psychology and Psychiatry, 38*, 581–586.

Hayslip, B., & Goldberg-Glen, R. (Eds.). (2000). *Grandparents raising grandchildren.* New York: Springer.

Hayslip, B., & Patrick, J. (2006). *Custodial grandparenting: Individual, cultural, and ethnic diversity.* New York: Springer.

Hayslip, B., Shore, J., Henderson, C., & Lambert, P. (1998). Custodial grandparents and the impact of grandchildren with problems on role satisfaction and role meaning. *Journal of Gerontology, 53*, 164–173.

Helgeson, V. S., Reynolds, K. A., & Tomich, P. L. (2006). A meta-analytic review of benefit finding and growth. *Journal of Consulting and Clinical Psychology, 74*, 797–816.

Henderson, T. L., & Stevenson, M. L. (2003, May). Grandparents rearing grandchildren: Rights and responsibilities. *Virginia Cooperative Extension.* Retrieved September 1, 2006, from http://www.ext.vt.edu/pubs/gerontology/350-255/350-255.html

Hetherington, E. M. (1989). Coping with family transitions: Winners, losers, and survivors. *Child Development, 60*, 1–14.

Jendrek, M. (1993). Grandparents who parent their grandchildren: Effects in lifestyle. *Journal of Marriage and the Family, 55*, 609–621.

King, J. (2004). *The assessment of caregiving style.* Unpublished master's thesis, University of North Texas, Denton.

Kropf, N., & Burnette, D. (2003). Grandparents as family caregivers: Lessons for intergenerational education. *Educational Gerontology, 29*, 361–372.

Lawton, M. P., Kleban, M. H., Moss, M., Rovine, M., & Glicksman, A. (1989). Measuring caregiving appraisal. *Journal of Gerontology, 44*, 61–71.

Lazarus, R. S., & Folkman, S. (1984). *Stress, appraisal, and coping.* New York: Springer.

Littleton, H., Horsley, S., John, S., & Nelson, D. V. (2007). Trauma coping strategies and psychological distress: A meta-analysis. *Journal of Traumatic Stress, 20*, 977–988.

Loeber, R., & Stouthamer-Loeber, M. (1986). Family factors as correlates and predictors of juvenile conduct problems and delinquency. In M. Tonry & N. Morris (Eds.), *Crime and Justice* (pp. 29–149). Chicago: University of Chicago Press.

Machac-Burleson, M., Henderson, C., Nelson, D., Hayslip, B., King, J., & Harman, M. (2008). The impact of caregiving style, coping, and benefit finding on the adjustment of caregivers of individuals with dementia. *The Gerongologist, 48 (Special Issue III)*, 165.

McCausland, J., & Pakenham, K. I. (2003). Investigation of the benefits of HIV/AIDS caregiving and relations among caregiving adjustment, benefit finding, and stress and coping variables. *Aids Care, 15*, 853–869.

McCord, J. (1982). A longitudinal study of the link between broken homes and criminality. In J. Gunn & D. P. Farrington (Eds.), *Abnormal offenders delinquency and the criminal justice system*. London: Wiley.

Minkler, M., & Fuller-Thomson, E. (1999). The health of grandparents raising grandchildren: Results of a national study. *American Journal of Public Health, 89*, 1384–1389.

Penley, J. A., Tomaka, J., & Wiebe, J. S. (2002). The association of coping to physical and psychological health outcomes: A meta-analytic review. *Journal of Behavioral Medicine, 6*, 551–603.

Robinson, C. C., Madleco, B., Olsen, S. F., & Hart, C. H. (1995). Authoritative, authoritarian, and permissive parenting practices: Development of a new measure. *Psychological Reports, 77*, 819–830.

Roth, S., & Cohen, L. J. (1986). Approach, avoidance, and coping with stress. *American Psychologist, 41*, 813–819.

Sands, R. G., & Goldberg-Glen, R. S. (2000). Factors associated with stress among grandparents raising their grandchildren. *Family Relations, 49*, 97–105.

Sheikh, J. I., & Yesavage, J. A. (1986). Geriatric depression scale (GDS): Recent evidence and development of a shorter version. In T. L. Brink (Ed.), *Clinical gerontology: A guide to assessment and intervention* (pp. 165–173). New York: Haworth Press.

Snyders, C. R., & Pulvers, K. M. (2001). Dr. Seuss, the coping machine, and "Oh, the Places You'll Go." In C. R. Snyder (Ed.), *Coping with stress: Effective people and processes* (pp. 3–29). Oxford, England: Oxford University Press.

Tomich, P. L., & Hegelson, V. S. (2004). Is finding something good in the bad always good? Benefit finding among women with breast cancer. *Health Psychology, 23*, 16–23.

U. S. Bureau of the Census. (2001). *Coresident grandparents and grandchildren*. Retrieved November 10, 2007, from http://www.census.gov

Ware, J. E. & Sherbourne, C. D. (1992). The MOS 36-item short-form health survey (SF-36). Conceptual framework and item selection. *Medical Care, 30*, 473–483.

3 Resourcefulness in Grandmothers Raising Grandchildren[1]

Jaclene A. Zauszniewski and Carol M. Musil

Abstract

This chapter explores resourcefulness: the theoretical basis of personal and social resourcefulness; measuring resourcefulness; the relationships of resourcefulness to mental and physical health status, adaptive functioning, and quality of life; and evidence based strategies for increasing resourcefulness in grandmothers raising grandchildren. Resourcefulness is a repertoire of cognitive-behavioral skills for coping with adversity (Rosenbaum, 1990; Zauszniewski, 1997, 2006). Our work in the area of resourcefulness has shown that while there are no differences in overall resourcefulness between grandmothers raising grandchildren and non-caregiving grandmothers, greater resourcefulness contributes to better family functioning and fewer depressive symptoms in these women. Therefore, teaching the skills constituting resourcefulness to grandmothers can be beneficial for reducing the effects of family life stress, minimizing depressive symptoms and promoting healthy functioning.

Over one million American grandmothers are primary caregivers for their grandchildren. Grandmothers raising grandchildren report more stress, strain, and depressive symptoms than grandmothers not living with grandchildren (Musil, Warner, Zauszniewski, Wykle, & Standing, 2009) and perceive more problems in family functioning (Musil, Warner, Zauszniewski, Jeanblanc, & Kercher, 2006). Raising grandchildren can be overwhelmingly stressful, and it may adversely affect the grandmother's physical and mental health, unless she is resourceful. Resourcefulness is a repertoire of cognitive-behavioral skills for coping with adversity (Rosenbaum, 1990; Zauszniewski, 1997) that involves the ability to perform daily tasks independently (i.e., personal resourcefulness) and to seek help from others when unable to function independently (i.e., social resourcefulness) (Zauszniewski, 2006). Resourcefulness is believed to bolster one's capacity to deal with stress, and thus can reduce the effects of family life stresses on grandmothers' depressive symptoms and overall functioning.

Conceptualization of Resourcefulness

Resourcefulness, as conceptualized here, grew out of the work of Rosenbaum (1980), who initially proposed that learned resourcefulness reflected verbal and non-verbal cognitive skills. These skills, which focus on self-control, include self-instructions to manage emotional and physiological responses to stress, problem-solving, delay of gratification, and belief that one can manage internal stimuli (Zauszniewski, 1995, p. 16). Zauszniewski's continued work (Zauszniewski, 2006) in the area of resourcefulness led to dropping the label of "learned" from the concept name, even though there is a learned component to resourcefulness as a skill. Secondly, a growing understanding of the value and limits of resourcefulness as originally conceptualized led to an expanded conceptualization of "resourcefulness," to include both *personal resourcefulness*, as described in Rosenbaum's original 1980 conceptualization, and *social resourcefulness*, to recognize the appropriateness and importance of seeking outside help when needed.

Personal Resourcefulness

Personal resourcefulness (PR) skills include verbal and non-verbal cognitive skills that are used to control the potentially disturbing effects that cognitions, emotions, and sensations may have on performing daily activities (Rosenbaum, 1980). Rosenbaum (1980) called these PR skills "learned resourcefulness." His theory says that individuals acquire throughout life a basic repertoire of cognitive-behavioral coping skills that enable them to achieve health goals independently (without help from others); these skills are learned through conditioning, modeling, and formal or informal instruction (Rosenbaum, 1990). Abilities to think positively and solve problems, which constitute PR, are personal strengths that are learned.

Since the early 1990s, researchers have described such behaviors as personal resources that are pivotal factors in achieving positive outcomes (McBride, 1993; Schuldberg, 1993). Although Rosenbaum (1980) suggested that resourcefulness is a relatively enduring personal characteristic, changes in resourcefulness have been found over time in response to health-related situations (Biren, 1990; Lewisohn & Alexander, 1990; Reachman, 1990) and in response to interventions that teach PR skills (Braden, 1991; Braden, McGlone, & Pennington, 1993; Braden, Mishel, & Longman, 1998; Kreulen & Braden, 2004; LeFort, Gray-Donald, Rowat, & Jeans, 1998; Rosswurm, Larrabee, & Zhang, 2002; Zauszniewski, 1997). Our longitudinal analysis of resourcefulness over 24 months indicates that resourcefulness does not differ between grandmothers based on caregiving group, and that resourcefulness is relatively stable over time (Musil et al., 2011), with autocorrelations of .69 across the first two waves of data one year apart, and .61 over five years (Musil, 2010). However, theoretically, it is possible that constructive intrapersonal and interpersonal experiences or other therapeutic interventions could positively affect one's resourcefulness (Rosenbaum, 1980, 1990; Zauszniewski, 2006), but these have not been scientifically evaluated, to our knowledge. Since research results indicate that resourcefulness can be improved with targeted resourcefulness training (Zauszniewski et al., 2006, 2007), this is an area for intervention development with grandmothers raising grandchildren, especially those who are experiencing depressive symptoms or who are having difficulty managing any of the many family issues that arise.

Social Resourcefulness

Social resourcefulness (SR) skills, or skills in seeking help from others, are strategies for overcoming difficulties associated with perceived stress (Nadler, 1990) and promoting physical and psychological health (Quayhagan & Quayhagan, 1988) and quality of life (Ruffing-Rahal & Wallace, 2000). Rapp, Schumaker, Schmidt, Naughton, and Anderson (1998) describe "social resourcefulness" as behaviors used to establish and maintain supportive relationships and obtain help from others. Help-seeking behavior, including the use of formal health services and informal help from family members, has been positively associated with health status (Blaum, Liang, & Liu, 1994; Jorm, Henderson, Scott, MacKinnon, Korten, & Christensen, 1993). In a study of functionally dependent elders, psychological symptoms were reduced with greater use of informal support (Mui & Burnette, 1994).

Measuring Resourcefulness Skills

Three measures of resourcefulness in adults have been described in the literature. The original measure of resourcefulness, the Self-Control Schedule (SCS), was developed by Rosenbaum (1980) to capture the cognitive-behavioral skills constituting what he called "learned resourcefulness." This 36-item measure, which used a 6-point Likert scale, included items reflecting the use of positive affirmations, delay of gratification, problem-solving, and belief in coping effectiveness. However, items on this scale that reflected the use of "outside help" are reverse-coded, implying that seeking the help of others is not characteristic of one who is resourceful. In 2006, Zauszniewski and colleagues published a measure, called the Resourcefulness Scale that reflected the two dimensions of resourcefulness: personal and social. This scale contains 28 items rated on a 6-point Likert scale with 16 items measuring self-help skills constituting personal resourcefulness and 12 items measuring help-seeking skills comprising social resourcefulness. The 16 items that make up the personal resourcefulness subscale were derived from Rosenbaum's SCS through psychometric testing (Zauszniewski, Lai, & Tithiphontumrong, 2006). The 12 social resourcefulness items were developed as parallel items for the 28-item RS scale and were supported by psychometric testing (Zauszniewski et al., 2006b). The scale has reported strong estimates of internal consistency reliability ($\alpha = .85$) and construct validity (Zauszniewski et al., 2006b).

Most recently, Zauszniewski and Bekhet (2011) developed an 8-item measure of the resourcefulness skills that are taught during resourcefulness training. Unlike the 28-item Resourcefulness Scale described above, which captures general use of resourcefulness skills within particular everyday situations, the Resourcefulness Skills Scale measures the use of the eight resourcefulness skills, including the three help-seeking and the five self-help skills, that are taught during resourcefulness training. This scale, which is a useful adjunct for assessing intervention fidelity, has reported estimates of reliability ($\alpha = .78$) and validity (Zauszniewski & Bekhet, 2011).

Resourcefulness Improves Family Functioning

Research in the area of resourcefulness with grandmothers has shown that lower resourcefulness is associated with worse family functioning (Musil et al., 2006) and increased frequency of depressive symptoms (Musil et al., 2009). Although no detectable differences in resourcefulness were found across different types of grandmothers, comparing primary caregivers (i.e., those raising grandchildren), multi-generational caregivers (i.e., shared responsibility in raising grandchildren), and non-caregivers (i.e., those with no ongoing responsibility for care of grandchildren) (Musil et al., 2006; Musil et al., 2011), greater resourcefulness has been found to contribute to better family functioning for grandmothers raising grandchildren (primary caregivers) and those in multigenerational homes (Musil et al., 2006).

Resourcefulness Associated with Lower Stress and Depressive Symptoms

We examined correlates of resourcefulness using data from Musil's study of grandmothers across five time waves. Stress and reward, measured as visual analog scales, showed cross-sectional correlations (inverse and positive, respectively), with resourcefulness ranging from $r = .15$ to $.22$; thus, although rather weak, more resourcefulness was associated with less stress and greater reward in the role of grandmother. Cross-sectional correlations between depressive symptoms and resourcefulness ranged from $-.32$ to $-.42$ across five time waves, with greater resourcefulness related to fewer depressive symptoms. Similarly, subjective support showed moderate cross-sectional correlations with resourcefulness, with the associations in a range of $r = .27$ to $.44$, whereby grandmothers reporting greater resourcefulness experienced more support from family and friends.

Personal Versus Social Resourcefulness

Taken together, these findings suggest that more resourceful grandmothers perform daily activities despite potentially stressful conditions, apply effective methods for managing daily activities, maintain confidence in their ability to cope effectively, report fewer depressive symptoms, and promote optimal family functioning. However, in these studies of grandmothers, resourcefulness was operationalized in a restricted way that focused only on measurement of personal or self-help skills, referred to in other literature as "learned resourcefulness" (Rosenbaum, 1980, 1990); help-seeking, or social resourcefulness skills, were not captured. Indeed, as previously described, in the earlier writings on learned resourcefulness, items on the resourcefulness measure that reflect seeking help from others were reverse coded (Rosenbaum, 1980), indicating that if one sought outside help, one was less resourceful. However, as previously mentioned, the more recent conceptualization of resourcefulness has been expanded to incorporate measurement of social or help-seeking skills (Zauszniewski, 2006). The closest proxy variable with the studies of grandmothers described above was the inclusion of measures of social support. In Musil's study of grandmothers across five time waves, (Musil et al., 2006, 2009), learned resourcefulness showed good to strong correlations with subjective support at each wave.

Social Support and Depressive Symptoms

When we compared grandmothers raising grandchildren, multi-generational home grandmothers, and non-caregiver grandmothers (Musil et al., 2009), both groups that lived with grandchildren reported more intra-family strains (interpersonal conflicts and difficulties) and financial stresses than non-caregivers to grandchildren. Interestingly, grandmothers raising grandchildren reported significantly less subjective support and more depressive symptoms than did non-caregivers. For all grandmothers, resourcefulness reduced the effects of strain on depressive symptoms; for primary and non-caregivers, but not those in multigenerational homes, subjective support also had an effect on depressive symptoms. Subjective support had an additional moderating effect on depressive symptoms for grandmothers raising grandchildren: high subjective support in the face of high strain contributed to fewer depressive symptoms (Musil et al., 2009). These findings underscore the importance of being able to call upon and use personal resourcefulness strategies such as positive self-talk, maintaining a positive attitude and trying new ways to manage problems, and also the importance of social resources, which includes knowing when to seek and accept the help and advice of family and friends.

Importance of Resourcefulness

The implication of these findings in relation to resourcefulness, specifically the personal resourcefulness skills of grandmothers, and the indicators of their social support, is that interventions to inspire and strengthen both personal and social resourcefulness skills may be beneficial. For example, encouraging grandmothers to use more positive self-statements and recalling past successes in difficult situations are simple exercises that can strengthen an individual's personal resourcefulness skills (Zauszniewski et al., 2006). In addition, encouraging and supporting grandmothers to seek help from others, including help from formal (i.e., health care professionals and other) and informal sources (i.e., family, friends, teachers, other grandmothers, etc.), may be beneficial in bolstering their social resourcefulness skills. Indeed, pervious research has shown that individuals who use both personal and social resourcefulness skills have the best quality of life outcomes (Zauszniewski, 1996). Thus, teaching both the personal and social skills constituting resourcefulness is of paramount importance. Interventions to teach grandmothers raising grandchildren to be resourceful in managing their stress may promote their optimal health so they can continue raising their grandchildren and avoid the need for institutional placement or foster care.

Group Versus Individual Methods to Teach Resourcefulness

The skills constituting personal and social resourcefulness skills are believed to be learned (Rosenbaum, 1980, 1990; Nadler, 1990; Rapp et al., 1998) and have been taught successfully to elders using a small group format (Zauszniewski, 1997; Zauszniewski, Bekhet, Lai, McDonald, & Musil, 2007; Zauszniewski et al., 2006). Although a small group format for teaching resourcefulness skills has been found to be effective in improving self-assessed health and functional status (Zauszniewski et al., 2006) and promoting positive affect and reducing depressive cognitions (Zauszniewski et al., 2007), convening groups for the grandmothers, which would take them away from their grandchildren, may not be feasible for teaching resourcefulness, and in general have been reported to be ineffective (Biegel & Song, 1995) for providing support in community settings.

In addition, meta-analyses of the effects of interventions on caregiver burden and psychological well-being have shown that group interventions had smaller effects than individual formats (Lorig, Sobel, Ritter, Laurent, & Hobbs, 2001; Yin, Zhou, & Bashford, 2002). However, although these studies were not conducted in samples of grandmothers, stronger effects for individual interventions have been reported for caregivers of children (Thomas & Corcoran, 2003). Finally, individualized interventions minimize sampling bias that might occur in clinical trials due to attrition of study participants who choose not to attend a group intervention (Gage & Kinney, 1995). Ongoing research with grandmothers is examining the effectiveness of teaching personal and social resourcefulness skills to grandmothers raising grandchildren using individualized, tailored methods.

Rationale for Both Personal and Social Resourcefulness

The negative impact of grandchild caregiving stress on quality of life may be preventable with appropriate intervention (Kelley, Whitley, Sipe, & Yorker, 2000; Musil, 1998; Musil & Ahmad, 2002; Musil et al., 2006). Grandmothers caring for grandchildren need not experience depressive symptoms or declines in their physical functioning or psychological well-being. Zauszniewski (1996) has demonstrated that adults who were high on both personal (PR) and social resourcefulness (SR) also had significantly less anxiety and depression, and better self-assessed health and adaptive functioning than those who had either high PR alone or high SR alone. Thus, it follows that if grandmothers are taught both PR and SR, their psychological and physical health should be positively affected.

As described previously, PR and SR consist of different sets of skills that have the potential to promote psychological, social, and physical functioning (Zauszniewski, 2006; Zauszniewski et al., 2006; Zauszniewski et al., 2007). Therefore, grandmothers should then be expected to benefit from the use of both PR and SR skills as they continue to care for their grandchildren. There is beginning evidence in ongoing research with grandmothers raising grandchildren that teaching the personal and social skills constituting resourcefulness has positive effects on decreasing perceived stress and depressive symptoms and enhancing their quality of life. (Zauszniewski, Au, Musil, & Standing, 2011).

Resourcefulness Training Intervention

Teaching the personal (self-help) and social (help-seeking) skills constituting resourcefulness involves implementation of three mnemonic strategies, use of an acronym, chunking, and practice through self-reinforcement, to help grandmothers remember and use the eight skills comprising the resourcefulness repertoire. The personal and social resourcefulness skills are taught to grandmothers during a single, one hour session with a trained intervention provider. Using the acronym and chunking strategies, each skill is described and examples of how each one may be used by grandmothers in their daily interactions with their grandchildren are discussed.

In general, an ***acronym*** is formed by the first letter of words or groups of words to form a new word (Nelson & Archer, 1972). In resourcefulness training (RT), the acronym uses the eight letters spelling **RESOURCE** to prompt recall of specific PR and SR skills as follows: **R**ely on family / friends; **E**xchange ideas with others; **S**eek professionals or experts; **O**rganize daily activities; **U**se positive self-talk; **R**eframe the situation positively; **C**hange from usual reaction; **E**xplore new ideas. The second mnemonic strategy to be used in RT is called ***chunking***, which refers to the common rule that an individual can remember between five and nine things at one time (Miller, 1956). In RT, the word **RESOURCE** contains eight letters, which is a reasonable "chunk" of ideas for the grandmothers to remember. In addition, SR skills are chunked in the first three letters and PR skills are chunked in the last five letters.

The third and final mnemonic strategy involves ***practice***. The individualized, tailored approach to teaching resourcefulness to grandmothers raising grandchildren involves the use of a daily written journal or digital voice recorder over a four-week period following the training session with the intervention provider. With either of the two self-reinforcement methods, the grandmothers review and reflect on their use of resourcefulness skills on a daily basis. Preliminary findings have shown that the two self-reinforcement strategies, currently being tested in ongoing research with grandmothers, are nearly equivalent in terms of feasibility, fidelity, and effectiveness (Zauszniewski, Au,

Musil, & Standing, 2011a,b,c; Zauszniewski, Musil, Au, & Standing, 2011.) If these findings hold up over continued analysis, then we can conclude that practice is a key component to reinforcing resourcefulness skills.

Intervention Development and Testing

We are currently analyzing data on the effectiveness of the resourcefulness training interventions. As we have the opportunity to analyze complete data from our ongoing studies, we will be better able to draw conclusions about the short and long-term outcomes of resourcefulness training interventions, as well as the factors that facilitate the use of personal and social resourcefulness skills. We are encouraged by the cross-sectional and longitudinal studies that show links between resourcefulness and mental health and positive health behavior. Further positive findings from our research about the applicability and effectivity of resourcefulness training with grandmother caregivers will contribute to a feasible and low-cost intervention to improve grandmother well-being, which promises to have a positive cascade on their ability to care for themselves, their grandchildren, and their families.

Implications for Helping Grandmothers

While we are optimistic about the potential of resourcefulness training as a strategy for helping grandmothers raising grandchildren to strengthen their ability to handle stressful situations and family challenges, we are cautious about prescribing this intervention until further evaluation of its efficacy and effectiveness occurs. In the interim, we encourage grandmothers to continue using a variety of active coping strategies, which are shown to reduce depressive symptoms (Musil & Ahmad, 2002), to attend to their health, and to engage with supportive others as often as possible.

Note

1 This research was supported by the following grants from the National Institute of Nursing Research/National Institutes of Health: "Intergenerational caregiving to youth at risk" and "Grandmothers, Families, Caregiving and Transitions" (PI: Musil; RO1-NR05067) and "Promoting resourcefulness in grandmothers raising grandchildren" (PI: Zauszniewski; R21 NR010581).

References

Biren, M. W. (1990). Resourcefulness and successful treatment of agoraphobia. In M. Rosenbaum (Ed.), *Learned resourcefulness: On coping skills, self-control, and adaptive behavior* (pp. 182–201). New York: Springer.

Blaum, C. S., Liang, J., & Liu, X. (1994). The relationship of chronic diseases and health status to the health services utilization of older Americans. *Journal of the American Geriatric Society*, *42*(10), 1087–1093.

Braden, C. J., McGlone, K., & Pennington, F. (1993). Specific psychosocial and behavioral outcomes from the systemic lupus erythematosus self-help course. *Journal of Health Education Quarterly, 20*(1), 29–41.

Braden, C. J., Mishel, M. H., & Longman, A. J. (1998). Self-help intervention project. Women receiving breast cancer treatment. *Journal of Cancer Practice, 6*(2), 87–98.

Gage, M. J., & Kinney, J. M. (1995). They aren't for everyone: The impact of support group participation on caregiver well-being. *Clinical Gerontologist, 16*(2), 21–34.

Henderson, A. S., Jorm, A. F., MacKinnon, A., Christensen, H., Scott, L. R., Korten, A. E., & Doyle, C. (1993). The prevalence of depressive disorders and the distribution of depressive symptoms in later life: A survey using Draft ICD-10 and DSM-III-R. *Journal of Psychological Medicine, 23*(3), 719–729.

Kelley, S. J., Whitley, D., Sipe, T. A., & Yorker, B. C. (2000). Psychological distress in grandmother kinship care providers: The role of resources, social support, and physical health. *Journal of Child Abuse and Neglect, 24*(3), 311–321.

Kreulen, G. J., & Braden, C. J. (2004). Model test of the relationship between self-help-promoting nursing interventions and self-care and health status outcomes. *Journal of Research Nursing Health, 27*(2), 97–109.

LeFort, S. M., Gray, D. K., Rowat, K. M., & Jeans, M. E. (1998). Randomized controlled trial of a community-based psycho-education program for the self-management of chronic pain. *Journal of Pain, 74*(2–3), 297–306.

Lewisohn, P. M., & Alexander, C. (1990). Learned resourcefulness and depression. In M. Rosenbaum (Ed.), *Learned resourcefulness: On coping skills, self-control, and adaptive behavior* (pp. 202–217). New York: Springer.

Lorig, K. R., Sobel, D. S., Ritter, P. L., Laurent, D., & Hobbs, M. (2001). Effect of a self-management program on patients with chronic disease. *Journal of Effective Clinical Practice, 4*(6), 256–262.

Miller, G. A. (1956). The magical number seven, plus or minus two. *Psychological Review, 63*(2), 81–97.

Mui, A. C., & Burnette, D. (1994). Long-term care service use by frail elders: Is ethnicity a factor? *The Gerontologist, 34*(2), 190–198.

Musil, C. M. (1998). Health, stress, coping, and social support in grandmother caregivers. *Health Care for Women International, 19*(5), 441–455.

Musil, C. M., & Ahmad, M. (2002). Health of grandmothers: A comparison by caregiver status. *Journal of Aging and Health, 14*(1), 96–121.

Musil, C. M., Gordon, N. L., Warner, C. B., Zauszniewski, J. A., Standing, T., & Wykle, M. (2011). Grandmothers and caregiving to grandchildren: Continuity, change, and outcomes over 24 months. *The Gerontologist, 51*(1), 86–100.

Musil, C. M., Warner, C. B., Zauszniewski, J. A., Jeanblanc, A. B., & Kercher, K. (2006). Grandmothers, caregiving, and family functioning. *Journal of Gerontology B Psychology Science and Social Science, 61*(2), 89–98.

Musil, C., Warner, C., Zauszniewski, J., Wykle, M., & Standing, T. (2009). Grandmother caregiving, family stress and strain, and depressive symptoms. *Western Journal of Nursing Research, 31*(3), 389–408.

Nadler, A. (1990). Help-seeking behavior as a coping resource. In M. Rosenbaum (Ed.), *Learned resourcefulness: On coping skills, self-control, and adaptive behavior*. New York: Springer Publishing.

Nelson, D. L., & Archer, C. S. (1972). The first letter mnemonic. *Journal of Educational Psychology, 63*(5), 482–486.

Quayhagen, M. P., & Quayhagen, M. (1998). Alzheimer's stress: Coping with the caregiving role. *The Gerontologist, 28*(3), 391–396.

Rapp, S. R., Shumaker, S., Schmidt, S., & Naughton, M. (1998). Social resourcefulness: Its relationship to social support and welling among caregiver of dementia victims. *Journal of Aging and Mental Health, 2*(1), 40–48.

Rosenbaum, R. (1980). A schedule for assessing self-control behavior: Preliminary finding. *Journal of Behavior Therapy, 11*(1), 109–121.

Ruffing-Rahal, M., & Wallace, J. (2000). Successful aging in a wellness group for older women. *Health Care Women International, 21*(4), 267–275.

Schuldberg, D. (1993). Personal resourcefulness: positive aspects of functioning in high-risk research. *Journal of Psychiatry, 56*(2), 137–152.

Thomas, C., & Corcoran, J. (2003). Family approaches to attention deficit hyperactivity disorder: a review to guide school social work practice. *Children and Schools, 25*(1), 19–34.

Zauszniewski, J. A. (1995). Learned resourcefulness: a conceptual analysis. *Issues in Mental Health Nursing, 16*, 13–31.

Zauszniewski, J. A. (1995). Theoretical and empirical considerations of resourcefulness. *Nursing Research, 27*(3), 177–180.

Zauszniewski, J. A. (1996). Self-help and help-seeking behavior patterns in healthy elders. *Journal of Holistic Nursing, 14*(3), 223–226.

Zauszniewski, J. A. (1997). Teaching resourcefulness skills to older adults. *Journal of Gerontological Nursing, 23*(2), 14–20.

Zauszniewski, J. A., Au, T. Y., Musil, C. M., & Standing, T. S. (2011a). *Resourcefulness training for grandmothers: Preliminary evidence for effectiveness.* American Academy of Nursing 37th Annual Meeting and Conference, Washington, DC, October, 2011.

Zauszniewski, J. A., Au, T. Y., Musil, C. M., & Standing, T. (2011b). *Resourcefulness training for grandmothers: Feasibility of two methods.* Midwest Nursing Research Society 34th Annual Scientific Conference, Columbus, OH, March, 2011.

Zauszniewski, J. A., Au, T. Y., Musil, C. M., & Standing, T. S. *Resourcefulness training for grandmothers: Establishing fidelity.* (2011c). Council for Advancement of Nursing Science special topics conference, Washington, DC, October, 2011.

Zauszniewski, J. A., & Bekhet, A. K. (2011). Measuring use of resourcefulness skills: Psychometric testing of a new scale. *Journal of International Scholarly Research Network*, e-pub June 7, 2011.

Zauszniewski, J. A., Bekhet, A. K., Lai, C. Y., McDonald, P. E., & Musil, C. M. (2007). Effects of teaching resourcefulness and acceptance on affect, behavior, and cognition of chronically ill elders. *Issues in Mental Health Nursing, 28*(6), 575–592.

Zauszniewski, J. A., Eggenschwiler, K., Preechawong, S., Roberts, B. L., & Morris, D. L. (2006a). Effects of teaching resourcefulness skills to elders. *Aging and Mental Health, 10*(4), 404–412.

Zauszniewski, J. A., Lai, C., & Tithiphontumrong, S. (2006b). Development and testing of the resourcefulness scale for older adults. *Journal of Nursing Measurement, 14*(1), 57–68.

Zauszniewski, J. A., Musil, C. M., Au, T. Y., & Standing, T. (2011). *Resourcefulness training for grandmothers raising grandchildren: Is there a need?* Midwest Nursing Research Society 34th Annual Scientific Conference, Columbus, OH, March, 2011.

4 The Role of Resilience in Mediating Stressor-Outcome Relationships Among Grandparents Raising Their Grandchildren

Bert Hayslip Jr., Shanna R. Davis, Craig S. Neumann, Catherine Goodman, Gregory C. Smith, Robert J. Maiden, and Gloria F. Carr

Abstract

The incidence of custodial grandparenting has increased over the last decade, and grandparents raise their grandchildren for a variety of reasons, i.e., the death, drug use, divorce, or incarceration of the child's birthparents. While it is commonly recognized that grandparents face added stress and much adversity that arises from caregiving, current research tends to be mixed regarding the effects of grandparents raising grandchildren. Indeed, while much research concludes that grandparent caregivers experience declines in over all health and well-being, other work suggests that grandparent caregiving may actually be a positive experience, leading to personal growth and to deeper, more satisfying relationships with a grandchild. That some studies paint a negative picture while others do not may be a consequence of varying levels of resilience among custodial grandparents. The model proposed and tested in this study centralizes resilience as an adaptive quality that grandparent caregivers possess in varying degrees, and examines resilience as a mediator of relationships between several antecedent grandchild-related and life situation-related (life resources) variables that affect custodial grandparents in both parental and well-being related ways. Based upon data gathered from 239 custodial grandparents, it was found that resilience, as well as its parental equivalent, parental efficacy, was significant in mediating the effects of grandparent caregiving. Thus, grandparent caregivers who vary in terms of personal resilience are likely to fare better or worse in coping with thedemands of raising a grandchild.

Introduction

Among those grandparents raising their grandchildren in the support group was a 38-year-old grandmother, clearly the youngest person in the group of adults in their 50s and 60s. Among those in the group, her outlook was the most optimistic

—she talked about how she had been blessed with the opportunity to raise her granddaughter, who was 6 years old. She looked toward the future, spoke positively about her life, and did not dwell on the past. It came to light that this woman assumed the care of her grandchild because her daughter had been brutally murdered. Six months after assuming the care of her granddaughter, her husband died of cancer. Within the same year, her granddaughter was also diagnosed with cancer. The other grandparents in the group were in awe of her—how had she been able to overcome such misfortune?

What caused this woman to look on the bright side of things, to say nothing of having survived such tragedies? Clearly this woman possessed something inside her that allowed her to overcome the trauma and loss that she had experienced. Such events would cause many of us to become depressed, hopeless, and at the least, pessimistic about the future. This grandmother was *resilient*—either she had always been so, or she learned to be so in light of the obstacles put in front of her in the context of the deaths of her daughter and husband as well as her granddaughter's cancer, to say nothing of the challenges associated with raising a grandchild.

Grandparents Raising Grandchildren: The Big Picture

One in ten children lives with a grandparent, and approximately 40% of such children are being raised primarily by this grandparent. According to the U.S. Census Bureau (2001), as of the year 2000, nearly 2.5 million children were being raised by their grandparents. This number has been steadily increasing over the past decades and has now reached epidemic proportions. Based on more recent Census data, according to a recent report released by the Pew Research Center (2010), 2.9 million children are now being raised by a grandparent, representing a 16% increase since 2000, with the number of such children increasing 6% from 2007 to 2008, largely due to the Recession. Interestingly, this sharp increase varied by ethnicity, where among Whites, there was a 9% increase, and a 2% increase was seen among African-Americans, in contrast to no increase among Hispanics. When the figures from 2000–2008 are analyzed, a similar picture emerges.

Grandparents are usually asked to take responsibility for the care of their grandchildren due to a variety of issues speaking to disruptive and often stigmatizing events within the family that include the death of a parent, a parent's divorce, incarceration, drug addiction or alcoholism, child abuse and neglect, teen pregnancy, or AIDS (Cox, 2000; Edwards, 1998; Bowers & Myers, 1999; Connealy & DeRoos, 2000; Hayslip & Kaminski, 2005; Hayslip & Page, in press; Park & Greenberg, 2007; Thomson, Minkler, & Driver, 2000).

The Challenges of Raising a Grandchild

There is no shortage of research on the effects of grandparents raising their grandchildren, and it clearly suggests that grandparent caregiving *can be* a highly stressful, isolating, and otherwise difficult experience (see Hayslip & Kaminski, 2005; Hayslip & Page, in press; Park & Greenberg, 2007 for reviews). Many, but not all grandparents who raise their grandchildren are at risk of social isolation, stress and issues related to it, and financial strain (Cox, 2000; Hayslip & Kaminski, 2005). Many such stresses associated with grandparents raising grandchildren are related to lack of social interaction, conflict with spouses and friends, lack of energy and time, fear about health issues and what will happen to the grandchildren if they are unable to care for them, concerns regarding not being able to spend their lives enjoying what they like, the strain on relationships with other non-resident grandchildren, and financial burdens (Giarrusso et al., 2000; Hayslip & Kaminski, 2005; Musil, Schrader, & Mutikani, 2000; Silverstein & Vehvilainen, 2000). Financial burdens are the most often cited issue of concern, especially among minority grandparents, and on average, government assistance covers only a quarter of the expense of raising a child (Brown & Mars, 2000). One-third of grandparent caregivers live below the poverty line (Pew Foundation, 2010). Brown and Mars reported the most stressful issue for grandparents was difficulty regarding their own health, followed by their ability to provide a good life for the grandchild. Additionally, many grandparent caregivers fear the biological parents' involvement with the child and often report considerable conflict over the relationship with the child's birthparent (Hayslip & Kaminski, 2005; Park & Greenberg, 2007).

Grandparents who provide care full-time for their grandchildren are more likely to be poor, on some form of welfare, less likely to have insurance, and more likely to have less education, relative to non-custodial grandparents (Cox, 2000; Thomson, Minkler, & Driver, 2000). Grandparents often are confused about and unsure of their role as a primary caretaker of their grandchildren, in part because the role of grandparent itself is ambiguous (Cox, 2000; Rosow, 1985). Not only is the role of parent new, but grandparents are often forced to take on such responsibilities in the wake of either family dysfunction or tragedy. Perhaps complicated by the often sudden nature of the decision to raise a grandchild, Cox (2000) has suggested that many grandparents may feel obligated to accept their grandchildren when they really do not want to do so. In contrast, Sands and Goldberg-Glenn (2000) reported that 40% of the grandmothers in their study felt that they actively and voluntarily sought out the caregiving role. Hayslip, Shore, Henderson, and Lambert (1998) noted that nearly a third of caregiving grandparents felt taken advantage of by their children and another third resented their children for putting them in the position of having to be a caregiver. Silverstein and Vehvilainen (2000) found that most grandparents perceived the arrangement of caretaker for their grandchildren as a permanent situation, whereas about 15% saw it as temporary until the parent was able to care for the child again.

Underscoring such ambivalence is the fact that only about half of caregiving grandparents have some form of legal responsibility (Brown & Mars, 2000). Caring for a grandchild also makes more difficult the task of redefining one's life as a middle aged or older person in society—friendship networks are disturbed, contact with one's other grandchildren diminishes, job and retirement plans must often be put on hold. Either due to the physical realities of aging or illness, grandparents are often physically challenged in carrying out duties of parenting a grandchild (Hipple & Hipple, 2008). Silverstein and Vehvilainen (2000) reported that nearly a quarter of their grandparent sample report worse health since taking on the caregiving role, and in this light, it is significant that grandparents often ignore their own health problems in attending to the physical and emotional well-being of their grandchildren (Baker & Silverstein, 2008).

Such problems affect other areas of a grandparent's life. For example, Rodgers-Farmer (1999) reported that grandmothers raising grandchildren did, in fact, experience elevated levels of parenting stress and that parenting stress was positively correlated with higher levels of depression, which, in turn, produced more inconsistent parenting practices. Musil (1998) also reported significantly higher levels of depression and anxiety in grandmother caregivers. Rodriguez and Crowther (2006) found that grandparents who felt they had no choice in raising their grandchildren had lower subjective views of their well-being and felt less self-efficacious.

The Other Side of Grandparent Caregiving: The Glass Half Full

Coexisting with the largely pessimistic view of parenting a grandchild is one that stresses the rewards of doing so. Grandparents report a sense of being needed, being able to improve the grandchild's life, establishing closer bonds to the child, all of which can enable them to better ensure the well-being of their grandchildren (Edwards & Daire, 2006). Indeed, 90% of custodial grandparents would choose to take on the caregiver role again if they were asked to make the decision a second time (Hayslip & Kaminski, 2005), and many grandparents perceive their new role as parent to their grandchild in very rewarding and positive terms (Brown & Mars, 2000; Cox, 2000; Giarrusso, Silverstein, & Feng, 2000; Marx & Solomon, 2000; Musil, Schrader, & Mutikani, 2000).

The mixed nature of the literature on grandparent caregiving is illustrated in the findings of Giarrusso, Silverstein, and Feng (2000) who found that roughly one-third of grandparents found parenting stressful, another third found it to be only mildly stressful, while the other third found it to be not stressful at all. These authors also reported that about half of their sample found caregiving to be equally stressful and rewarding, 27% found it mostly rewarding, and only 19% found it to be mainly stressful. Giarrusso et al. also found no differences in reported levels of stress across grandparents who varied from one another demographically.

These findings at once suggest that while the stress experienced by a grandparent as a caregiver to grandchildren is universal, some can apparently find the resources to enable them to overcome the challenges associated with parenting a child in middle age and later life, leading them to perceive the experience of raising a grandchild as indeed rewarding and fulfilling.

A similarly inconsistent picture of the impact of custodial grandparenting is painted by work with the children being raised by their grandparents. Some studies have shown that children raised by their grandparents have worse physical health, increased behavioral problems, and lower academic scores than children raised by biological parents (Bowers & Myers, 1999; Edwards & Daire, 2006; Edwards, 1998; Hayslip, Silverthorn, Shore, & Henderson, 2000). Furthermore, children who are raised by their grandparents are often at risk for psychological problems, especially insecurity and trust issues which can be compounded by fears that their grandparents may not be able to care for them forever (Cox, 2000). Edwards (1998) stated that on average, grandchildren raised by their grandparents only made up about 10% of the school population, yet they accounted for nearly 70% of the behavior problems. One reason why this may be true is that these children experience an almost total loss of their social support network at a young age (Edwards & Daire, 2006). Contrary to these rather grim findings, some work reports that children raised by grandparents actually perform better in school, show more autonomy in decision making, and exhibit fewer deviant behaviors (Solomon & Marx, 2000).

Even the physical and psychological costs of grandparent caregiving are not agreed upon. Indeed, not all grandparents' health is negatively impacted by raising a grandchild (Hayslip, Shore, & Emick, 2006). Caregivers who are married, in good health, and have a satisfactory income are more satisfied with their caregiving role than are those who are single, of low income, and poorer health (Goodman, 2006). Goodman also found that role satisfaction among grandmothers increased with age. Hayslip, Temple, Shore, and Henderson (2006) found that grandparents caring for only one child experienced less stress than those caring for multiple children and that the more meaning and value a grandparent associated with the caregiving role, the greater their satisfaction was in taking on that role.

Personal Resilience and Custodial Grandparenting

Resilience is generally defined in terms of positive adaptation in the face of adversity, and can be conceived as a trait-like attribute that persons possess in varying degrees, as a dynamic process in dealing with change, and as an outcome, derived from one's experience in dealing with stress and adversity (Smith & Hayslip, in press). Indeed, resilience may mediate (or connect) *exposure* to stressful experiences—*responses* to such experiences relationships, and is typically discussed in terms of either (1) a person's *characteristics or qualities of the environment* that in varying degrees, may or may not put a person at risk for a given negative outcome, (2) *protective factors* that insulate persons from negative outcomes, to include relationships with others and social support, and (3) *outcomes* that are either negative (e.g., health difficulties, depression) or positive (the acquisition of a skill or greater well-being) (Smith & Hayslip, in press). In this light, Coon (in press) stresses the fact that resilient caregivers maintain a positive orientation to the future and find a way to persevere in the face of the stresses of caregiving.

As these approaches to resilience apply to grandparent caregivers, the above literature clearly suggests that the demands of caregiving are real for many grandparents. It is important to note that how one deals with stressful caregiving experiences may reflect ongoing resilience or they may bring about resilience. This resilience may develop in the face of difficulties associated with raising a problematic grandchild, grief at the loss of a relationship with an adult child or at the loss of the normalcy and predictability of one's life as planned for, isolation from others, life disruption, or poor health and depression (see Emick & Hayslip, 1999; Hayslip & Kaminski, 2005; Hayslip, Shore, Henderson, & Lambert, 1998; Park & Greenberg, 2007).

Bonanno (2004) suggests that resilience can be viewed as a form of psychological immunity all people possess, and like the physical immune system, psychological immunity (resilience) varies greatly from individual to individual, and indeed resilience may protect one from further health-related and/or psychosocial damage (Fagundes et al., in press; Smith & Hayslip, in press). A similar view is expressed via the concept of salutogensis, or the origin of health, wherein resilience is not built up through avoiding stress and trauma, but rather through active coping, problem solving, and the use of resources to manage and deal with a stressor appropriately (Almedon, 2005). This mirrors the way in which the human physical immune system is exposed to disease and illness and grows stronger from limited exposure to pathogens.

A grandparent's ability to "weather the storm" in raising grandchildren would likely increase his/her ability to adequately parent and provide a loving and stable home for the child. This, in turn, might foster better behavior in the child by allowing the child to develop secure attachments to a grandparent, which, in turn, could also positively contribute to the well-being of the grandparent. Indeed the relationship between a grandchild's behavior and a grandparent's mental health is bidirectional (Edwards, 1998; Goodman & Hayslip, 2008; Rogers & Henkin, 2000).

Clearly, as the majority of work with grandparent caregivers suggests that the negatives might outweigh the positives, it often seems that discussing grandparent caregivers' strengths is almost an afterthought. Rather than consider such resources as the exception to the rule, we argue that the role of personal resilience should be *central* to any discussion of custodial grandparenting. Importantly, dependent upon the nature of the questions one asks about grandparent caregivers, the portrait painted by one's findings can either be optimistic (stressing resourcefulness or resilience) or pessimistic (stressing depression and poor health) in nature.

In this light, what might account for this contradictory picture speaking to the impact of raising a grandchild? We argue that such a picture is influenced by the extent to which grandparents are resilient in the face of loss and trauma. Indeed, because not all grandparents are overwhelmed by the challenges of raising a grandchild suggests that such persons are in varying degrees, personally resilient.

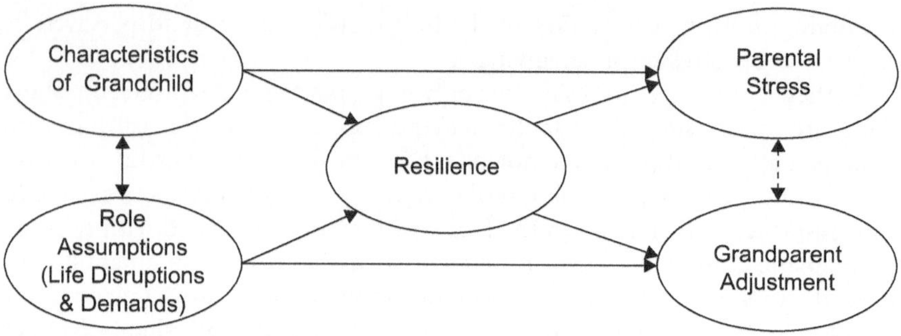

Figure 4.1 Resilience as Mediator

Purpose of the Present Study

The purpose of the current study was to explore the role of personal resilience in enabling grandparents to be better able to deal with the demands of raising a grandchild than are others. A secondary purpose was to explore the potential mediating role that beliefs about one's parenting skills might play in linking grandchild characteristics and parental stress. Confidence in one's parental skills may grow out of efforts to raise a grandchild (especially one who is experiencing emotional or behavioral problems), leading to less parental stress (Almedon, 2005; Cox, 2000; Musil, 1998; Rodgers-Farmer, 1999). For purposes of this study, we are treating parental efficacy as parallel to personal resilience as it is thought to mediate stress-outcome relationships.

The model explored here (Figure 4.1) illustrates how personal resilience may mediate (or connect) the effects of grandchild-specific stressors, role demands, and life disruption on parental stress and personal adjustment. This model suggests that resilience may mediate these negative effects, wherein grandparents with greater resiliency will be less prone to experience the negative effects of raising a grandchild, while those who are less resilient will be more susceptible to the effects of grandchild difficulties and life disruption. As an exploratory endeavor, we are also exploring whether parental efficacy will act in a similar manner, wherein those grandparents whose efficacy beliefs about their parenting skills are more positive may experience less parental stress. In contrast, persons whose parental efficacy is more negative will experience more parental stress, brought about by their relative inability to deal with a problematic grandchild (see Almedon, 2005). It could also be that parental stress precedes grandchild adjustment difficulties (see Smith & Dolbin-MacNab, this volume).

Method

Sample and Procedure

The sample consisted of 42 male participants and 196 female grandparent caregivers (one participant omitted gender). Seventy-nine percent of the sample was comprised of Caucasian grandparent caregivers, with African-American grandparents making up 13.8% of the total sample. Grandparent caregivers' ages ranged from 38 to 90 years in age, with the mean age being 58.06 (*SD* = 8.17). The number of grandchildren being cared for by a grandparent caregiver ranged from 1 to as many as 13, with the average number of grandchildren being cared for being 1.61 (*SD* = 1.19). The mean age of the grandchild in care was 9.44 (*SD* = 4.65); their ages ranged from less than a year to 24 years of age. The average length of time that a grandparent had been caring for his/her grandchild was 6.44 years (*SD* = 4.68), and the length of time in care ranged from less than a year to 24 years.

Grandparent caregivers were recruited from within and around the Dallas-Ft. Worth, Texas area, as well as from other states and Canada, using available resources that included grandparent organizations (e.g., grandparents.com, Generations United, the Brookdale Foundation), support groups, the community at large, and contacts through undergraduate students. In all cases, strict criteria were defined to ensure the reliability of all survey data; all surveys were sealed and signed by participants and each was contacted and responses verified by telephone. Grandparents qualified for the study if they were currently caring for a grandchild on a full-time basis. Grandfamilies in the present study were predominantly skipped-generation families, meaning that the child's biological parents were not currently residing with the grandparent and child, although the child and grandparent may still have been in regular contact with the parent(s). A minority was co-parenting in nature, where the biological parent lived with the grandparent and grandchild, but was not the only caretaker.

Two hundred and seventy survey packets were mailed to grandparent caregivers who indicated an interest in the project, described in terms of studying resilience among such persons. Two hundred and thirty-nine grandparents returned a completed survey, yielding a response rate of 88.1%. A letter of invitation, an informed consent form, a demographic information sheet, and the survey packet were mailed to each participant. Participants signed and returned by mail the consent form separate from the demographic information sheet and the survey packet.

Measures

Participants completed a basic Demographic Information Form (DIF) that assessed variables such as gender, age, education level, and SES; in addition to the DIF, participants were asked to complete the following surveys.

Life Disruption Scale: The extent of life disruption experienced was measured by items proposed by Jendrek (1993) in research relative to grandparents raising grandchildren. The scale consists of 20 items addressing the extent to which caring for a grandchild has affected the caregiver. The items were rated on a 5-point Likert scale ranging from 1 = *Not at all* to 5 = *A great deal.* An internal consistency reliability coefficient of .93 was reported (Hayslip, 2003). Examples of items in this scale include: "doing things for fun or recreation," "worrying about thing," and "having contact with friends." Higher scores indicated more life disruption.

Strengths and Difficulties Questionnaire: The Strengths and Difficulties Questionnaire (SDQ; Goodman, 2001; Palmieri & Smith, 2007) is a self-report measure that consists of 25 items answered along a 3-point Likert scale, with 1 = *not true* and 3 = *certainly true*. The SDQ was used to assess psychological adjustment of children and adolescents. The 25 items are organized into five subscales that look at prosocial behavior, emotional symptoms, conduct problems, hyperactivity-inattention, and peer relationship problems. Satisfactory internal consistency reliability has been demonstrated for all scales except peer relationship problems, (alphas ranging from .41 to .62). Retest stability was found to have a lower bound estimate of .62 at 4 to 6 months. Overall SDQ scores (summed across the 25 items) were used here, with higher such scores indicating more dysfunction.

Extent of Grandchild Problems: Each grandparent rated along a 5-point Likert scale (1 = *no problem* to 5 = *severe problem*) the extent to which the grandchild was experiencing difficulties in a variety of areas (e.g., abusing alcohol, depression, drug abuse, oppositional behavior, learning or school difficulties). Total scores across 10 potential areas of difficulty represented greater perceived grandchild behavioral/emotional difficulties, and such scores differentiated grandparent caregivers who experienced more psychosocial distress from those who did not (Emick & Hayslip, 1999; Hayslip, Shore, Henderson, & Lambert, 1998). Based upon this sample, the alpha for this scale was .70.

Parental Role Strain: Custodial grandparent's parental role strain was assessed via a 17-item measure derived from the Structure of Coping Scale (Pearlin & Schooler, 1978) and used to identify potential strains in grandparent's roles as parents, as well as to identify emotional stress experienced by grandparents connected to this role. Each item is scored on a 4-point Likert scale, where 1 = *never*, to 4 = *very often*. Higher scores (alpha = .89) indicted the grandparent experienced more stress and strain associated with the caregiving role.

Resilience. The Resilience Scale (RS) (Neill & Dias, 2001) is a 15-item self-report survey modified from Wagnild and Young's (1993) Resilience Measure used to measure themes of personal resilience. All items are worded positively and responses are on a 4-point Likert scale. Concurrent validity has been supported by significant correlations between RS scores and measures of morale, life satisfaction, and depression. The scale's Cronbach's alpha was .91. Higher scores represented higher levels of resilience.

Hardiness-Personal Views Survey (PVS): Hardiness was assessed via the PVS (Kobasa, 1985), a 50-item scale assessing hardiness which is comprised of three subscales: Control (feeling that all events are a consequence of one's own actions), Commitment (active attempts to infuse meaning into one's life), and Challenge (where changes in life are defined as exciting and stimulating, rather than stressful experiences). Each item is scored in a Likert-type manner, where 1 = *not at all true*, to 4 = *completely true*. Higher scores indicated higher levels of hardiness. The Cronbach alpha of the PVS composite score is .88 (Funk, 1992).

Parental Efficacy: To measure parental efficacy, a 9-item scale (Bachicha, 1997) assessing generalized parental efficacy assessed grandparents' perceptions of their ability as parents to solve problems and understand their grandchild. Each of the nine items were answered on a 5-point Likert-type scale, where 1 = *strongly disagree*, to 5 = *strongly agree*. Higher scores (alpha = .88) indicated greater parental efficacy. This scale has been successfully used to assess the impact of a psychosocial intervention targeting grandparent caregivers (Hayslip, 2003).

Grandparents Perceptions of Relationships with Grandchildren: Grandparents' perceptions of their relationships with grandchildren were measured by the Positive Affect Index (10 items) and Negative Affect Index (10 items) (Thomas, 1990). The Positive Affect Index asked grandparents to describe the extent of their mutual understanding with, trust in, respect for, and affection for their grandchildren, whereas the Negative Affect Index measured the extent of the grandparents' negative feelings toward irritating behaviors of the grandchild (alpha = .79). An additional question asked the participants to rate the quality of the grandchild relationship (Likert 5-point scale, with 1 = *none* and 5 = *a great deal*). Higher scores indexed greater Positive and Negative Affect.

Parental Stress. Parenting Stress Index/Short Form (PSI/SF): The PSI/SF (Abidin, 1990) is a 36-item self-report measure consisting of three subscales: the Parental Distress Factor, the Parent-Child Dysfunctional Interaction Factor, and the Difficult Child Factor. The Parental Distress Factor measured parental distress; the Parent-Child Dysfunctional Interaction Factor evaluated whether the parent derives satisfaction from interactions with the child and whether the child meets parental expectations. The Difficult Child Factor measured the child's ability to self-regulate. The PSI/SF demonstrates high internal consistency (alpha = .91), high test-retest stability (r = .84), adequate construct, discriminant and predictive validity, acceptable concurrent validity with clinical and self-report criteria, and acceptable cross cultural validity (Abidin, 1990). PSI/SF Total scores were used here. All PSI/SF items were reframed to apply to "my grandchild." Items were responded to on a 5-point Likert scale ranging from 1 = *strongly disagree* to 5 = *strongly agree*. Custodial grandparents completed the PSI/SF as it related to their acquired roles as the grandchild's functional parent.

Grandparenting Satisfaction: Satisfaction with grandparenting was assessed using 15 questions (alpha = .79) used in the Thomas (1990) study. Each question was answered on a 5-point Likert-type scale (1 = *strongly disagree* to 5 = *strongly agree*), and higher scores indicated greater satisfaction.

Psychological and Physical Health. Short Form-36 (SF-36) General Health Survey: The SF-36 (Ware, 1993) is a 36-item self-report measure that was used to assess physical and mental health. The SF-36 has scales measuring physical functioning, role disability due to physical health problems, bodily pain, general health perceptions, vitality, social functioning, role disability due to emotional health problems, and general mental health. Estimates of internal consistency reliability for the SF-36 scales exceed .80.

Psychological Well-Being: Psychological Well-Being (Liang, 1985) was assessed via a 15-item self-report scale that was designed to measure respondents' feelings about their lives. The scale integrated items from the Bradburn Affect Balance Scale (Bradburn, 1969) and the Life Satisfaction Index A (Neugarten, Havighurst, & Tobin, 1961). The Liang scale allows for the assessment of positive and negative affect (transitory affective components), happiness (long-term affective component), and congruence (long-term cognitive component) (alpha = .68).

Center for Epidemiologic Studies Depression Scale (CES-D): Psychological distress/depression was assessed via the CES-D (Radloff, 1977) a 20-item self-report scale designed to measure current level of depressive symtomatology with an emphasis on depressed mood. Participants were asked to endorse the response that best describes how often they feel a particular way in the past week. Questions were answered on a 4-point Likert-type scale, where 1 = *rarely or some of the time* to 4 = *most or all of the time*. Higher scores indicated more health problems. The scale exhibits high internal consistency (alpha = .85), adequate test-retest stability (correlations range from .45 to .70), exceptional concurrent validity with clinical and self-report criteria, and substantial construct validity (Radloff, 1977).

Mental Health Attitudes: Attitudes towards psychological help (Hayslip, Temple, & Currin, 2007) were assed using two scales. The first measured *openness to seeking psychological help*; this is assessed using a list of 24 problems such as deep depression, forgetfulness, and arguments with children. Participants were asked whether they would seek help from a counselor or therapist for each problem. The number of items each participant endorsed is then summed to give an openness score, wherein higher scores indicated greater openness towards seeking mental health services. Alpha coefficients in the 1991 and 2000 samples were .81 and .85 for younger adults, and .87 for older adults (Hayslip et al., 2007). The second scale measured *professional and mental health bias*; this was measured on a 5-point Likert scale (1 = *strongly disagree* and 5 = *strongly agree*) where items described various negative attitudes one might hold towards mental health care issues. Agreement with the statements indicated a negative attitude towards the value of mental health care, the stigma attached to seeking mental health services, and to mental health care professionals themselves. Higher scores indicated more negative attitudes (less positive biases), where the relationship between openness and bias was negative. For bias, alpha coefficients ranged from .67 to .84 (Hayslip et al., 2007).

Statistical Analysis of the Data

A regression analysis was conducted to explore the meditational role that resilience may play in explaining the relationship between for example, child demands and parental stress (see Figure 4.1). As per the recommendation of Baron and Kenny (1986), hierarchical regression was used to establish relationships between, for example, (a) child demands and parental stress, (b) resilience and child demands, and (c) parental stress and resilience. In this case, if resilience serves as a mediator, then controlling for it will lessen the relationship between child demands and parental stress. Doing so will also increase the variance accounted for (R^2) in the outcome variable, and was assessed via an F test ($p < .05$). This regression analysis was repeated for each measure of child difficulties, parental stress, life resources, resilience and adjustment-dysfunction. A path analysis was then conducted to examine whether the model illustrated in Figure 4.1 was consistent with the data we gathered from this sample of grandparent caregivers.

The regression analysis was repeated to also explore the mediating role of parental efficacy. Based upon our model (see Figure 4.1), tests of the mediating roles of personal resilience and parental efficacy were consistent with the distinctions made by Emick and Hayslip (1999) and Hayslip, Shore, Henderson, and Lambert (1998) in terms of the dual set of difficulties faced by grandparent caregivers: (1) challenges associated with raising a problematic grandchild per se, and (2) overall lifestyle and adjustment-related challenges associated with raising grandchildren without problems.

Factor Structure of Measured Variables

Prior to the regression and path analyses, exploratory factor analyses were carried out for measures relating to the above constructs to examine if each were better described by a common factor(s). Factor scores were used here to avoid the attenuation of relationships that accompany measurement error (Baron & Kenny, 1986). In order to examine the factor structure defining key components in the model, principle component analysis with varimax rotation to a terminal solution was carried out in each case.

Independent (Antecedent) Variables: Grandchild Difficulty and Life Resources

Grandchild Difficulties

This was composed of three components (rated grandchild problems, SDQ grandchild difficulty score, and SDQ overall difficulty score) and produced one factor titled Child Difficulties (loadings exceeded .87). This factor had an eigenvalue of 2.45, accounting for 81.8% of total variance shared among the measures; higher scores indexed more difficulties.

Life Resources

The next two factors derived were composed of five measures: grandparent satisfaction, life disruption, overall physical health, mental health, and physical health limitations. The two factors derived from these measures were labeled *Life Resources 1* and *Life Resources 2*, with Life Resources 1 (less life disruption, better physical health, more positive mental health attitudes, fewer health limitations, where loadings exceeded .42) had an eigenvalue of 2.69, accounting for 53.8% of the shared variance, while Life Resources 2 (greater role satisfaction, less life disruption, where loadings exceeded .68) had an eigenvalue of 1.06 and accounted for 21.3% of the shared variance. Greater scores indexed *more* life resources.

Resilience as a Mediator

A resilience factor was formed using the three subscales from the PVS of hardiness, challenge, commitment, and control, as well as the above additional measure of personal resilience. The resilience factor (where all loadings exceeded .66) had an eigenvalue of 2.33, and accounted for 58.4% of the shared variance among the measures.

Dependent Variables—Outcomes

Parental Stress

The factor derived was labeled *Parental Stress*, and was comprised of four measures (more parental strain, less positive affect, more negative affect, and more parental stress, with loadings exceeding .68), and had an eigenvalue of 2.57, accounting for 64.5% of the shared variance among measures.

Adjustment/Dysfunction

The outcome variable *Adjustment* was composed of five measures: mental health openness, mental bias, mental health breadth, the CESD, and well-being. Two factors were created, Adjustment Factor 1 (*Negative Well-Being*—less mental health openness, more depression, less well-being, with loadings exceeding .31) and Adjustment Factor 2 (*Negative Mental Health Attitudes*—less mental health openness, more negative mental health bias, less mental health breadth, with loadings exceeding .33). Negative Well-Being had an eigenvalue of 1.61, with total shared variance among measures accounted for being 32.33%, and Negative Mental Health Attitudes had an eigenvalue of 1.45, accounting for 29.2% of the shared variance among measures. *Higher* such scores in each case represented *greater* grandparent dysfunction.

Table 4.1 suggests that both personal resilience and parental efficacy are correlated with most antecedents and parental/personal outcomes and that personal resilience and parental efficacy are at best, moderately related to one another.

Hierarchical regression analyses (see Table 4.2) were then conducted by first entering the antecedent variable and then entering either resilience or parental efficacy as a mediator to examine what roles each may play in explaining the relationships between the antecedent and the outcomes in this study.

Table 4.1 Correlations among Derived Factors (*$p \le .05$ **$p \le .01$)

	Child Difficulty	*Parental Stress*	*Life Resor I*	*Life Resor II*	*Adjustment I*	*Adjustment II*	*Resilience*
Resilience	−.178*	−.413**	.494**	−.144	−.604**	−.130	—
Parental Efficacy	.121	−.646**	.263**	−.242**	−.269**	−.103	.396**

Table 4.2 Regression Analyses: Resilience (top) and Parental Efficacy (bottom) as mediator

Antecedent	*Outcome*	*Beta*[1]	*Beta*[2]	*Beta*[3]	R^{2a}	R^{2b}	R^2_{chng} [c]	F_{chng} [d]
Child Diff	Par. Stress	.64	.58	−.25	.41	.47	.06	14.66**
Child Diff	Adj. I	.63	.56	.18	.39	.42	.03	6.41*
Child Diff	Adj. II	.63	.63	.03	.39	.39	.00	NS
Life Resor1	Par. Stress	−.50	−.39	−.23	.25	.29	.04	8.23**
Life Resor1	Adj. I	−.70	−.54	−.33	.49	.57	.08	27.71**
Life Resor1	Adj. II	.19	.31	−.25	.04	.08	.04	6.70**
Life Resor2	Par. Stress	.47	.43	−.38	.22	.36	.14	30.13**
Life Resor2	Adj. I	.06	−.03	−.59	.01	.35	.34	73.08**
Life Resor2	Adj. II	.06	.05	−.08	.00	.01	.01	NS
Child Diff	Par. Stress	.64	.56	−.55	.40	.70	.30	153.09**
Child Diff	Adj. I	.29	.19	.25	.08	.15	.07	11.89**
Child Diff	Adj. II	−.20	−.20	−.11	.04	.05	.01	NS
Life Resor1	Par. Stress	−.50	−.34	−.53	.25	.51	.26	78.65**
Life Resor1	Adj. I	−.67	−.64	−.13	.45	.47	.02	4.78*
Life Resor1	Adj. II	.16	.19	−.10	.03	.04	.01	NS
Life Resor2	Par. Stress	.45	.31	−.55	.21	.49	.28	85.92**
Life Resor2	Adj. I	.02	−.04	−.30	.00	.08	.08	14.17**
Life Resor2	Adj. II	.05	.04	−.05	.00	.00	.00	NS

1—direct; 2—adjustment for mediator; 3—mediator/outcome; a—direct; b—with mediator; c—R^2 change with mediator; d—F value with mediator; *$p \le .05$; **$p \le .01$.

Overall, thirteen of 18 regressions conducted suggested that resilience (seven of nine comparisons) does in fact play ($p \le .05$) a meditational role and, in addition, also supports the role of parental efficacy as a mediator (six of nine comparisons) in understanding antecedent-outcome relationships among grandparent caregivers. Where the F change is significant ($p < .05$), this suggests that the mediating role of personal resilience or parental efficacy is substantial.

Last, path analysis tested the model (Figure 4.1) focusing on the role that personal resilience may play in understanding the relationship between the antecedents and the outcomes measured here. This model simultaneously incorporates antecedents, the mediator, and outcomes, using the *Life Resource 1* and

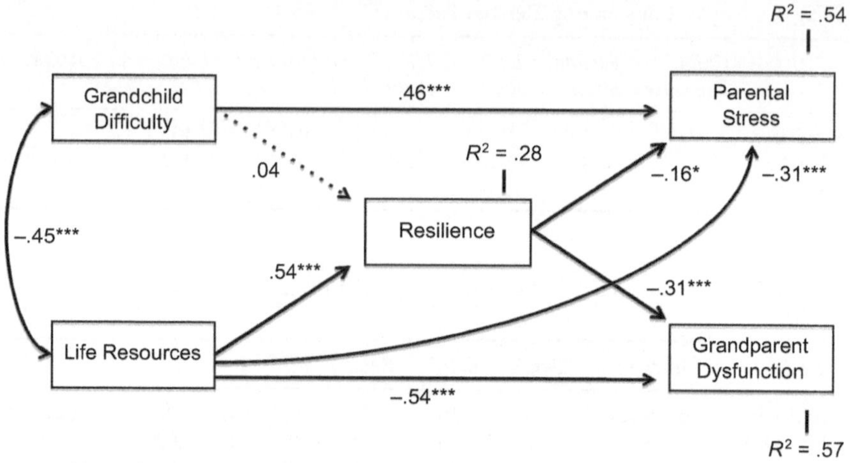

Figure 4.2 Path Analytic Findings

Adjustment 1 factor scores (see Table 4.1). This model (Figure 4.2) fits the data well (X^2, 1 = 2.94, p = .08, *CFI* = .99, *SRMR* = .01), where resilience helps to explain the connection between life resources and grandparent dysfunction, but not the connection between grandchild difficulty and parental stress. More life resources are linked to greater resilience and to less dysfunction, greater grandchild difficulty is associated with greater parental stress, and greater resilience is associated with less grandparent dysfunction and less parental stress. This model does not suggest that grandchild difficulty and resilience are related, taking into consideration the relationship between life resources and grandchild difficulty (less grandchild difficulty is associated with more life resources).

Discussion

Our observations about the mixed nature of available findings regarding the stressfulness of grandparent caregiving as well as the need to centralize the concept of personal resilience in understanding grandparent caregivers in a more positive light gave rise to the present study. Indeed, studies to date have been split fairly equally regarding whether raising one's grandchild has predominantly negative or positive effects on the grandparent caregiver (see above). There are a number of reasons as to why studies have found such mixed results; *one* of those reasons may be sampling differences in resilience among grandparent caregivers, as well as the fact that some grandparent caregivers are more resilient than others. We acknowledge that our approach to resilience, i.e., that it is a trait-like attribute that may correlate with one's coping skills, social support (see Figure 4.2), that is not shared by many, who believe that resilience is derived from experience, brought about by environmental resources (e.g., social support) or that resilience is a dynamic process, understood in terms of the person's ongoing efforts to gain control over or actively engage the environment (for a review, see Smith & Hayslip, in press).

Staudinger, Marsiske, and Baltes (1995) suggested that because older individuals are more likely to experience intense stressors (i.e., the deaths of family members and friends, illness, chronic pain and discomfort, and facing one's own mortality), they are also more likely to call on their own resilience to help maintain normal functioning in everyday life. Because older individuals may be forced to call upon their resilience qualities more regularly, it is important to equip such persons with ways in which to help them enhance and add to their existing resiliency reserve (Staudinger, Marsiske, & Baltes, 1995). Bergeman and Wallace (1999) argued that because adversity is unavoidable, especially in later life, optimal functioning can only be achieved through the development and enhancement of resiliency. This might be achieved in many ways, such as providing more support from others, encouraging persons to attend to their health, making environmental changes (i.e., in moving from a crime ridden neighborhood to a safer one), or in developing new coping skills.

The primary purpose of the current study was to examine the mediating role of personal resilience to help understand why some grandparent caregivers are better able to adjust to and handle the added stresses of caring for their grandchild, while others experience more negative effects. A secondary purpose was to explore the role that parental efficacy, viewed here as a domain-specific aspect of resilience may play in this respect. This study was based on the assumption that resilience may possibly mediate the negative effects of caring for a grandchild on parental and personal adjustment, where grandparents who were more resilient should report fewer negative such effects than those who were less resilient. As Oburu (2005) has suggested that social support and adaptive coping styles may possibly mediate the effects of raising one's grandchild, it may be that both could be linked to one's level of resilience.

Collectively, these findings indicate that resilience does appear to at least partially mediate the relationship between antecedents (grandchild difficulties and life resources) and both grandparent adjustment difficulty and parental stress. Of the outcome measures here, mental health attitudes may be least likely to be affected by personal resilience as a mediator. The path analytic findings do however, generally reinforce the central role of resilience in buffering the effects of stress on grandparent caregivers and in addition suggest that fewer rated child difficulties are related to more life resources. We reached a similar conclusion regarding parental efficacy as a mediator, though it should be made clear that alternative models regarding the role of parental efficacy are possible, i.e., that parental stress precedes grandchild difficulties, mediated by dysfunctional parenting skills (Smith & MacNab, this volume).

These results support our hypothesis that resilient attributes grandparents possess in varying degrees mediate the negative impact of raising one's grandchild, and thus suggest that individuals with more resilience likely experience less personal difficulties and less parental stress in caring for a grandchild.

They also indicate that parental efficacy *may* also act as a mediator to buffer the negative impact that caregiving may have on grandparent caregivers. Thus, individuals with higher levels of resiliency as well as individuals with higher parental efficacy report less parental stress as well as fewer overall adjustment difficulties.

Implications for Enhancing Resilience in Grandparent Caregivers: How Can We Help?

Knowing that resilience and parental efficacy help to mediate the effects of negative experiences of raising a grandchild may have beneficial implications for both grandparent caregivers and their grandchildren. As Rogers and Henkin (2000) proposed that grandparent caregivers' emotional stability and outlook were related to the grandchild's behavior, and Goodman and Hayslip (2008) found that the effects of better grandparent mental health and grandchild behavior were bidirectional—each influenced the other, more resilient and/or more parentally efficacious grandparents should be better able to cope with a changed life situation and/or deal with the impact of managing a problem grandchild and therefore, be more able to maintain a more positive outlook on life. Being more efficacious as a parent should lead to experiencing less strain and stress in parenting a grandchild, enabling grandparents to provide a more caring and stable atmosphere for their grandchildren as well as better equip them to foster valued positive behaviors in those grandchildren. Again, it may also be that parental distress leads to more grandchild problematic behaviors (Smith, Palmieri, Hancock, & Richardson, 2008).

Given the work linking stress and illness among grandfamilies (e.g., Marx & Solomon, 2000), if grandparents are able to modify the negative effects of caregiving, then they could reduce the stress they are experiencing and, in turn, possibly ward off future health declines and illness. This is say nothing of the fact that resiliency, as an indicator of mental health, can add years to a person's life, wherein those with good mental and emotional health tend to outlive those with poor mental and emotional health (Hayslip, Patrick, & Panek, 2011). Thus, grandparent caregivers may live longer and enjoy better health as they age if they are more resilient (Coon, in press; Fagundes et al., in press).

Clearly, older adults can enhance their resilience (Bergeman & Wallace, 1999). In this light, grandparents can do a multitude of things to help improve their resiliency as caregivers of their grandchildren by either increasing their own personal resilience or minimizing the adverse effects of caring for a grandchild on them (Hayslip, 2009):

- Grandparents can educate themselves about the challenges of raising a grandchild; knowledge is power and strength. They can learn to assess their own strengths and weaknesses, and learn to ask for help when necessary.
- Grandparents can seek out the support of others and not allow themselves to become isolated from friends, as they are a source of strength in the

face of adversity. Talking with others who are also raising grandchildren, creating a weekly get together or perhaps joining a support group can be very helpful.

- Grandparents should pay special attention to the importance of taking care of themselves physically and emotionally; grandparents cannot care for their grandchild unless they are caring for themselves too. While a grandchild's welfare is important, one cannot ignore his or her own health and well-being (Baker & Silverstein, 2008).
- If the grandparent is married or is in a committed relationship, this relationship should be nurtured. Purposefully make time for both to spend alone time together. Do not ignore the impact that raising a grandchild may have on a marriage or relationships with friends, neighbors, or co-workers.
- Grandparents should not ignore their own needs; they should strive to discover what gives them pleasure and commit to having "alone time" where such things can be enjoyed.
- Grandparents should take every opportunity to enroll in classes or programs that teach assertiveness and decision making skills, new methods of coping, as well as programs that improve one's parenting skills.
- Grandparents should do things every day that empower them personally. Even small things—helping someone else, solving a practical problem, or fixing something around the house—can be empowering (see Cox, 2000).
- Grandparents should become their own advocates, letting others know about their needs.
- Grandparents should approach the challenges of raising a grandchild as something that they *can* deal with, i.e., developing an attitude of confidence in one's ability to nurture both oneself and one's grandchild. Both the grandparent and the grandchild will benefit.
- Grandparents should develop a "never give up, I can see this through" attitude—having a sense of humor about life's challenges is also very helpful.
- Grandparents should be their own best friends, forgiving themselves for not being perfect—everyone makes mistakes!
- Grandparents should strive to be hopeful and optimistic about the future, setting goals that they can achieve, even goals that can be met in a day.
- Grandparents should draw upon their life experience—that they have probably been able to cope with difficult situations in the past. How did they do this? What can they learn from those experiences, particularly those that are beyond their control (e.g., an adult child's choices)? They should take comfort in the serenity prayer. Identifying what qualities helped them get through tough times in the past and striving to maintain and/or develop such qualities is an important aspect of personal resilience.
- Grandparents should actively think about what makes them and their grandchild happy, and set out to do those very things. In this context, the availability of community resources and supportive services is important in supporting such efforts.

Limitations and Future Directions

Despite the value of our findings for understanding and improving resilience in grandparent caregivers, several limitations regarding the present study should be kept in mind: self-report measures were used here; they are subject to the effects of reporting bias. As the sample was composed of grandparent caregivers who chose to participate, they may be more resilient to begin with. The sample was also composed of predominantly Caucasian grandmothers; grandparents of different ethnicities as well as grandfathers may experience the impact of resilience on the caregiving role differently.

As the present data are correlational, future work examining resilience in grandparent caregivers may benefit from exploring its longitudinal aspects as it relates to both grandparents and grandchildren, wherein causal links might be more easily established. Consequently, findings from alternative models tested in this manner may or may not be consistent with findings based upon the model tested here. Moreover, it is entirely possible that relationships between resilience and adjustment as well as between parental efficacy and either parental stress or grandchild problem behaviors are bidirectional. Likewise, differences in the mediating roles of resilience and parental efficacy across grandparent gender, ethnicity, and socioeconomic status remain to be explored, as do the role of other risk factors (e.g., poverty, social isolation, being divorced or widowed, nature of the relationships among the grandparent, the birthparent, and the grandchild) in concert with resilience in predicting adjustment among grandparent caregivers.

References

Abdin, R. (1990). *Parenting stress index/short form.* Charlottesville, VA: Pediatric Psychology Press.

Almedon, A. M. (2005). Resilience, hardiness, sense of coherence, and post traumatic growth: All paths leading to "light at the end of the tunnel"? *Journal of Loss and Trauma, 10*, 253–265.

Bachicha, D. (1997). *A validation study of parental self-efficacy scale.* Unpublished doctoral dissertation, University of New Mexico.

Baker, L., & Silverstein, M. (2008). Preventative health behaviors among grandmothers raising grandchildren. *The Journal of Gerontology: Social Sciences, 63B*, S304–S311.

Barron, R. M., & Kenny, D. A. (1986). The moderator-mediator variable distinction in social psychological research: Conceptual, strategic, and statistical considerations. *Journal of Personality and Social Psychology, 51*, 1173–1182.

Bergeman, C., & Wallace, K. (1999). Resiliency in later life. In T. Whitman, V. Thomas, & R. White (Eds.), *Life-span perspectives on health and illness* (pp. 207–225). Mahwah, NJ: Lawrence Erlbaum.

Bonnano, G. (2004). Loss, trauma, and human resilience: Have we underestimated the human capacity to thrive after extremely aversive events? *American Psychologist, 59*, 20–28.

Bowers, B. F., & Myers, B. J. (1999). Grandmothers providing care for grandchildren: Consequences of various levels of caregiving. *Family Relations, 48*, 303–311.

Bradburn, N. M. (1969). *The structure of psychological well-being.* Chicago: Aldine.

Brown, D. R., & Mars, J. (2000). Profile of contemporary grandparenting in African American families. In C. Cox (Ed.), *To grandmother's house we go and stay* (pp. 203–217). New York, NY: Springer Publishing Company, Inc.

Connealy, M., & DeRoos, Y. (2000). Grandparenting and family preservation. In B. Hayslip & R. Goldberg-Glen (Eds.), *Grandparents raising grandchildren* (pp. 23–33). New York: Springer.

Coon, D. (in press). Resilience and family caregiving. In B. Hayslip & G. Smith (Eds.), *Annual review of gerontology and geriatrics: emerging perspectives on resilience in adulthood and later life*. New York: Springer.

Cox, C. B. (2000). Why grandchildren are going to and staying at grandmother's house and what happens when they get there. In C. Cox (Ed.), *To grandmother's house we go and stay* (pp. 3–19). New York: Springer.

Edwards, O. W. (1998). Helping grandkin—Grandchildren raised by grandparents: Expanding psychology in the schools. *Psychology in the Schools*, *35*, 173–181.

Edwards, O. W., & Daire, Andrew P. (2006). School-aged children raised by their grandparents: Problems and solutions. *Journal of Instructional Psychology*, *33*, 113–119.

Emick, M., & Hayslip, B. (1999). Custodial grandparenting: Stresses, coping skills and relationships with grandchildren. *International Journal of Aging and Human Development*, *58*, 35–61.

Fagundes, C. P., Gillie, B., Derry, H., Bennett, J., & Keicolt-Glaser, J. (2012). Resilience and immune function in older adults. In B. Hayslip & G. Smith (Eds.), *Annual review of gerontology and geriatrics: emerging perspectives on resilience in adulthood and later life* (pp. 29–48). New York: Springer.

Funk, S. C. (1992). Hardiness: A review of theory and research. *Health Psychology*, *11*, 335–345.

Giarrusso, R., Silverstein, M., & Feng, D. (2000). Psychological costs and benefits of raising grandchildren: Evidence from a national survey of grandparents. In Carole B. Cox (Ed.), *To grandmother's house we go and stay* (pp. 71–90). New York: Springer.

Goodman, C. C. (2006). Grandmothers raising grandchildren: The vulnerability of advancing age. In B. Hayslip & J. Patrick (Eds.), *Custodial grandparenting: Individual, cultural, and ethnic diversity* (pp. 133–150). New York: Springer.

Goodman, C. C., & Hayslip, B. (2008). Mentally healthy grandparents' impact on their grandchildren's behavior. In B. Hayslip & P. Kaminski (Eds.), *Parenting the custodial grandchild: Implications for clinical practice* (pp. 41–52). New York: Springer.

Goodman, R. (2001). Psychometric properties of the strengths and difficulties questionnaire. *Journal of the American Academy of Child and Adolescent Psychiatry*, *40*(11), 1337–1345.

Hayslip, B., Jr. (2003). The impact of a psychosocial intervention on parental efficacy, Grandchild relationship quality and well being among grandparents raising grandchildren. In B. Hayslip Jr. & J. Hicks Patrick (Eds.), *Working with custodial grandparents* (pp. 163–178). New York: Springer.

Hayslip, B., Jr. (2009). *Final Report: University of North Texas resilient grandparent project*. Denton, TX: University of North Texas.

Hayslip, B., Jr., & Kaminski, P. L. (2005). Grandparents raising their grandchildren: A review of the literature and suggestions for practice. *The Gerontologist*, *45*, 262–269.

Hayslip, B., & Page, K. (in press). Grandparent-grandchild/great-grandchild relationships. In R. Blieszner & V. H. Bedford (Eds.), *Handbook of aging and the family*. New York: Praeger.

Hayslip, B., Patrick, J., & Panek, P. (2011). *Adult development and aging* (5th edition). Malabar, FL: Krieger.

Hayslip, B., Jr., Shore, R. J., & Emick, M. A. (2006). Age, health, and custodial grandparenting. In B. Hayslip & J. Patrick (Eds.), *Custodial grandparenting: Individual, cultural, and ethnic diversity* (pp. 75–87). New York: Springer.

Hayslip, B., Shore, R. J., Henderson, C. E., & Lambert, P. L. (1998). Custodial grandparenting and grandchildren with problems: Their impact on role satisfaction and role meaning. *Journal of Gerontology: Social Sciences, 53B*, S164–S174.

Hayslip, B., Jr., Silverthorn, P., Shore, R. J., & Henderson, C. E. (2000). Determinants of custodial grandparents' perceptions of problem behavior in their grandchildren. In B. Hayslip & R. Goldberg-Glen (Eds.), *Grandparents raising grandchildren* (pp. 255–268). New York: Springer.

Hayslip, B., Temple, J. R., & Currin, J. B. (2007). The development of a multidimensional attitude toward mental health scale: Preliminary findings from two cohorts of younger and older adults. *Clinical Gerontologist, 30*, 65–73.

Hayslip, B., Jr., Temple, J. R., Shore, R. J., & Henderson, C. E. (2006). Determinants of role satisfaction among traditional and custodial grandparents. In B. Hayslip Jr. & J. Patrick (Eds.), *Custodial grandparenting: Individual, cultural, and ethnic diversity* (pp. 21–35). New York: Springer.

Hipple, L., & Hipple, J. (2008). Raising a granddaughter: Sharing our experience. In B. Hayslip & P. Kaminski (Eds.), *Parenting the custodial grandchild: Implications for clinical practice* (pp. 93–100). New York: Springer.

Jendrek, M. (1993). Grandparents who parent their grandchildren: Effects on lifestyle. *Journal of Marriage and the Family, 55*, 609–621.

Kobasa, S. C. (1985). *Personal views survey*. Chicago: Hardiness Institute.

Liang, J. (1985). A structural integration of the Affect Balance Scale and the Life Satisfaction Index A. *Journal of Gerontology, 40*, 552–561.

Marx, J., & Solomon, J. C. (2000). Physical health of custodial grandparents. In C. Cox (Ed.), *To grandmother's house we go and stay* (pp. 37–55). New York: Springer.

Musil, C. M. (1998). Health, stress, coping, and social support in grandmother caregivers. *Health Care for Women International, 19*, 441–455.

Musil, C. M., Schrader, S., & Mutikani, J. (2000). Social support, stress, and special coping tasks of grandmother caregivers. In C. Cox (Ed.), *To grandmother's house we go and stay* (pp. 56–70). New York: Springer.

Neill, J. T., & Dias, K. L. (2001). Adventure education and resilience: the double edged sword. *Journal of Adventure Education and Outdoor Learning, 1*, 35–42.

Neugarten, B. L., Havighurst, R. J., & Tobin, S. (1961). The measurement of life satisfaction. *Journal of Gerontology, 16*, 134–143.

Oburu, P. O. (2005). Caregiving stress and adjustment problems of Kenyan orphans raised by grandmothers. *Infant and Child Development, 14*, 199–210.

Palmieri, P. A., & Smith, G. C. (2007). Examining the structural validity of the strengths and difficulties questionnaire (SDQ) in a U.S. sample of custodial grandmothers. *Psychological Assessment, 19*, 189–198.

Park, H., & Greenberg, J. (2007). Parenting grandchildren. In J. Blackburn & C. Dumus (Eds.), *Handbook of gerontology: Evidence-based approaches to theory, practice, and policy* (pp. 397–425). New York: John Wiley.

Pearlin, L., & Schooler, C. (1978). The structure of coping. *Journal of Health and Social Behavior, 19*, 2–21.

Pew Research Center (2010). Since the Great Depression, more children raised by grandparents. http://pewresearch.org/pubs/1724/sharp-increase-children-with-grandparents. Retrieved January 21, 2012.

Radloff, L. (1977). The CES-D Scale: A self report depression scale for research in the general population. *Applied Psychological Measrement, 1*, 385–401.

Rodgers-Farmer, A. Y. (1999). Parenting stress, depression, and parenting in grandmothers raising their grandchildren. *Children and Youth Services Review, 21*, 377–388.

Rogers, A., & Henkin, N. (2000). School-base interventions for children in kinship care. In B. Hayslip & R. Goldberg-Glen (Eds.), *Grandparents raising grandchildren* (pp. 221–238). New York: Springer.

Rodriguez, R. L., & Crowther, M. R. (2006). A stress process model of grandparent caregiving: The impact of role strain and intrapsychic strain on subjective well-being. In Bert Hayslip Jr. & Julie Hicks Patrick (Eds.), *Custodial grandparenting: Individual, cultural, and ethnic diversity* (pp. 287–302). New York: Springer.

Rosow, I. (1985). Status and role change through the life cycle. In R. Binstock & E. Shanas (Eds.), *Handbook of aging and the social sciences* (pp. 693–710). New York: Academic Press.

Sands, R., & Goldberg-Glen, R. (2000). Using a microanalysis of a videotaped interview to understand the dynamics of a grandparent-headed household. In B. Hayslip & R. Goldberg-Glen (Eds.), *Grandparents raising grandchildren* (pp. 239–254). New York: Springer.

Silverstein, N. M., & Vehvilainen, L. (2000). Grandparents and schools: Issues and potential challenges. In C. Cox (Ed.), *To grandmother's house we go and stay* (pp. 268–282). New York: Springer.

Smith, G. C., & Hayslip, B. (in press). Resilience in adulthood and later life: What does it mean and where are we heading? In B. Hayslip & G. Smith (Eds.), *Annual review of gerontology and geriatrics: emerging perspectives on resilience in adulthood and later life*. New York: Springer.

Smith, G. C., Palmieri, P., Hancock, G., & Richardson, V. (2008). Custodial grandparents' psychological distress, dysfunctional parenting, and grandchildren's adjustment. *International Journal of Aging and Human Development, 67*, 327–358.

Solomon, J., & Marx, J. (2000). The physical, mental, and social health of custodial grandparents. In B. Hayslip & R. Goldberg-Glen (Eds.), *Grandparents raising grandchildren* (pp. 239–254). New York: Springer.

Staudinger, U. M., Marsiske, M., & Baltes, P. B. (1995). Resilience and reserve capacity in later adulthood: potentials and limits of development across the life span. In D. Cicchetti & D. J. Cohen (Eds.), *Developmental psychology* (pp. 801–849). New York: Wiley.

Thomas, J. L. (1990). The grandparent role: A double blind. *International Journal of Aging and Human Development, 31*, 169–177.

Thomson, E. F., Minkler, M., & Driver, D. (2000). A profile of grandparents Raising grandchildren in the United States. In Carole B. Cox (Ed.), *To grandmother's house we go and stay* (pp. 20–33). New York: Springer.

United States Census Bureau (2001). Census 2000 Supplementary Survey: Profile of selected social characteristics. Avalible: http://www.census.gov/c2ss/www/products... les/2000/tabular/c3sstable2/01000us.htm.

Wagnild, G., & Young, H. (1993). Development and psychometric evaluation of the Resilience Scale. *Journal of Nursing Measurement, 1*, 165–178.

Ware, J. E. (1993). *SF-36 Health Survey: Manual and Interpretation Guide*. Boston, MA: The Health Institute, New England Medical Center.

5 Resilient Grandparent Caregivers

Pathways to Positive Adaptation

Sandra J. Bailey, Bethany L. Letiecq, Minde Erickson, and Rebecca Koltz

Abstract

Guided by the Double ABCX Model and McCubbin and McCubbin's Resiliency Model, the current study explores the characteristics of grandparent caregivers emblematic of resilience as well as those characteristics that appear to hinder movement toward resilience or positive adjustment and adaptation. Using qualitative methods, we analyze life history interviews conducted with 26 grandparent caregivers. Results reveal six overarching themes that characterized resilient grandfamilies, including (1) positive appraisal and acceptance of their family as newly configured; (2) narratives of survival and never giving up; (3) healthy boundary maintenance within their families; (4) commitment to newly established routines and rhythms; (5) social connectivity; and (6) commitment to their grandchildren. Implications for educators, counselors, and other helping professionals are discussed.

Resilient Grandparent Caregivers: Pathways to Positive Adaptation

Grandparents rearing grandchildren often confront both normative, expected challenges facing aging individuals and non-normative, unexpected challenges facing grandfamilies that can make their lives more complex, and physically and psychologically more stressful, than those of their non-parenting counterparts (Musil, Gordon, Warner, Zauszniewski, Standing, & Wykle, 2011). Beyond finding themselves unexpectedly parenting their grandchildren, grandparent caregivers often must deal with the repercussions of the events leading up to this change in their family life, including the death of an adult child (i.e., the grandchild's parent), substance abuse, mental illness, incarceration, teenage pregnancy, divorce, and abandonment (Waldrop & Weber, 2001). Adjusting to the role of caregiver, many grandparents experience increased stress, intra-family strain, and depression symptoms; and decreased perceived rewards, supports, family functioning and physical well-being (Jooste, Hayslip, & Smith, 2008; Letiecq, Bailey, & Kurtz, 2008; Musil et al., 2010). As grandfamilies adapt to their new family configuration, many of these challenges persist, and some, such as self-rated health, have been found to worsen with time (Musil et al., 2010).

Given the growth of grandparent caregiving over the past decade—nationwide, there are now an estimated 2.5 million grandparents providing sole care for at least one grandchild (U.S. Census, 2009)—it is imperative that the elements of resilient grandfamilies be discovered, examined, and promoted. The aim of this chapter is to identify characteristics related to resilient grandparents parenting a second time around as well as those characteristics illustrative of grand-families who are struggling to positively adjust and adapt. Understanding such characteristics may be useful to those working with grandparent caregivers to promote their resilience and to ameliorate some of the challenges to positive adaptation commonly faced by these grandparents.

Conceptual Model of Resilience

McCubbin and McCubbin (1988) conceptualize resilient families as those who are "resistant to disruption in the face of change and adaptive in the face of crisis situations" (p. 247). Resilient families endure even when faced with adversity. The study of family resilience took hold in the 1970s when researchers began examining why some children growing up in adverse conditions fared better than others (Luthar, Cicchetti, & Becker, 2000; Rutter, 1979) and today it is a prominent concept in the fields of psychology (Black & Lobo, 2008), health (Tak & McCubbin, 2002), and family science (McCubbin & McCubbin, 1988). According to Masten (2001) resilience is an ordinary family process, not one that is extraordinary. Masten explains that resilience is a basic human adaptation to circumstances that occur in one's life. If the individual is secure and functioning well then adversity typically can be tolerated. On the other hand, if the individual is not functioning well when faced with adversity, then the risk for maladaptation and poor outcomes increases.

In their early work on resilient families, McCubbin and McCubbin (1988) identified two typologies—rhythmic families and regenerative families. The construct of rhythmic families is based on family time and routines as well as how much the family values time and routines. Rhythmic families have predictable plans of activities, a shared sense of togetherness, and a rhythm of family interactions. The construct of regenerative families includes family cohesion and hardiness. These families cope with crises through trust, maintaining calmness, and maintaining family stability. They pull together during adversity and believe they have control to get through crises. Rhythmic and regenerative families engage in processes of adjustment and adaptation that McCubbin and McCubbin (1991) have identified in their model of resiliency.

Based on Hill's (1949) ABCX model and McCubbin and Patterson's (1983) Double ABCX model, McCubbin and McCubbin's (1991) Resiliency Model of Family Stress, Adjustment, and Adaptation was developed "to explain why some families are more resilient than others and are better able to adjust and adapt to stress, distress and crises by examining the family system as a unit" (Tak & McCubbin, 2002, p. 192). The model is comprised of two distinct parts: the adjustment phase and the adaptation phase. Each phase describes the family's ability to cope with stressors, given family demands, resources, strengths, and problem-solving skills (McCubbin, 1993). The severity of the stressor is determined by the degree to which the stressor threatens to destabilize the family or puts significant demands on its resources and abilities (McCubbin & McCubbin, 1993). Family demands are defined as the stimulus that puts pressure on the family system to change. In this model, McCubbin and McCubbin recognize that demands, such as financial problems, health problems, or other changes in the family's structure or life cycle, can pile-up over time. Resources refer both to existing resources (e.g., individual, family and community support systems) and to new resources that may be developed and strengthened in response to the family stressors (Tak & McCubbin, 2002). The family's problem solving skills and capabilities refer to the strengths (e.g., what the family has) and coping behaviors (e.g., what the family does) as they adjust and adapt to the stressor event (McCubbin & McCubbin, 1993). In this model, resilience is conceptualized as a dynamic and complex process and not an attribute of a given individual. As Masten (2001) notes, it is essential to recognize that the adaptation process is not only complicated, but it takes time.

According to McCubbin (1993), there are five propositions that describe relationships within the resiliency model, including: (1) the pile-up of demands (e.g., stressors, strains, and transitions) is negatively related to family adaptation; (2) family strengths (cohesion, adaptability, hardiness, family time, and routines) are positively related to adaptation; (3) the availability of resources are positively related to adaptation; (4) the family's positive appraisal of the situation is positively related to family adaptation; and (5) the range and depth of the family's skills and capabilities is related to adaptation, such that a healthy repertoire of coping skills can enhance family resilience. In her work to identify the aspects of resilience among families coping with a chronic illness, Patterson (1991) found that balance, healthy boundary maintenance, competent communication, positive appraisals, flexibility, commitment to the family unit, active coping, social connectivity, and engagement with professionals all signaled resilience.

Factors Related to Resilient Grandfamilies

The Resiliency Model has not been extensively applied to grandparents rearing their grandchildren (Musil, Warner, Zauszniewski, Wykle, & Standing, 2009; Musil, Warner, Zauszniewski, Jeanblanc, & Kercher, 2006); however, a number of studies have begun to identify the characteristics, dimensions, and properties of resilient grandfamilies (McCubbin & McCubbin, 1988). For example, in 2009, Bailey, Letiecq, and Porterfield examined the coping strategies of grandparent caregivers as they adjusted and adapted to taking on the sole caregiving of their grandchildren. Bailey and her colleagues found that grandparents employed five strategies, including shifting their roles, identity, relationships, resources, and perceptions of the situation to positively adapt and meet the needs of grandchildren. Briefly, grandparents who were deemed to be positively adjusting to their new family configuration had successfully been able to redefine their work and family roles and their identity from grandparent to parent. These grandparents also experienced shifts in relationships within and outside their families, moving away from traditional grandparenting relationships in their family and social systems to those of parent-child. Grandparents also discussed grappling with resources, as many shifted out of retirement-mode and into wage earner-mode, or sought new resources from their social networks or government agencies. Lastly, and perhaps most importantly, grandparents who positively adjusted shifted their perceptions from a crisis-orientation to a positive orientation, where they worked to reframe the situation and often found joy and satisfaction in parenting a second time around (Boss, 2002).

Other research also sheds light on positive adjustment and adaptation among grandparent caregivers. For example, researchers have found that the attitude adopted when parenting a second time around can be indicative of the outcome of the situation. While some grandparents feel that by raising their children's children, they are enabling the "parents" to continue down an unhealthy, often destructive path in life, others reframe and embrace the experience as a chance to improve upon prior parenting inadequacies (Pinson-Millburn, Fabian, Schlossberg, & Pyle, 1996). When viewing their circumstance, those grandparents who accepted the situation for what it was and used it as an opportunity for growth and increased fulfillment in life were more willing to reach out to others for support, as well as develop and implement a specific plan of action, indicative of active coping (Lumpkin, 2007).

Similarly, grandparent resourcefulness was found to decrease the likelihood of depressive symptoms (Musil et al., 2009) while spirituality was shown to increase a family's ability to cope with unfavorable life events (Juby & Ryecraft, 2004). In a study examining the ups and downs of being the primary caregiver of one's grandchild/ren, prayer, meditation, and faith were cited as important coping mechanisms, allowing the grandparents the strength to handle anxiety and uncertainty (Waldrop & Weber, 2001).

Although this review is not extensive, in each of the studies mentioned, we begin to see characteristics of grandfamily resilience. In this chapter, we further explore these characteristics to better understand the ways in which grandparent caregivers positively adjust and adapt to their new family configuration. We also examine certain characteristics of grandfamilies that appear to be less resilient and discuss possible strategies to support movement to bonadaptation.

Method

Sample

For this study, we conducted 26 face-to-face life history interviews with grandfamilies rearing grandchildren in a rural western state. Interviews were conducted with a grandparent ($n = 19$) or with a married couple dyad ($n = 7$).

In all, we heard from 23 grandmothers and 10 grandfathers. Grandparents ranged in age from 36 to 71 years, with a mean age of 56 years. Most (69%) participants were married at the time of the interview. The remainder was single, separated, divorced, or widowed. Grandfamilies in this study cut across all income levels, with annual household incomes ranging from less than $15,000 to more than $70,000. Participant education levels were also diverse, with four grandparents having less than a high school diploma, nine having a high school diploma or general equivalency diploma, and 20 having some postsecondary education. Grandparents had been the primary caregivers of their grandchildren for an average of 5.5 years, with a range from 5 months to 24 years. The sample was primarily White, with the exception of one Native American grandparent.

Of the 26 grandfamilies interviewed, the majority ($n = 18$) had informal or private care arrangements. Of these families, 10 had hired attorneys to draw up documents establishing guardianship of the grandchildren in their care (but had not gone to court), five had no legal ties to their grandchildren, one couple had privately adopted their grandchild, and two had "mixed" informal arrangements, where one couple had privately adopted their granddaughter and had no legal ties to two other grandchildren under their care, and one couple had legal guardianship of two grandsons and no legal ties to another grandson under their care. The remaining eight grandfamilies were involved in the formal child welfare system as kin foster families, but only one couple had gone through foster care licensure.

Procedure

Family life history interviews (Goodley, Lawthom, Clough, & Moore, 2004) were conducted to better understand how grandparent caregivers came to be, the quality of their intergenerational relationships, and how they navigated social systems (e.g., health care, schools) to meet the needs of their grandchildren. Interview questions also documented legal issues facing grandparents, child welfare involvement, and receipt of state-based financial assistance and services. We used purposive and snowball sampling strategies to recruit grandparent caregivers. We limited the geographic distance between the location of the grandparents and the university to approximately 90 miles due to resource and time constraints. Participants were solicited through local newspaper ads, radio stations, and support groups. Other grandparents then heard about our study by word of mouth and contacted the research team. Inclusion criteria stated that grandparents were the sole, full-time care providers of their grandchild(ren), and biological parents of the grandchildren did not reside in the grandparent's home. Only one interested grandparent was not included in the study because she provided part-time care for her grandchildren. All interviews were conducted by two trained interviewers, were held in the grandparents' home, and lasted about two hours. Participants received $100 for their time.

Data Analysis

To explore resiliency in the grandfamilies, two steps were used to analyze the data. Analytic induction (Patton, 2002), was used to explore resilient characteristics, properties and dimensions of the families or the lack thereof. This form of analysis begins deductively when the researcher develops hypotheses about a topic and then explores the data case by case to determine if the hypotheses are supported. If a case—an interview—does not support the hypotheses then the hypotheses are revised. The goal is to explain a phenomenon using qualitative methodology. We identified recurrent codes that emerged in the data that reflected positive and negative adjustment and adaptation among the grandparent caregivers. Two of the authors met to discuss the coding and resolve discrepancies found in the coding. Next, we collapsed codes into more general recurrent themes that reflected characteristics of resilience. Grandfamily pseudonyms were used throughout this study and no identifying information was included to maintain participant anonymity.

Results and Discussion

The current study explored the characteristics of grandparent caregivers that appeared to be emblematic of resilience as well as those characteristics that appeared to hinder movement toward resilience or positive adjustment and adaptation. In accordance with McCubbin and McCubbin's Resiliency Model, all the grandfamilies in this study were faced with numerous stressors and demands (e.g., financial challenges in meeting the needs of their grandchildren; mental and physical health burdens experienced by caregivers) that necessitated significant shifting of perceptions, roles, identities, relationships, and resources as their families morphed into grandfamilies (see Bailey et al., 2009). Resilient grandfamilies were able to tap into their individual, familial, and community-based resources and engaged in active coping and healthy problem solving to deal with their stressors and to meet the demands—old and new—on their families. Resilient families talked about establishing daily rhythms of their new families and discussed the importance of engendering such regenerative characteristics as family cohesiveness and calm. More specifically, in our analysis, we found six overarching themes that characterized resilient grandfamilies, including (1) positive appraisal and acceptance of their family as newly configured; (2) narratives of survival and never giving up; (3) healthy boundary maintenance within their families; (4) commitment to newly established routines and rhythms; (5) social connectivity; and (6) commitment to their grandchildren. Although some grandparent caregivers articulated poor coping and adaptation as they discussed certain circumstances of their lives, all grandfamilies shared "resilience narratives" and helped remind us that resilience is indeed not an end point, but a process of positive adjustment and adaptation as life's stressors and demands throw us out of balance and challenge us to regain stability.

Positive Appraisal and Acceptance of the Situation

According to Boss (2002), perhaps the most important component of positive adaptation is how one perceives life stressors and demands. All grandparents in our study were faced with familial crises necessitating their involvement in their grandchildren's lives, and nearly all seemed to struggle to regain their footing as they transitioned to sole caregiver of their grandchildren. Many held out hope early on that their adult children would eventually return and become responsible parents. This hope seemed to keep some grandparents from adjusting to their roles as primary caregivers as they were in a state of "wait and see." However, over time, most came to accept that this would not happen and they began to make the adjustments necessary to function as a family unit. As this grandmother stated:

> I think we did [have hope]. Well, you know, I think the hope was always there, but, down inside, we knew it would never happen, just because we know [our daughter].

When asked if the hope was still there she continued:

> Not anymore. No. Not after this last little encounter. I think that has really pushed us to trying to do something legally with the courts and maybe, you know, prevent her from seeing them unless it's planned, and she's going to need some counseling on what she can and cannot say to them, you know, not to screw them up any more than their poor little minds can handle.

This scenario of holding out hope that their adult children would get it together and resume parenting of the grandchildren was heard by many grandparents. Yet most appeared to transition, from hopefulness to acceptance, coming to terms with the fact that their adult children were not willing or able to take care of the children, and that their role as grandparent caregiver was not going to be temporary. This acceptance and shift in perception of the situation was critical to many grandparent narratives of resilience.

When grandparents were ambivalent about this shift and lacked acceptance of their newfound responsibilities, we found the grandparents to be less positive in their appraisal of the situation and less resilient. For example, one grandmother discussed her struggle with roles:

> Well, we have to play both roles. I play mom and then I play grandma, and it's hard for me, because grandmas are supposed to be funner [sic]. The grandma-thing, you know, is, "Let's go shopping. Let's go spoiling your ass and send you home." Well we don't get that. So he has to—he gets both worlds at one time, which is confusing sometimes, probably for him, because it is for us. We want to be grandparents but we are parents.

This role of ambiguity and ambivalence may get in the way of grandparents' ability to intentionally foster rhythmic and/or regenerative qualities in their families that likely would result in more positive outcomes (Boss, 1999; McCubbin & McCubbin, 1988).

Narratives of Survival and Never Giving Up

In our analysis, beyond positive (or negative) appraisals of the situation, we also found narratives of grandparent strength in the face of familial adversity, hardship, and strife. Many grandparents, even if they accepted that their adult children weren't coming back, were unsure of their own ability to carry out the business of rearing their grandchildren and weathering the family challenges over the long haul. For one grandmother who was disabled and did not have the use of one arm, such doubts were strong, but so was her resolve to do what she needed to do for her grandchild:

> It's really funny, because if you'd told me that I would have been raising a baby disabled like I am when I hardly could take care of myself I would have told you, you were crazy. I didn't know how I'd put a sock, a baby sock on, I didn't know how you bathe him, but it's funny. I have a fake hand. I've never ever used it, I just dabbled with it. It's funny because it might take me ten times longer, but I have figured out a way to do everything I have needed to do. I guess it's kind of one of those "you do what you've got to do."

Another grandmother talked about the death of her son and her perspective on life that seemed to help pull her through the tough times. She said,

> I'm pretty strong, pretty stubborn, you know. But I believe in getting out there and going after something if you want it. I really wanted my music degree, and it wasn't easy and so I got it done and now I pay all the school loans . . . I have no regrets about doing it but it's tough. Life's tough, but I figure the death of my son is the worst thing that could happen to anybody and I survived that so I tell people that. I said, "If you survive the death of a child, you can survive anything."

And when discussing the stress that had occurred on their marriage since parenting a second time around, this grandfather stated:

> We don't, either one of us, believe in giving up. We would never ever do that to one another. I did at one point, I did offer Sally the chance to move home with her mother and stay there a couple of months if she wanted to. I mean you go through things, I mean, we've been married 32 years and there are ups and downs. I grew up in a family and so did Sally where you don't give up.

Throughout the interviews, we heard many stories of grandparents gearing up to do whatever it takes to ensure their grandchildren's needs were met. For many grandparents, their faith, whether general spirituality, faith in God, or faith in the system, was found to be a source of strength. As one grandmother shared, her religious faith helped her through the crisis and adaptation: "I would not have gotten near as far if I didn't have my Lord to talk to and take care of me, you know?" Whether faith-based or derived from another source, grandparents who embraced a "never give up" attitude appeared to engender a sense of control over the situation that ameliorated any sense of hopelessness or helplessness and likely helped them to promote a family feeling of solidarity and cohesion important to resilience.

Healthy Boundary Maintenance

Beyond positive appraisals, acceptance of the situation, and strength narratives, grandparents who demonstrated characteristics of resilience also figured out how to function in ways that promoted the health, safety, and well-being of themselves and their grandchildren. Particularly in grandfamily constellations where there were issues with substance abuse and/or mental illness, grandparents who were able to maintain healthy boundaries within their family system were more resilient. For example, a 46-year-old grandmother, Sharon, who was parenting her husband's grandson, shared how she no longer engages with her stepdaughter and chose to focus on the child. The stepdaughter was a diagnosed schizophrenic and in prison for methamphetamine sales. When asked about her stepdaughter's problems Sharon stated:

> I kind of stay away from her anymore. I broke myself off. It can't be fixed. [I told her,] "Let the prison system deal with you. I can't deal with you no more." I can't deal with it no more. I got him to raise. I can't deal with her.

But maintaining boundaries when that means keeping your own daughter or son from her or his child can be very difficult and throughout our analyses, we found many grandparents who struggled with these boundaries. Sometimes, one grandparent was better at boundary maintenance than his or her spouse or partner. For the following couple who were rearing two teenage grandchildren, this lack of boundary agreement in the family system led to marital discord and frustration as the grandmother felt that her husband enabled their adult daughter and was not as involved with the grandchildren as she would like. She shared, "I am sure she [adult daughter] gets the VA money the kids are supposed to have, but my husband doesn't want to, you know . . . 'rock the boat.'" She went on to say, "It's just that I'd like to have a little time of my own, you know? It's not my whole life. I try and not make it my whole life."

Commitment to Routines and Rhythms

McCubbin and McCubbin (1991) suggest that families who are rhythmic—that is, have routines, plan for family time, and share a sense of togetherness—are likely to be more resilient in the face of adversity. As many grandparents in our study shifted in their roles from "grandparent" to "parent," they discussed the importance of getting into a routine and stabilizing the family system. For one grandmother (Greta), who was a widow on disability, rearing her nine-month-old grandson, her commitment to such routines was evident even as she struggled with a highly acrimonious relationship with her adult daughter and no legal ties to her grandson. She shared:

> You know, she [her daughter] doesn't want to take time to put him in a high chair and teach him how to eat with a spoon, so she's still throwing bottles at him. I have him on a great schedule, you know, babies thrive on schedules, and now Nana thrives on schedules too, because it's pretty rigid. It's not horribly rigid, I mean, but, you know, we wake up, we have cereal [about] at a certain time, naps at certain times, and we sit in the high chair and eat food, you know it all varies, and if I go somewhere it varies, but he knows that when he gets put in his crib it's sleep time. He doesn't yell or cry or fuss, and it works out so good for me, and it makes him ten times easier to care for.

While this grandmother demonstrates a resilient characteristic in the form of routines and rhythms, her situation was still highly stressful and demanding given her daughter's constant threats to take back her son. McCubbin and McCubbin (1991) suggest that such high levels of stress within the family put them at risk for less positive adaptation.

Social Connectivity

Patterson (1991) suggests that social connectivity is important for family resilience. In our study of 55 rural grandparent caregivers, those grandfamilies with positive support networks or access to child care or some form of respite care appeared to better able to adjust and adapt to the stressors and demands in their families (Letiecq, Bailey, & Kurtz, 2008). Those grandparent caregivers living in more rural areas—where there are fewer resources for support—had higher levels of depressive symptoms.

For some grandparents, accessing child or respite care was a significant hindrance that challenged their positive coping and adaptation. In the case of Greta (mentioned above), her social network was limited to her mother and few others. One type of assistance that she voiced would be helpful was respite so that she could get out into the community more. She would like to volunteer again and stated, "Well it would be nice if I could get some sort of childcare to go volunteer or, you know, have a life, or whatever." She also articulated how her severely limited income due to her disability caused a great deal of stress for her.

Another grandmother also expressed great anger at her situation and felt she had "no life." She stated:

> We don't have nobody to watch him no more. We don't have our own time, let alone, you know, time by yourself. We don't have that no more, so it's not like, "Oh, we feel like going to get [grandson]. Let's go and hang out for the day or the weekend," or whatever. We don't—it's not that way at all. It's—sometimes it's like we are forced inside to ourselves to go do these things because he's our kid, not just a grandkid . . . It's kind of hard for all of us, actually.

This grandmother does not have the social support she needs or that she and her husband need as a couple. The couple shared that their grandson's father has promised to help with child care but has yet to follow through, leaving the grandparents frustrated and isolated. Such circumstances seem to be hindering the grandparents from establishing a sense of family cohesion or control over the situation. Indeed, their shared time together does not appear to be promoting a "rhythmic" family, but instead a frustrated and tired family unit.

Another grandparent couple (Tom and Tina) also struggled with the lack of social connectivity. Tom and Tina shared with us that they were experiencing financial pressures, lacked social support, and that Tina was in need of respite care. Tina's family was complex—her grandfamily unit was comprised of her two-year-old grandson and her third husband Tom, to whom she had been married two years. Tina's daughter from her first marriage was the parent of her grandson and she was serving 15 years in prison for armed robbery. Both parents of the grandson had been involved with methamphetamine. When asked about the transition to parenting a second time around, Tina stated:

> I'm depressed, frustrated . . . because there's just nobody, you know? We don't have no family, no nothing here in [this town] and it's just very frustrating. I don't have patience, so it goes all day every day, you know and there's some days that I just need a break, and there's no one to give me a break.

Tina continues,

> It's just, you know, I don't have a babysitter and he's never been with day care, and it just keeps me busy 24/7, and sometimes, there's times when I just need a break. Tom works eight to eight and he works six days a week.

Tina shared that her grandson was also difficult to manage and she felt he had anger problems. She admitted that she too would get angry. Compounding the issue is that her current husband, Tom, has never been a parent before and has a very close relationship with the grandson. Tina finds it difficult to communicate her needs and to be validated by her husband. Again, the lack of social connectivity and support appears to be a significant impediment to promoting qualities more characteristic of healthy, functional, resilient families.

Commitment to Their Grandchildren

Commitment to family, and perhaps more specifically, to the well-being of grandchildren, was found in this study to be an important characteristic of resilience. Grandparents who focused on the needs of their grandchildren and the joy that their grandchildren brought to their lives had trajectories that appeared to lead toward resilient outcomes. As one grandparent stated:

> I was so glad that we had him because had he gone to Family Services, who knows what would have happened. We'd have probably never seen him, and it was kind of fun and then when [his father] died, it was like "Oh my gosh now I really have to do this." So I felt like it was a gift because I was getting to do this again.

Grandparents who found the joy and positive aspects of parenting also demonstrated more resilient characteristics.

> The good stuff is when they come and they give you hugs and they tell you they love you and when you can see—you can see that you've made a difference, you know. Joey, he's got heart. He's got so much heart that it's just unreal, and Jordan, she is a beautiful little girl. She's a—I call her my drama queen, you know, and I tell her, "You can be anything you want to be," because she can come in and light up your, you know, just—but then she has this attitude that can go the other way too, but she puts her arms around and says, "Mom, I love you. You've done a good job. You're my Mom, you know?" Those are rewards enough.

When asked what has worked well since parenting a second time around, this grandmother stated:

> Having to get up with them, having to do something, having a purpose because, like I said, I don't—a lot of times I don't feel good. I cannot not feel good and have kids. You need, you know, so they give me a reason to get up every day, make my bed, get out of bed.

This grandmother demonstrated how a commitment to her grandchildren fostered a rhythmic family quality, and likely helped her and her grandchildren adapt to their new family configuration.

Another grandmother spoke about the adjustments that were made when she took in her granddaughters. These were changes from being in an "empty nest" back to having children in the home. "I think in a way you might say it's faith-strengthening for us because it's—you find out very soon—it's not about you or your agenda anymore . . . your priority list is changed." Again, for grandparents who appeared able to transition from "grandparent" to "parent," to reframe their situation to the positive, and summon up the strength and will to rise to the challenges of rearing their grandchildren, they appeared more resilient and more able to grapple with adversity. Likewise, for grandfamilies who were able to establish and maintain healthy boundaries, to utilize social networks of support, and commit to their grandchildren, we tended to see more positive adaptation. When grandfamilies were overwhelmed by the stressors and demands of their circumstances, we tended to see more negative coping and less resilient characteristics. These findings hold implications for practitioners and helping professionals working with grandfamily constellations to support their bonadaptation and resilience.

Implications for Practitioners

The life stories of these grandparent caregivers reveal that there is no single pathway to positive adaptation. Furthermore, resiliency is dynamic in nature and not an "either/or" status (Masten, 2001). The data do suggest ways in which practitioners might respond to the needs of grandparent caregivers to assist them in moving towards more positive coping and adaptation. First, we will address how agency staff such as parent educators, Extension staff, and child care workers can work towards supporting these grandfamilies. Second, we will discuss how licensed counselors and other helping professionals might apply these findings in their professional practice.

Findings suggest that practitioners can help bolster grandfamily resilience by supporting their positive appraisals of their familial situations, encouraging acceptance of grandparents' newfound roles, helping grandparents reframe their family narratives as stories of survival and endurance in the face of adversity, and encouraging their commitment to their grandchildren as a family good as well as a social good. Grandparents who step up to the plate to rear their grandchildren in the face of family adversity provide a critical function within society that would likely overwhelm the child welfare system should grandparents choose to not get involved (Letiecq, Bailey, & Porterfield, 2008).

Beyond supporting "resilience narratives" among grandfamilies, practitioners likely can provide significant support by increasing grandparent social connectivity (Patterson, 1991). Many grandparents discussed how the lack of respite and social support—the lack of social connectivity—hindered their ability to effectively parent and function as healthfully as desired. We are continually told that parenting a second time around is tiring! For those grandparents who are physically exhausted it is difficult to maintain a positive outlook on the situation and develop necessary routines and traditions for their new family. Child care advocates can work towards changing rules regarding income levels so that grandparent-headed households can access subsidized child care. Non-profit groups might fundraise to have specially designated funds to assist grandfamilies who do not qualify for subsidized child care opportunities.

Parent educators and Extension staff can offer parenting classes designed specifically for grandparent caregivers. Parenting today is different than it was a generation ago and because parenting a second time around is off time this compounds the stressors that accompany parenting. Parenting classes that emphasize the need for routine and tradition (rhythmic families) and the cohesiveness and flexibility needed as the child develops (regenerative families) may assist grandfamilies in reaching a sense of stability, a sense of control, and resilience. Such classes should also key in on maintaining healthy boundaries within the grandfamily unit and provide grandparents with a repertoire of skill sets often needed to establish clear boundaries and maintain them, especially when adult children are struggling with substance abuse and mental health issues that often create confusion, instability, and chaos for families.

In addition to parenting classes, support groups (Cohen & Pyle, 2000) have also been found to assist grandparent caregivers. Having an opportunity to share one's experience with others and realize that he/she is not alone can assist in reducing stress and potentially change perceptions of the situation and support the reframing of family narratives. Support groups also provide the setting where social networking can begin for grandparents who feel isolated. Information about local resources can be shared as grandparents discuss issues related to school, access to food banks, and child care. Our own evaluation of support groups finds that grandparents become more comfortable in reaching out to others and finding services as the result of participation in the group.

Studies have indicated that a lack of social support, both tangible and emotional, can have detrimental effects on a grandparent's ability to effectively manage stress (Hayslip & Kaminski, 2005). While support groups have proven beneficial, O'Reilly and Morrison (1993) pointed out that there are often other needs that cannot be appropriately attended to via a support group alone. Therefore, support groups should be looked at as one piece of a multi-faceted approach taken when dealing with grandparents parenting a second time around (Smith, 2003). For example, some grandparents suffering from emotional problems such as depression or anxiety may benefit from individual counseling while those suffering from fatigue or physical ailments may benefit from respite or other professional services (Waldrop & Weber, 2001). One caveat to this, however, is that other research has alluded to the fact that some grandparents either do not have access to services they would actually welcome or are reluctant to depend on outside help such as that from government agencies, professionals, or community organizations (Gerard, Landry-Meyer, & Roe, 2006). Practitioners must be sensitive to grandparents' boundaries and seek ways to increase connectivity that fits within grandparents' ways of knowing.

Future research to help us understand these relationships is needed to continue to inform our practice.

Implications for Counselors and Helping Professionals

For counselors and helping professionals working within the support group context, it seems important that they understand that the needs of grandparents raising grandchildren are unique given the generational differences between themselves and their grandchildren. With regard to resilience, counselors and helping professionals can benefit grandparents by attending to two themes identified in this study: acceptance of change and a positive appraisal of the situation.

First, grandparents noted that an acceptance of the change in the family dynamic needed to occur. For counselors working with grandparents, this seems like an important transition to attend to. Scholossberg, Waters, & Goodman (1995) identified transitions such as this as "surprise transitions," or a transition that was unexpected. Counselors who have an understanding of transition theory may be able to highlight the notion of surprise transitions and explore the thoughts, feelings, and behaviors that are associated with the transitions. Helping professionals might also utilize psychoeducational materials that reinforce resilience within grandfamilies, including materials that promote positive coping skills, positive parenting skills, the establishment of routines and rhythms, and healthy and functional crisis management.

In our study, resilient grandparents shared that a positive appraisal of their situation which included a positive outlook, hope, and faith was imperative. Grandparents stated that they had initial hope that their children would change and parent again, but that they needed to let that perception go, in order for new perceptions to emerge. This is known as an ambiguous loss. Boss (1999, 2002) describes ambiguous loss as a loss that is not as clearly defined as death. In the case of grandfamilies, their own children (the child's parents) may be present, but unable or unwilling to parent their children. For counselors and helping professionals who find themselves working with grandparents experiencing ambiguous losses, they might need to incorporate grieving in the support group context, as well as specifically address ambiguous loss and working towards acceptance of loss. Moreover, this study suggests that these helping professionals can support grandparents' ambivalence towards rearing their grandchildren and help grandparents make sense of their new roles within their families.

Once grandparents have had time to grieve and accept the new family dynamic, this study indicated that resilient grandparents appreciated assistance in regaining hope that is aligned with a more realistic perception of their unique situation. Positive outlook and hope seemed to be an important factor in helping these grandparents move forward. With that, counselors may look to and help grandparents reconnect with sources of hope, such as their faith, especially given that grandparents identified their faith as being instrumental in easing the transition to grandparent caregiving. Counselors can also be instrumental is assisting grandparents' reconnection with the joys of parenting. For these helping professionals working with grandfamilies, our research suggests that helping these families reframe their situation, and connect with more realistic expectations of themselves and others, may result in more positive adaptations and resilient outcomes.

Conclusion

Resiliency is a dynamic process rather than a static state or something that, once achieved, is constant. The narratives of these grandfamilies illustrate how fluid resiliency is in their lives. Although we were only able to capture their life stories at one point in their journey through parenting a second time around, we were able to capture the process of resiliency and identify themes that either supported or hindered their efforts of positive adaptation.

What can be learned from these stories is that there are several characteristics of resiliency for grandparent caregivers, including: positive appraisals and acceptance of their family as newly configured; a commitment to surviving and never giving up; maintaining health boundaries within their families; establishing routines and rhythms; developing social connectivity; and commitment to their grandchildren. While all six themes were not present in the life histories of each family interviewed, the frequency and pronouncement of these themes indicate their salience in the study of grandfamily resilience. Future research should continue to shed light on the resilience process within grandfamily constellations to support the health and well-being of these families.

References

Bailey, S. J., Letiecq, B. L., & Porterfield, F. (2009). Family coping and adaptation among grandparents rearing grandchildren, *Journal of Intergenerational Relationships, 7,* 144–158.

Black, K., & Lobo, M. (2008). A conceptual review of family resilience factors. *Journal of Family Nursing, 14,* 33–55.

Boss, P. (2002). *Family stress management: A contextual approach*, Thousand Oaks, CA: Sage Publications, Inc.

Boss, P. G. (1999). *Ambiguous loss: Learning to live with unresolved grief.* Cambridge, MA: Harvard University Press.

Cohen, C. S., & Pyle, R. (2000). Support groups in the lives of grandmothers raising grandchildren. In C. B. Cox (Ed.), *To grandmother's house we go and stay: Perspectives on custodial grandparents* (pp. 235–252). New York: Springer Publishing.

Gerard, J. M., Landry-Meyer, L., & Roe, J. G. (2006). Grandparents raising grandchildren: The role of social support in coping with caregiving challenges. *International Journal of Aging and Human Development, 62,* 359–383.

Goodley, D., Lawthom, R., Clough, P., & Moore, M. (2004). *Researching life stories: Method, theory, and analyses in a biographical age.* London: Routledge.

Hayslip, B. & Kaminski, P. L. (2005). Grandparents raising their grandchildren, *Marriage and Family Review, 37*, 147–169.

Hill, R. (1949). *Families under stress*. New York: Harper Publishing.

Jooste, J. L. Hayslip, B., & Smith, G. C. (2008). The adjustment of children and grandparent caregivers in grandparent-headed families. In B. Hayslip, Jr. & P. Kaminski (Eds.), *Parenting the custodial grandchild: implications for clinical practice* (pp. 17–40). New York: Springer.

Juby, C., & Ryecraft, J. R. (2004). Family preservation strategies for families in poverty. *Families in Society, 85*, 581–587.

Letiecq, B. L., Bailey, S. J., & Kurtz, M. A. (2008). Depression among rural Native American and European American grandparents rearing their grandchildren, *Journal of Family Issues, 29*, 334–356.

Letiecq, B. L., Bailey, S. J., & Porterfield, F. (2008). "We have no rights, we get no help": The legal and policy dilemmas facing grandparent caregivers. *Journal of Family Issues* (Special Collection: Transforming the discussion on diversity: The influence of policies and law on families), *29*(8), 995–1012.

Lumpkin, J. R. (2007). Grandparents in a parental or near-parental role: Sources of stress and coping mechanisms, *Journal of Family Issues, 29*, 357–372.

Luthar, S. S., Cicchetti, D., & Becker, B. (2000). The construct of resilience: A critical evaluation and guidelines for future work. *Child Development, 71*, 543–562.

Masten, A. S. (2001). Ordinary magic: Resilience processes in development. *American Psychologist, 56*, 227–238.

McCubbin, M. A. (1993). Family stress theory and the development of nursing knowledge about family adaptation. In S. L. Feetham, S. B. Meister, J. M. Bell, & C. L. Gillis (Eds.). *The Nursing Family* (pp. 46–58). Newbury Park: Sage.

McCubbin, H. I. & McCubbin, M. A. (1988). Typologies of resilient families: Emerging roles of social class and ethnicity. *Family Relations, 37*, 247–254.

McCubbin, M. A. & McCubbin, H. I. (1991). Family stress theory and assessment: The resiliency model of family stress, adjustment and adaptation. In H. I. McCubbin, & A. I. Thompson (Eds.), *Family assessment inventories for research and practice* (pp. 3–32). Madison, WI: University of Wisconsin-Madison.

McCubbin, M. A., & McCubbin, H. I. (1993). Family coping with health crisis: The resiliency model of family stress, adjustment and adaptation. In C. Danielson, B. Hamel-Bissell, & P. Winstead-Fry (Eds.), *Families, Health, and Illness* (pp. 21–63). St. Louis: Mosby.

McCubbin, H., & Patterson, J. (1983). Family transitions: Adaptation to stress, *Marriage & Family Review, 6*, 7–37.

Musil, C. M., Gordon, N. L., Warner, C. B., Zauszniewski, J. A., Standing, T., & Wykle, M. (2011). Grandmothers and caregiving to grandchildren: Continuity, change, and outcomes over 24 months. *The Gerontologist, 51*, 86–100.

Musil, C., Warner, C., Zauszniewski, J., Jeanblanc, A. B., & Kercher, K. (2006). Grandmothers, caregiving and family functioning. *The Journals of Gerontology: Series B, 61*(2), S89–S98.

Musil, C., Warner, C., Zauszniewski, J., Wykle, M., & Standing, T. (2009). Grandmother caregiving, family stress and strain, and depressive symptoms. *Western Journal of Nursing Research, 31*, 389–408.

O'Reilly, E., & Morrison, M. L. (1993). Grandparent-headed families: New therapeutic challenges. *Child Psychiatry and Human Development, 23*, 147–159.

Patterson, J. M. (1991). Family resilience to the challenge of a child's disability. *Pediatric Annals, 20*(9), 491–499.

Patton, M. Q. (2002). *Qualitative research and evaluation methods (3rd ed.)*. Thousand Oaks, CA: Sage Publications.

Pinson-Millburn, N. M., Fabian, E. S., Schlossberg, N. K., & Pyle, M. (1996). Grandparents raising grandchildren, *Journal of Counseling & Development, 74*, 548–554.

Rutter, M. (1979). Protective factors in children's responses to stress and disadvantage. In M. W. Kent & J. E. Rolf (Eds.), *Primary prevention of psychopathology: Vol. 3. Social competence in children* (pp. 49–74). Hanover, NH: University Press of New England.

Schlossberg, N. K., Waters, E. B., & Goodman, J. (1995) *Counseling adults in transition* (2nd ed.). New York: Springer Publishing.

Smith, G. C. (2003). *Working with custodial grandparents*. New York, NY: Springer Publishing Co.

Tak, Y. R. & McCubbin, M. (2002) Family stress, perceived social support and coping following the diagnosis of a child's congenital heart disease, *Journal of Advanced Nursing, 39*(2), pp. 190–198.

US Census (2009). 2005–2009 American Community Survey 5-Year Estimates. http://www.factfinder.census.gov/servlet/STTable?_bm=y&-geo_id=01000US&-qr_name=ACS_2009_5YR_G00_S1002&-ds_name=ACS_2009_5YR_G00_&-redoLog=false

Waldrop, D. P., & Weber, J. A. (2001). From grandparent to caregiver: The stress and satisfaction of raising grandchildren. *Families in Society, 83*, 461–472.

6 Grandparent Caregivers' Self-Care Practice

Moving Towards a Strengths-Based Approach

Christine A. Fruhauf and Kimberly Bundy-Fazioli

Abstract

It is well documented in the literature that grandparents often experience difficulties and challenges when assuming responsibility for rearing grandchildren. Despite the fact this area of inquiry received much attention, it is necessary for researchers and practitioners to move towards a strengths-based practice approach when researching and working with grandparent caregivers. As a result, data from 15 grandparent caregivers who participated in face-to-face interviews or focus group discussions about their health were analyzed utilizing the constant comparison approach. Analysis resulted in patterns and codes supporting grandparent caregivers' self-care practices. For example, grandparents did not dwell on health related challenges. Instead, they emphasized their self-care practices as they relate to physical and emotional health, and social support. Grandparents spoke about the importance of proper diet and exercise and healthy lifestyle choices, such as sobriety. They also believed they had a positive attitude and reflected this when they stated they were happy and upbeat. Many grandparents spoke of the fact they were blessed to have a second chance at parenting and that they recognized other grandparents they knew had it more difficult than they did. Following the strengths-based approach, when practitioners work with grandparents it is important that they work collaboratively and in partnership with grandparents and their grandchildren. This is perhaps one of the most basic principles, yet practitioners often overpower the narratives of grandparents with their expertise. We propose in our chapter that the strengths-based practice approach focuses on partnering with grandparents in order to support existing self-care practices, coping skills, fostering their hopes and dreams, and promoting positive health and wellness.

Grandparent Caregivers' Self-Care Practice: Moving Towards a Strengths-Based Approach

It is well documented in the custodial grandparenting literature that grandparents often experience challenges when assuming responsibility for parenting grandchildren (Fuller-Thomson & Minkler, 2000; Hayslip & Kaminiski, 2005).

In particular, researchers have focused their attention on negative impacts related to physical and mental health of grandparent caregivers. In these studies, researchers concluded grandparents experience negative health outcomes (Goodman, 2006; Soloman & Marx, 2000) as they delay seeking medical attention (Burnette, 1999), engage in risky health behaviors (Roberto, Dolbin-MacNab, & Finney, 2008) and are at risk for increased stress and depression (Minkler, Fuller-Thomson, Miller, & Driver, 2000; Musil & Standing, 2006) as a result of full-time caregiving for grandchildren.

Although emphasis is placed on the negative impact raising grandchildren has on the lives of grandparents, few researchers have highlighted positive outcomes (Hayslip & Kaminiski, 2005; Goodman, 2006) and thus, advances in meeting grandparents' needs through service provision are not solely supported through positive attributes. As a result, we believe it is necessary for researchers and practitioners to move towards building a strengths-based practice approach when working with grandparent caregivers. Drawing from our research with grandparents who assume primary care responsibilities to their grandchildren, in this chapter we will discuss grandparent caregivers' self-care practices as they relate to their overall health and well-being. We assume physical, mental, and social health are three components of overall health (Soloman & Marx, 2000; Whitelaw & Liang, 1991). For this research, we used Soloman and Marx's (2000) definition: (a) physical health as chronic and acute diseases, functional ability, and self-ratings of health; (b) mental health aspects including depression, anxiety, psychological problems, and life satisfaction; and, (c) social health as interactions with friends and family. We draw our insights from focus groups and interviews with grandparent caregivers.

Grandparent Caregiver Self-Care

Self-care focuses on personal health maintenance and is often described as the ability of individuals to improve or restore their health and even prevent future health challenges through positive lifestyle practices (Connelly, 1993). Self-care has been of interest among health related professionals since the 1980s when it first surfaced as an integral part of successful disease management (Becker, Gates, & Newson, 2004; Riegel & Dickson, 2008). The self-care literature is rooted in the medical field with more than 25,000 articles on the topic (Riegel & Dickson, 2008) usually focusing on self-care behavior when individuals are diagnosed with a chronic disease (i.e., heart failure, loss of kidney functioning, diabetes, etc.).

Orem (2001) and Orem and Vardiman (1995) are credited with developing the Self-Care Deficit Nursing Theory (SCDNT); a theory widely used and cited in the self-care literature. Orem (2001) states individuals have the ability to develop practical and intellectual skills and motivation for self-care. Further, the SCDNT involves three key components (Orem, 2001) important to understanding grandparent self-care practices. Self-care practices include an individual's: (a) investment in "continued existence, health, and well-being"; (b) maintaining "life, health, and well-being"; and, (c) awareness of self-care deficits when he/she is no longer able to care for him/herself (Rafii, Shahpoorian, & Azarbaad, 2008, pp. 35–36).

Despite the growth of self-care articles in the medical literature, the concept of self-care as it applies to grandparent caregivers has received minimal attention. Researchers who addressed self-care and grandparent caregivers provide insights into their challenges as grandparents' have less time and energy for self-care (Pruchno, 1999; Roe, Minkler, Saunders, & Thomson, 1996). This empirical work, however, does not present positive ways grandparents engage in their self-care. For example, Wohl, Lahner, and Jooste (2003) discuss findings from their work developing and evaluating support groups with grandparent caregivers. Of particular interest to our research, Wohl and colleagues reported grandparents were unable to take the time to engage in self-care practices. They stated that, "the idea of self-care is so foreign to these overworked caretakers that many had difficulty even generating a wish list of self-pampering activities during one of the groups" (Wohl et al., 2003, pp. 204–205). Possibly the only positive aspect associated with Wohl and colleagues' (2003) account, was to reframe self-care of grandparents to better meet their grandchildren's needs (i.e., if you are not healthy, then your grandchild's needs cannot be met). As a result, it is necessary to further explore self-care as an important component to the positive qualities of grandparent caregivers' experiences.

Purpose of the Study

The purpose of this study is to report findings from a larger qualitative research investigation addressing grandparent caregivers' physical, mental, and social health. We focus our report on grandparents' self-care as a way to highlight their approach to maintaining positive overall health. Further, we provide implications for practitioners using the strengths-based practice approach (Saleeby, 2011) towards helping individuals who are responsible for raising grandchildren.

Sample and Methods

The participants in this study were 15 grandparent caregivers who were raising their grandchildren full-time. Grandparents were predominantly female ($n = 13$) and ranged in age from 49 to 78 years old ($M = 61$). All grandparents were Caucasian expect for one grandmother who self identified as Latina. Most grandparents were raising one grandchild ($n = 10$) and grandchildren's ages ranged from 3 to 15 years old ($M = 10$). Grandparents reported raising their grandchildren because of parental neglect, drug and/or alcohol use/misuse, parental abandonment, emotional abuse of the grandchildren, parent incarceration, physical abuse of the grandchild, and parental death.

Grandparent caregivers were recruited through local support groups and word of mouth from a county kinship navigator and grandparents (i.e., grandparents who participated or were planning on participating in a focus group session told other grandparents about the research study). Grandparents participated in either one focus group session or a face-to-face interview. We encouraged grandparents to participate in the focus group discussion as focus groups are a way to understand individuals' shared phenomenon (Morgan, 1997). Three grandparents had scheduling conflicts with the time and date for the focus group discussions and wanted to still participate; therefore, we conducted face-to-face interviews with these grandparents.

We used the same semi-structured protocol for both the focus groups and face-to-face interviews to understand grandparent caregivers' health and well-being. We asked questions addressing physical, mental, and social health, and particular attention was paid to having grandparents describe positive aspects of their health. Questions included, "Tell us about what you are most proud of related to your physical, mental, and social health?" , "What activities help you deal with your health concerns?" , "How do you take care of yourself?" All interviews and focus groups were audio-recorded and transcribed verbatim.

Data analysis utilizing the constant comparison approach (Charmaz, 2010) resulted in patterns and codes (Saldaña, 2009) addressing grandparent caregivers' overall health and well-being. We read the transcripts in their entirety and made notations about patterns (i.e., words that are similar, frequent, and mention how and when things happen) in reference to what the data were describing (Saldaña, 2009). After patterns were established, we broke them down into codes which is "a word or short phrase that symbolically assigns a summative, salient, essence-capturing, and/or evocative attribute for a portion of . . . data" (Saldaña, 2009, p. 3). We then engaged in a constant comparison method of sorting through our notations into "like minded codes" or codes that were similar by linking an idea or pattern together (Saldaña, 2009). A line-by-line analysis of the data was then conducted (Charmaz, 2010) to refine the codes (Saldaña, 2009) resulting in emerging categories addressing health and well-being of grandparent caregivers within each health related area (i.e., physical, mental, and social). In this chapter, we only report the findings related to grandparent caregivers' self-care practices.

Findings and Discussion

Guided by concepts of Orem's Self-Care Deficit Nursing Theory and previously discussed literature on grandparent caregivers' health and well-being, this research attempted to expand the understanding of self-care practices of grandparent caregivers. In this section, we provide findings from our data and discuss grandparents' self-care as it relates to their physical, mental, and social health. We do so using direct quotes from grandparent caregivers to elucidate meanings. Participants' names have been changed to protect their identity.

From our data and supported by previous work, we found grandparents spoke about having their grandchildren in their home as "a blessing" and "an opportunity for a second chance" at raising children (Hayslip, Shore,

Henderson, & Lambert, 1998; Wohl et al., 2003). When grandparents discussed the impact of being a full-time caregiver, they often agreed that they "just do it" and that they have to take it "one day at a time." Furthermore, grandparent caregivers said at times they need to "surrender" as they can only do so much. Surrendering was not related to giving up, but as Orem (2001) suggests a component of self-care, it was grandparents' way to take time for themselves and permission to slow down and better care for their family. These findings provide a foundation of self-care practices of grandparent caregivers from our work and for the discussion in this chapter.

Physical Health

As described earlier, physical health refers to self-ratings of health, daily functioning, and both acute and chronic diseases. Despite the plethora of literature demonstrating health challenges of grandparents who rear grandchildren, a majority (67%) of grandparent caregivers in our study described their health as excellent ($n = 3$) or good ($n = 7$) and five participants (33%) described their health as fair. When asked about their physical health, none of the grandparents stated their health was poor. This was an interesting finding considering two grandparents shared their struggle with cancer, two grandparents disclosed having diabetes, and one grandparent shared he had heart disease. For future research it would be helpful to ask grandparents: "What does excellent health look like?" and, "What does poor health look like?" It is possible that grandparents did not want to label themselves as having "poor" health for fear that their ability to raise their grandchild might be questioned. In this section, we discuss self-care practices in regards to physical health by describing lifestyle choices and medical attention and tensions.

Lifestyle Choices

Included in grandparent caregivers' discussion of daily functioning were the importance of a proper diet and "eating right" while also including time for exercise (i.e., walking, biking, time outdoors, and strength training). Grandparents credited keeping up with their grandchildren as a way to maintain an exercise routine. This was explained by Candice when she said, "I walk. I like to walk . . . And, my eight year old, you know, they're really active and energetic so following them around is good exercise." Molly supported this when she said, "I have been grateful [to my grandson]. He has really helped keep me active." In addition to exercise, grandparents spoke towards needing (although, not necessarily always receiving) "a massage", "grandparent spa day", and relaxing in a "hot tub". These wish lists of things that they do and want to do for themselves is the opposite of what Wohl and colleagues (2003) discovered in their research. Possibly the fact that our interview guide probed grandparents to share the activities they do to maintain their health, prompted them to also add a "wish list" of self-care items they hoped to one day receive.

Other healthy lifestyle choices grandparents discussed included addressing everything from needing to lose weight to maintaining their sobriety. Grandparents' ability to engage in self-care and change negative lifestyle behaviors admittedly at times is "not easy" as they often are "drained" due to lack of sleep and parenting responsibilities. Deborah stated, "honestly, I'm exhausted at the end of the day and I'm lucky if I can, you know, get to bed and I know, get more energy . . ." for what is to come next. It is well known that getting enough, well rested sleep is a useful way to maintain a healthy lifestyle; grandparents' ability to engage in positive care-related routines (such as sleep) possibly allowed them the ability to cope with their chronic illnesses and physical health, as well as, the daily challenges of parenting children. Grandparents' investment towards maintaining their health and well-being supports Orem's (2001) components of self-care.

Medical Attention and Tensions

Maintaining a healthy lifestyle, however, was complicated for grandparents who spoke about engaging in self-care practices around their chronic illnesses. It was clear that grandparents experienced an internal tension between doctors' orders, knowing what they should be doing related to their self-care, and actually taking better care of themselves. This is best illustrated when Marla discussed being diabetic and that her husband, Scott, had a previous heart attack. Marla stated, "we try to maintain the visits with the doctor, but my blood sugar's not doing real well. . . . I know I [should] be eating better. I know I should be exercising. It's like I know . . ." but the reality of raising grandchildren often takes over their needs and self-care is often put after grandchildren (Wohl et al., 2003). Further, despite Loise having a blood pressure problem and "under all this stress, when [she is] in a lot of pain, that just keeps [her] blood pressure up a lot of times and [she deals] with it in holistic ways" because she does not have the financial resources to pay for her health care. Her resourcefulness in finding unique ways to care for herself is laudable, yet it was not determined if these holistic practices appropriately managed her blood pressure. Finally, from Dina's cancer diagnosis and treatment she found the strength to "really want to live and have a vengeance for [life] . . ." after a lifetime of suffering from depression and suicidal attempts beginning at age 13. Despite facing chronic illnesses, grandparents self-care related to their physical health was supported by their positive approach to mental health.

Mental Health

Grandparent caregivers' engagement in self-care practices can be characterized by "behavior based on insight and reflective judgments from which [they] can infer something about [their] mental health" (Orem & Vardiman, 1995, p. 165). Although we did not systematically measure grandparents ability to judge their mental health status, their comments related to depression, psychological problems, and life satisfaction illustrated the complexity of the impact raising grandchildren has on mental health. These factors were discussed by grandparent caregivers in our research and support positive life satisfaction. Positive solutions, working through feelings, and wisdom of time are three areas we will focus our attention on in this section.

Positive Solutions

Grandparents' believed they were "happy" and "upbeat" despite many of them agreeing with Silvia, when she stated, "I'm also on the balance beam and kind of flipping off the balance beam . . . happy though." Similarly, Candice reiterated her approach to mental health when she discussed daily challenges related to raising her grandchildren, "finding ways to solve things positively and turning it around and having a positive attitude from there I think that makes your health and your life a lot better" and Dina consciously made a decision to stay positive when she shared, "I decided that I would be positive and smile and give the world a different perception of disabled people. I call it 'building bridges to the heart.'" It appears that grandparents who participated in this study, discovered finding solutions to problems was more proactive than being reactive and feeling powerless. Grandparent caregivers' approach to their mental health may be the foundation for positively working through their emotions.

Working Through Feelings

Although grandparent caregivers engaged in self-care practices related to mental health, similar to previous research, many grandparents discussed the process of confronting feelings of anger, fear, resentment, frustration and denial (Giarrusso, Silverstein & Feng, 2000). Scott displayed this when he stated, "for a long time I harbored a lot of hate. I mean, I have a pretty hot temper when it comes to abuse . . . I finally had to put it to the man upstairs and He finally took care of that." For grandparents to recognize and work through feelings of anger and rage appeared to be an important step in their healing and self-care. Grandparent caregivers in this study discussed that they found support groups to be a place to share their emotions along with the pain of watching their grandchildren struggle with trauma-related feelings and behaviors. It was not determined, however, if grandparents' willingness to discuss their feelings at support groups was actually beneficial or potentially detrimental to them, as previous researchers have suggested (Strom & Strom, 1993; Szinovacz & Roberts, 1998).

Wisdom of Time

Grandparents' reliance on their own resourcefulness, resilience, and knowledge gained over time was apparent. Grandparents discussed using music, their faith, meditation practices, and books (although it was not determined if these were self-help books or pleasure reading) as a way to care for themselves. Like many participants, Dina's thoughts are similar when she stated, "my strengths are, my faith and my positive attitude. I always felt that it was more of just a positive attitude about things. . . . it is really my faith. . . . by the grace of God I am sitting her in front of you . . ." Periods of silence (i.e., reading, listening to music, deep breathing, reminiscence with friends and spouses, and just taking time for themselves) and spiritual guidance for purposes of reflection, is part of a larger process that enables grandparents to have time for greater self-knowledge (Orem & Vardiman, 1995). Possibly with time, grandparents' resilience may develop as indicated when Molly stated, "Well life is a learning [process], all the way through. No one said this world is easy." Grandparents discussed utilizing support from mental health professionals and other community services, including grandparent support groups, to assist them when they were experiencing depression or sadness. This further supports Orem's (2001) key component of grandparents' ability to know their deficits and when they are no longer able to properly care for themselves.

Social Health

Social health refers to the friends and family members who provide comfort and support to individuals. In addition to these areas, we found grandparents discussed the importance of community connections to their social health. As it relates to social health, we discuss grandparents' important connections, fostering new relationships, and support groups in this section.

Important Connections

Grandparents reported receiving support from friends through monthly lunches and talking over the phone. For some grandparents in our study, however, e-mail was a way to maintain connections with friends who lived in other states. Molly discussed not only a friend supporting her emotionally but also motivating her to go to the gym and exercise. This was evident when she said, "Yes, two mornings a week we go together. . . . She does the walk and the Pilate stretches with me. The other two days, I have [the] heart promotions [class] . . . it's in the water; in the pool exercise." Spouses also helped grandparents maintain their overall health. For example, Candice stated, "I think I have pretty good mental health . . . when I get stressed out or tired, I'll let my husband know . . . Say, Keith will go . . . and he kind of helps any way [he can]" and Ryan indicated his social network is Belinda, his wife, when he stated, "You're looking at it . . . we're here for each other." The importance of friends and spouses/partners are not only a way for grandparent caregivers to maintain and possibly improve their social health, but it is also a way for them to be physically healthy. This is further supported when Deborah stated that she "surround[s] [her]self with positive people . . ." which is important to grandparent caregivers as many of them stated that, "We've lost friends on account of because their kids [are] gone and they didn't want us to bring him [grandchild] over . . . well, he don't come, we don't come" as Scott confirmed.

Fostering New Relationships

From our research, we found that when grandparents' friends were not willing to have grandchildren over their house (Ehrle, 2001), it often resulted in grandparent caregivers "feeling isolated" and even "withdrawing" from social support networks (Shore & Hayslip, 1994). Yet, most grandparents showed resilience through their self-care when they found new friends who were compassionate and supportive of their decision to assume parental responsibility for their grandchildren. Some of their friends came from support groups as Jennifer stated, "I still have a lot of friends. I formed a lot of friendships in the grandparents support group" and both Emily and Susan agreed grandparents should, "Get in a support group . . . those ladies can pull you through anything." As a result, grandparents in our research found that support groups were not only beneficial in maintaining their social health, but they also benefited from the psychoeducational approach of the support groups (Smith, 2003).

Support Groups

The importance of support groups was discussed by grandparents as providing an avenue and opportunity to connect with other grandparents about raising grandchildren. Further, another benefit of support groups was the opportunity to build skills and knowledge as a way to better take care of their grandchildren. Not only did grandparent caregivers reflect building friendships with grandparents whom they met during support groups, they received valuable information about accessing community supports for children's activities, health stipends, and even encouragement to seek health care related assistance. Deborah shared that she followed-up on a resource that she learned about in the grandparent support group when she said, "I went to the Fort Collins Health Clinic and they did a lot for me. They really did . . ." Lonetta shared a similar story about getting "clothes from a lady in her church" and Emily said "the support . . . I mean the 4-H [club]. There's kind of a lot of the people involved in that club are foster kids or foster parents . . ." who not only helped her grandchildren but also was a way for her to connect with other people in similar situations. Connecting with grandparents and services/service providers through support groups is important for grandparents' success in raising grandchildren and for their overall health and well-being.

Implications for Direct Practice

Grandparent caregiver's self-care is vital for optimal physical, mental, and social health. Based on our data, many grandparents have the ability to identify and share their self-care practices, while other grandparents may not have the same ability. When assessing grandparent caregivers' self-care abilities it is important for practitioners to take into account both internal cognitive processes as well as available external resources within the grandparents' environment. Internal resources include a grandparent's ability to cognitively process social, emotional, cognitive, and physical cues within his/her living environment (Corcoran, 2006). In particular, how does a grandparents think, feel, and act in response to his/her living situation? How does a grandparent express his/her emotions in regards to life events? How does a grandparent respond to stress? External resources include taking into account social environmental factors such as housing, finances, familial relationships, and social supports. McQuaide and Ehrenreich's (1997) seminal work, referenced in both strengths-based and resiliency literature, argued that social environmental factors could either "augment strengths and [or] vulnerabilities" (p. 205). For example, if a grandparent finds that her long-term friend no longer wants to get together with her because there is now a child in tow, this loss could potentially contribute towards the grandparent's sense of isolation and loneliness. Or, if the grandparent by nature is determined and solid in her decision to raise her grandchild, this passion could propel the grandparent to seek out new supportive relationships. How grandparents make sense of their internal thoughts and feelings, and external environment is individualistic. This is important, as McQuaide and Ehrenreich (1997) state that "being able to access one's strengths effectively contributes not only to solving an immediate problem, but may also augment the [grandparent's] ability to deal with future problems" (p. 202). Therefore, we believe that self-care practices of grandparent caregivers are a process that grandparents actively engage in as a response to their changing health and their grandchildren's arrangement in the home. Yet, the self-care process is often overlooked in the grandparent caregiver literature and should be further explored.

Grandparents who exercise self-care and have incorporated self-care practices into their daily routine have usually drawn from internal and external resources that have supported and reinforced healthy coping skills. Practitioners can help to foster or reinforce positive coping and self-care practices of grandparent caregivers. We provide four focal areas practitioners should consider when supporting grandparents' self-care practices. In general, these include working from a strengths-based approach as well as learning about a grandparent's social environment, coping mechanisms, and self-care practices.

Strengths-Based Practice Approach

The first focal area is the concept of working from a strengths-based approach. Often, in practice, assessing for strengths is easier said than done (McQuaide & Ehrenreich, 1997; Saleebey, 2011). In a simplistic view, the strengths-based approach is the interrelationship between the practitioner's philosophical stance as well as the practitioner's depth of understanding on how each individual perseveres in the face of adversity. To fully practice from a strengths-based perspective, the practitioner must embrace the philosophy of working *with* grandparents as partners and truly fostering mutual collaboration. Saleeby (2011) states, "the strengths approach obligates us to understand—to believe

—that everybody (no exceptions here) has external and internal assets, competencies, and resources" (p. 127). Thus, it would be counterproductive for a practitioner to tell grandparent caregivers how they can better take care of themselves. Instead it behooves the practitioner to believe that every person who is challenged by struggles will learn from them and, therefore, has intrinsic knowledge and skills about themselves (Saleebey, 2011). As a result, practitioners need to be cognizant of how they interact with grandparents. If a practitioner finds that a grandparent is resistant or difficult to engage, then it is the practitioner's responsibility to evaluate his/her beliefs, approach and demeanor. For example, we suggest the practitioner ask colleagues and supervisors for feedback. Practitioners should also ask themselves: "Do I believe this grandparent is capable of raising his/her grandchild?" and, "Do I believe in the grandparent's strengths and abilities?" The answers to these questions will help pinpoint what the grandparent is sensing in his/her interaction with the practitioner.

Social Environment

The second focal area is learning about the grandparent in the context of his/her social environment. In order to learn about a grandparent's self-care practices it is imperative that the practitioner take time to listen and learn about internal and external resources. Conducting an eco-map is a valuable tool in learning how grandparents view their familial resources (Hartman, 1995) and practitioners should consider bringing this into their practice with grandparents. An eco-map is a diagram visually portraying familial resources (strengths and challenges) that is constructed with the grandparent. This visual diagram places the grandparent's household members in a circle in the middle of the page (i.e., lists each family member separately in the circle). The practitioner then asks questions of the grandparent that help identify supports and challenges for each family member within the social environment. For example, Shaefor and Horejsi (2006) suggest asking the following questions: Does the family have sufficient income to cover needs such as food, shelter, transportation, child care, health care, school supplies? Is the grandparent caregiver employed? If so, does he/she enjoy his/her job? Does the family feel safe in their neighborhood? What is the grandparent's relationship with other family members, relatives, and neighbors? What social, cultural, or religious activities within the community does the grandparent participate in? Does the grandparent caregiver perceive conflicts within his/her community relating to his/her values and beliefs? (Shaefor & Horejsi, 2006, pp. 257–258). The answers to each question are portrayed in a smaller separate circle outside of the family circle and a line is drawn between the family member and the identified resource illustrating strength (double lines ═) or a conflict (a single line with slash marks +++). Visually the eco-map helps the practitioner and grandparent see strengths and challenges of resources within the grandfamily's social environment. As a result, the eco-map exercise has the potential for the practitioner and grandparent to discuss areas they can work on together to help fix challenges that may occur.

Coping Mechanisms

The third focal area is learning about a grandparent's coping mechanisms. Utilizing strengths and conflicts identified in the eco-map, the practitioner is able to ask questions that seek more depth and understanding into the grandparent's self-care practices. When grandparent caregivers are having difficulty identifying self-care practices, due to perhaps feeling overwhelmed and exhausted, coping related questions derived from solution-focused therapy can help identify what they are "doing to survive their pain and circumstances" (De Jong & Berg, 2008, p. 220). Coping questions such as "How have you managed to cope?" and "Given the conflicts you are juggling, how have you kept things from getting worse?" help to emphasize a grandparent caregiver's strengths (Shulman, 2009, p. 623). Grandparent caregivers' answers to the coping questions open up the door for possibilities and exceptions to presenting problems and conflicts. By focusing on times when conflicts are less problematic the practitioner is able to explore exceptions, such as "What do you suppose you did to make that happen?" (De Jong & Berg, 2008, p. 367). A practitioner's awareness and acknowledgment of how a grandparent helps his/her family survive each day, provides information on potential sources of coping, resilience, and self-care (McQuaide & Ehrenreich, 1997). Awareness can be emphasized in practice, reinforcing the grandparent's management of his/her own health and well-being while also supporting his/her self-care process.

Self-Care Practices

The fourth focal area is learning about grandparents' self-care practices. There are many grandparents who are able to easily identify self-care practices and share what helps them to relax and what provides relief from day-to-day stress. However, there will also be grandparents who feel overwhelmed with the task of day-to-day activities related to childrearing and, thus, can easily neglect any focus on their self-care. The task for practitioners and grandparent caregivers is to not only identify current self-care practices, but also identify self-care obstacles. What interferes with daily self-care? How can these obstacles be addressed? One way to help grandparents who are overwhelmed by a myriad of obstacles and problems is the practitioner's use of the skill of partializing.

Breaking Down Obstacles

Partializing is a useful problem-managing skill when obstacles appear insurmountable (Shulman, 2009). Together, the practitioner and grandparent can work to break down obstacles into "manageable proportions" (Shulman, 2009, p. 150). Manageable proportions are smaller pieces of the larger problem (Shulman, 2009). For example, a grandparent may share, "I get so much out of support groups but there is no way I can attend as I do not have money for child care. I do not have reliable transportation and I am too tired by the end of the day to go and sit for an hour." This grandparent has identified three overarching obstacles: money for child care, reliable transportation, and her exhaustion. The aim of partializing is to address each issue one by one. The goal is not for the practitioner to solve the problem, but instead work with the grandparent caregiver to identify smaller, manageable steps in resolving or coping with each issue. It is important for the practitioner to believe that the problem is manageable and that there is a next step (Shulman, 2009). The next step may be the culmination of creative brainstorming and perhaps, learning about community resources. Or, the next step may be the enduring belief, by the practitioner, that the grandparent caregiver can persevere and not only survive, but thrive. As a result, the act of problem solving obstacles using the skill of partializing helps to promote healthy coping skills and support self-care practices of grandparents regardless if they present themselves as already engaging in positive practices.

Working with Grandparents

The focal areas for direct practice can help guide practitioners' work with grandparents using a strengths-based approach in identifying and supporting grandparent caregivers' self-care practices. Practitioners provide a key role in ensuring a focus on grandparents' strengths versus deficits. The challenge is to consciously and intentionally incorporate a strengths-based perspective in every interaction. Supervisors can promote this approach by paralleling this process during supervision. The supervisor's ability to role model a strengths-based perspective helps build a practitioner's competence and skill level. Often, time availability can limit supervision to focus on what is not working. Instead, we recommend supervisors and practitioners focus on what is working and brainstorm possibilities for tackling obstacles. Through this process, practitioners' belief in and support of grandparent caregivers has the potential to promote grandparents' confidence in themselves. This in turn, may promote grandparents' self-efficacy and a better quality of life for themselves as well as their grandchildren.

Conclusion

Our research highlights the capacity of grandparents to exercise awareness and choice in their self-care practice. Grandparents in our study demonstrated the importance of self-care in respect to physical, mental, and social health. Drawing on Orem's (2001) model of self-care, grandparents appeared invested in positive living, and thus were aware of lifestyle choices, medical decisions, solutions to providing care to themselves and their grandchildren, their feelings, and the importance of positive, healthy relationships.

The potential limitation of this research is that many grandparents were actively involved in grandparent support groups within their community. This raises the question as to whether grandparents who are more resourceful and resilient are the same grandparents who focus on the "glass half full" versus the "glass half empty" mantra. Is there something about this population where the wisdom of their years has contributed towards resilience? Has time strengthened a grandparent's resolve to weather changes and transitions? Has involvement in support groups encouraged grandparent caregivers to explore positive self-care practices? And, do grandparent caregivers realize they are engaging in self-care? Grandparent caregivers in this study demonstrated an impressive level of self-care, insight, and determination to do what it takes to provide the best care to their grandchildren while maintaining their health. As a way of encouraging and maintaining grandparents' self-care, practitioners should direct services to grandparents from a strengths-based approach.

References

Becker, G., Gates, R. J., & Newsom, E. (2004). Self-care among chronically ill African Americans: Culture, health disparities, and health insurance status. *American Journal of Public Health, 94*, 2066–2073.

Burnette, D. (1999). Custodial grandparents in Latino families: Patterns of service use and predictors of unmet needs. *Social Work, 44*(1), 22–34.

Charmaz, K. (2010). *Constructing grounded theory: A practical guide through qualitative analysis*. Thousand Oaks, CA: Sage.

Connelly, C. (1993). An empirical study of a model of self-care in chronic illness. *Clinical Nursing Specialist, 7*, 247–253.

Corcoran, J. (2006). *Cognitive-behavioral methods for social workers*. Boston, MA: Pearson Education.

De Jong, P., & Berg, I. K. (2008). *Interviewing for solutions*. Belmont, CA: Brooks/Cole.

Ehrle, G. M. (2001). Grandchildren as moderator variables in the family: Social, physiological, and intellectual development of grandparents who are raising them. *Family Development and Intellectual Functions, 12*, 223–241.

Fuller-Thomson, E., & Minkler, M. (2000). The mental and physical health of grandmothers who are raising their grandchildren. *Journal of Mental Health and Aging, 6*, 311–323.

Giarrusso, R., Silverstein, M., & Feng, D. (2000). Psychological costs and benefits of raising grandchildren: Evidence from a national survey of grandparents. In C. Cox (Ed.), *To grandmother's house we go and stay: Perspectives on custodial grandparents* (pp. 71–90). New York, NY: Springer.

Goodman, C. C. (2006). Grandmothers raising grandchildren: The vulnerability of advancing age. In B. Hayslip, Jr., & J. H. Patrick (Eds.), *Custodial grandparenting: Individual, cultural, and ethnic diversity* (pp. 133–150). New York, NY: Springer.

Hayslip, B., & Kaminski, P. (2005). Grandparents raising their grandchildren: A review of the literature and suggestions for practice. *The Gerontological Society of America, 45*, 262–269.

Hayslip, B., Shore, R. J., Henderson, C., & Lambert, P. (1998). Custodial grandparenting and grandchildren with problems: Their impact on role satisfaction and role meaning. *Journal of Gerontology: Social Sciences, 53B*, S164–S174.

Hartman, A. (1995). Diagrammatic assessment of family relationships. *Families in Society: The Journal of Contemporary Human Services, I*, 111–122.

McQuaide, S., & Ehrenreich, J. (1997). Assessing client strengths. *Families in Society: The Journal of Contemporary Human Services, 2*, 201–212.

Minkler, M., Fuller-Thomson, E., Miller, D., & Driver, D. (2000). Grandparent caregiving and depression. In B. Hayslip, Jr. & R. Goldberg-Glen (Eds.), *Grandparents raising grandchildren: Theoretical, empirical, and clinical perspectives* (pp. 207–219). New York, NY: Springer.

Morgan, D. L. (1997). *Focus groups as qualitative research* (2nd ed.). Thousand Oaks, CA: Sage.

Musil, C. M., & Standing, T. (2006). Grandmother's diaries: A glimpse at daily lives. In B. Hayslip, Jr. & J. H. Patrick (Eds)., *Custodial grandparenting: Individual, cultural, and ethnic diversity* (pp. 89–104). New York, NY: Springer.

Orem, D. E. (2001). *Nursing: Concepts of practice* (6th ed.). St. Louis, MO: Mosby.

Orem, D. E., & Vardiman, E. M. (1995). Orem's nursing theory and positive mental health: Practical considerations. *Nursing Science Quarterly*, *8*(4), 165–173.

Pruchno, R. (1999). Raising grandchildren: The experiences of black and white grandmothers. *The Gerontologist*, *39*, 209–221.

Rafii, F., Shahpoorian, F., & Azarbaad, M. (2008). The reality of learning self-care needs during hospitalization: Patients' and nurses' perceptions. *Self-Care, Dependent-Care, & Nursing: The Official Journal of the International Orem Society*, *16*(2), 34–39.

Riegel, B., & Dickson, V. V. (2008). A situation-specific theory of heart failure self-care. *Journal of Cardiovascular Nursing*, *23* (3), 190–196.

Roberto, K. A., Dolbin-MacNab, M. L., & Finney, J. W. (2008). Promoting health for grandmothers parenting young children. In B. Hayslip, Jr. & P. Kaminiski (Eds.), *Parenting the custodial grandparent: Implications for clinical practice* (pp. 75–89). New York, NY: Springer.

Roe, K. M., Minkler, M., Saunders, F., & Thomson, G. E. (1996). Health of grandmothers raising children of the crack cocaine epidemic. *Medical Care*, *34*, 1072–1084.

Saldaña, J. (2009). *The coding manual for qualitative researchers*. Los Angeles, CA: Sage.

Saleebey, D. (2011). *The strengths perspective in social work practice* (6th ed.) New York, NY: Allyn & Bacon.

Shaefor, B., & Horsjsi, C. (2006). *Techniques and guidelines for social work practice*. Boston, MA: Pearson Education.

Shulman, L. (2009). *The skills of helping individuals, families, groups, and communities*. Belmont, CA: Brooks/Cole.

Shore, R. J., & Hayslip, B. (1994). Custodial grandparenting: Implications for children's development. In A. Gottfried & A. Gottfried (Eds.), *Redefining families: Implications for children's development* (pp. 171–218). New York, NY: Plenum.

Soloman, J. C., & Marx, J. (2000). The physical, mental, and social health of grandparents. In B. Hayslip, Jr. & R. Goldberg-Glen (Eds.), *Grandparents raising grandchildren: Theoretical, empirical, and clinical perspectives* (pp. 183–205). New York, NY: Springer.

Smith, G. C. (2003). How caregiving grandparents view support groups: An exploratory study. In B. Hayslip, Jr. & J. H. Patrick (Eds). *Working with custodial grandparents* (pp. 69–91). New York, NY: Springer.

Whitelaw, N. A., & Liang, J. (1991). The structure of the OARS physical health measures. *Medical Care*, *29*, 332–347.

Wohl, E. C., Lahner, J. M., & Jooste, J. (2003). Group process among grandparents raising grandchildren. In B. Hayslip, Jr. & J. H. Patrick (Eds). *Working with custodial grandparents* (pp. 195–211). New York, NY: Springer.

Part II

Interpersonal Aspects of Resilience and Resourcefulness in Grandparent Caregivers

7 Raising Grandchildren as an Expression of Native Hawaiian Cultural Values[1]

Loriena A. Yancura and Heather Greenwood

Abstract

Cultural values are an important source of resilience for Native Hawaiian older adults. This chapter uses information from scholarly literature on Native Hawaiian families, as well as qualitative comments from a survey of Native Hawaiian grandparents raising grandchildren (GRG) to describe how these values may also be an important resource for practitioners working with this population. Two aspects of Native Hawaiian culture are described: traditional cultural practices relevant to grandparenthood and relatively recent historical events that have influenced contemporary GRG. The chapter concludes with specific recommendations to assist service providers in fostering resilience in Native Hawaiian GRG.

Introduction

The research and clinical literature contains very little information about Native Hawaiian GRG, particularly recommendations for fostering resilience. Some information relevant to fostering resilience in GRG may be drawn from a small body of work in the public health literature, which focuses on *kūpuna*, or Native Hawaiian older adults in general. This work suggests that they are often reluctant to seek assistance from outsiders because their experiences have been tempered by cultural trauma (Browne, Mokuau, & Braun, 2009) and misunderstandings based on stereotyped notions about their way of life (Imada, 2004; Kaomea, 2004). However, when assistance is provided in a sensitive manner, they benefit from value-based interventions emphasizing the positive attributes of Native Hawaiian culture (Browne, Mokuau, & Braun, 1998; Mokuau, 2011). The notion that cultural values are important sources of resilience may be especially relevant to Native Hawaiian GRG due to the traditional role of grandparents as caretakers of children and guardians of cultural practices. This chapter draws upon information in the literature, as well as a survey of Native Hawaiian GRG, to describe these cultural values and discuss how they may serve as a source of resilience for Native Hawaiian GRG.

Resilience is particularly important for Native Hawaiian and Pacific Islander (NHPI) grandparents. In the United States, the percentage of NHPI grandparents living in the same household as their grandchildren is five-times that of non-Hispanic White grandparents. The percentage reporting that they are responsible for raising their grandchildren is similarly large, nearly four times that of non-Hispanic White grandparents (Simmons & Dye, 2003). This fact is relevant to practitioners working with grandparents raising grandchildren (GRG) in a surprising number of places. There are more individuals of NHPI descent living in the Western United States than in Hawai'i, particularly in California, Washington, Texas, Nevada, and Oregon (U.S. Census Bureau, 2011). A basic understanding of Pacific Island cultures can benefit service providers who work with GRG in these and other states. Paying attention to cultural influences on grandparenting practices can help practitioners develop programs that foster resilience in GRG (Cox, 2002; Cox, 2011, Hayslip & Kaminski, 2005). At this point, it is important to note that the term NHPI, as used by the U.S. Census Bureau, encompasses a variety of peoples indigenous to islands in the Pacific Ocean. However, Native Hawaiians are by far the largest ethnic group represented in the NHPI category (Grieco, 2001). The discussion to follow will focus on Native Hawaiian culture.

Our discussion will begin with a brief introduction to features of traditional Hawaiian/Pacific culture that pertain to contemporary families. We will then use data collected from a survey of GRG whose grandchildren attend public schools in Hawaii to illustrate two particularly relevant aspects of culture in the lives of Native Hawaiian GRG: symbolic meaning of grandparenthood and socio-historical experience. We will conclude with specific recommendations for how this information can be used to foster resilience in Native Hawaiian GRG.

The Native Hawaiian Culture

The traditional lifestyle of Native Hawaiians began with the arrival of settlers from the Kahiki/Marquesas Islands to Hawai'i in about 100 A.D. and lasted until Western contact, marked by the arrival of Captain James Cook to the Hawaiian Islands in 1773. This lifestyle centered on farming and fishing and emphasized living in balance and harmony with spirits, nature, and mankind (Hope & Hope, 2003). Traditional Hawaiians were in constant communication with the Gods. Spirituality, or *ho'omana*, was at the center of their relationships with both physical and social environments. Ho'omana has been described as the fundamental value from which all others derive (Mokuau et al., 1998). Another basic value is *aloha 'āina*, which means to care for the land. It reflects the deep spiritual connection and sense of responsibility that Native Hawaiians have with nature (Mokuau, 2011). Stewardship for the land and its people is also reflected in another important concept, *pono*, which refers to correct, righteous, moral behavior. Pono describes the balance and harmony in the relationship with nature that is at the center of well-being (Ka'Opua, 2008). Pono is also the key to healthy social relationships, particularly among members of the extended family, or *'ohana* (McCubbin, 2006).

Traditionally, Native Hawaiians worked *lo'i* (taro fields) in land segments called *ahupua'a*, within which labor, goods, and services were shared (Hope & Hope, 2003). This practice of communally working the land greatly influenced traditional worldviews. Values of *laulima* (cooperation), *kōkua* (helping), and *lōkahi* (unity) reflect the importance of working together and remain central to Native Hawaiian culture (Mokuau, 2011). These values are still evident in much of what practitioners have observed to foster resilience in Native Hawaiian families and older adults. Decisions are typically made by group consensus with special attention to making sure that everyone has a voice in the process (McCubbin, Ishikawa, & McCubbin, 2008). Practitioners and group leaders are members of the group. They must keep a humble attitude to indicate their respect for the group (Duponte, Martin, Mokuau, & Paginawan, 2010). The tone of communication is important as well. The spoken word should be gentle and optimistic (Hope & Hope, 2003) to reflect a group dynamic of harmoniously working together for common good.

By far the most important social group in traditional Native Hawaiian culture was the 'ohana. 'Ohana is an inclusive term that includes individuals linked by marriage and adoption as well as blood (Handy & Pukui, 1998). The practice of *hanai* is an example of the flexible nature of family in Native Hawaiian culture. Hanai is a term that may be used as a verb or noun to represent the adoption of a baby into a household other than its biological parents. Hanai children were encouraged to keep ties with both biological and hanai 'ohana; and children who were hanaied (or hanai'd) were considered to be fortunate to have support from many sources (Wood, 2007). Hanai relationships are still practiced. References to hanai relationships between individuals, such as "hanai mother" or "hanai granddaughters," are common in local media, particularly obituaries. Ties among hanai family members are often equivalent to those among biological family members (Handy & Pukui, 1998).

All family relationships are at the *pico*, or center of well-being, in the Hawaiian worldview (McCubbin, 2006). The collective needs of the 'ohana are often placed above the needs of its individual members. Because harmony between family members is critical to health, efforts aimed at reducing physical health disparities in Native Hawaiian populations frequently focus on restoring family harmony (Browne, Mokuau, & Braun, 2009; Ka'Opua, Mitschke & Kloezeman, 2008). Similarly, reminding kūpuna that taking care of themselves allows them to take better care of others is believed to be an effective way to promote self-care behaviors (Yancura, 2010). Including family members in important health care decisions, such as end-of-life planning, is also very important to Native Hawaiian families (Kataoka-Yahiro, Yancura, Page, & Inouye, 2011).

The leaders and most respected members of traditional Native Hawaiian families were kūpuna. Traditional Hawaiian knowledge, such as *hula* (i.e., songs, chants, and dances), prayers, and genealogical records, were passed through non-written channels. Because kūpuna learned these practices from ancestors, kūpuna play a particularly important role in perpetuating cultural traditions

(Kaomea, 2004). They are still considered to be keepers of spiritual and cultural knowledge. Because of this, respect for kūpuna represents respect for Native Hawaiian culture (Mokuau et al., 1998).

Grandparenthood From a Native Hawaiian Perspective

The above discussion indicates that kūpuna are vital to the continuation of traditional Hawaiian culture. They are guardians of cultural practices grounded in hoʻomana (spirituality), which symbolize deep connections to ʻohana (family) and ʻāina (land). However, culture is not a static concept, but a process. It is continually evolving and adapting to changing social, economic, and political circumstances. In the modern world, Native Hawaiian kūpuna maintain relatively weakened societal power to that of their ancestors. Social and political factors have led to what many scholars have referred to as cultural trauma for Native Hawaiians. Over a comparatively short historical period, traditional culture was nearly destroyed by outside forces (Duponte et al., 2010; Kaomea, 2004; McCubbin et al., 2008). This state of affairs is echoed in the collective experiences of GRG. Traditionally their role was an elemental one, with social and political power as well as support from a strong and extended ʻohana. However, factors related to cultural trauma have weakened both their political power and family support networks. The following section summarizes the academic literature on features of Native Hawaiian culture particularly relevant to resilience in GRG. It focuses on two aspects, the symbolic meaning of grandparenthood and socio-historical context. It then turns to a discussion of how cultural values may lead to resilience in Native Hawaiian GRG. Both sections are illustrated by comments from a survey of Native Hawaiian GRG in Hawaiʻi.

Data Source for Illustrative Comments

The comments used in this study were drawn from a survey of grandparents raising grandchildren who attend public schools in Hawaii. The survey was conducted as part of the GRG Task Force of the Joint Legislative Committee on Family Caregiving of the Legislature of the State of Hawaiʻi and sponsored by the State of Hawaii Executive Office on Aging. Data were collected by the ʻOhana Caregivers research project of the University of Hawaii at Manoa (ʻOhana Caregivers, 2011) with cooperation from the Queen Liliʻuokalani Children's Center and the State of Hawaiʻi Department of Education (DOE).

Of the 259 grandparents responding to the survey, 114 stated that their ethnicity was Native Hawaiian or Part-Hawaiian. The ages of these Native Hawaiian grandparents ranged from 28 to 80 years ($X = 57.42$, $sd = 9.41$). The number of grandchildren they were raising ranged from 1 to 9 ($X = 2.54$, $sd = 1.67$). The most common legal status was "legal guardianship" (49.6%) followed by "no formal legal relationship" (18.4%), "legal adoption" (13.6%), "power of attorney" (11.2%) and "foster parent" (in the foster care system,

4.0%). These GRG were prompted to circle multiple reasons for why they were raising their grandchildren. The most common were that the children's biological parents were "on drugs" (39.2%), followed by "in jail" (27.2%), "divorced" (16.8%), "deceased" (11.2%) and "work long hours" (10.4%).

The survey contained forced-choice response options for all questions except the last one, which prompted respondents to "Please share any comments in the space below." Surprisingly, nearly half (48%) of the Native Hawaiian GRG who returned the survey wrote in the space provided. Many wrote several sentences, sharing information about their circumstances and needs. Although the survey was not originally designed to collect qualitative data, we regarded the responses they provided as a rich and serendipitous source of information on their beliefs about grandparenting. We then sorted and analyzed their comments into categories and used them to illustrate what the literature suggests about the symbolic meaning of grandparenthood and the influence of social and historical circumstances as well as indicate how these incorporating these beliefs into clinical and community practices may be used to foster resilience in Native Hawaiian GRG.

Symbolic Meaning of Grandparenthood

In Native Hawaiian culture, grandparenthood has a distinct meaning which appears to stem from two traditional values; the centrality of ʻohana, and the function of kūpuna as leaders of family and society. This meaning can be broken into three interrelated beliefs about grandparenthood: communal responsibility for all children, specific responsibility for the well-being of their family, and the responsibility for overseeing the cultural development of future generations. These beliefs were evident in the comments of the GRG responding to our survey.

The first of these beliefs is that kūpuna have communal responsibility for children. This is related to Ikel's (1998) discussion of kinship flexibility, which is the degree to which societies provide alternatives to biological linkages for creating family ties. The practice of hanai by grandparents or other adults in the ʻohana demonstrates the flexible nature of kinship in Native Hawaiian culture. Ayers-Counts (2007) states that the communal responsibility for children from older adults is common to many Pacific Island cultures. This notion was illustrated in several comments made by the GRG in our survey. The quote below shows that many members of the ʻohana are involved in raising a child.

> *We care for our grandchild, due to his mother abandoned him and his father chose drugs and fooling around, better than raising his children. So my son couldn't raise him, so my husband and I took over. And he's our baby, even though it's hard at times, due to our ages. We have our other children and only daughter helps us to raise him. And that's why Hillary Clinton, says it best, It takes a village to raise a child! So True! Mahalo* [Thank you] *to you too! I enjoyed filling this survey out and everything is true.*

A comment made by another grandparent expands upon this notion by expressing that taking care of grandchildren is essential to the well-being of all children.

> *If all of us grandparents try and save our mo'opuna's* [grandchildren] *they no doubt will know what it feels like to have someone who loves them unconditionally 24/7.*

These comments illustrate that the meaning of grandparenthood in Native Hawaiian culture expands beyond biological bonds. It includes ties between older adults and all children. Many kūpuna appear to accept responsibility of providing care for all children.

The second belief is that kūpuna carry a specific responsibility to represent the interests of the members of their 'ohana. Among Polynesian cultures, it was common for older adults to assume child-rearing responsibilities while their younger parents "engaged in the pleasures of labor, travel, & sociability" (Handy & Pukui, 1998, p. 179). These child-rearing responsibilities took forms from ranging from helping their children raise their grandchildren to hanai relationships, where grandparents took a baby into their own households. This practice was described in the following comment by one of our respondents.

> *I take care of my grandson because of I love him and I am helping my daughter out. She became a mother at a young age. And she was raised by my mom. I was a young mother at one time.*

This belief also appears to include grandparents' strong notion of responsibility for taking care of their grandchildren as illustrated in the following comment.

> *As you can see, what I have selected and wrote is because my grandchildren has no fault in having dead beat parents. I couldn't see them in no foster care. So I took them from birth until now and forever till the day I die.*

The responsibility expressed by grandparents indicates their desire for grandchildren to be taken care of, as well as taught to take care of themselves. The following comment illustrates grandparents' concern for grandchildren's futures.

> *We are ages 65 and 69. How do we provide for a 6 year old's future? We have retired income, comfortable, but what about her future and guidance . . . Thank you for giving us voice.*

These comments reflect the symbolic role of grandparents as kūpuna, wise elders and family leaders who feel a deep responsibility is to keep the family safe as well as guide generations into the future.

The third belief about the symbolic meaning of grandparenthood takes the notion of grandparent responsibility a step further. In addition to the responsibility of providing physical care, Native Hawaiian grandparents take responsibility for guiding the cultural development of younger generations (Mokuau, 2011). This belief was evident in many of the grandparents' comments, which contained strong sentiments about the possibility of their grandchildren being brought up by outsiders. Several GRG referred to their grandchildren as "blood family", "flesh and blood", and "blood relatives".

> *The children are my flesh and blood, and I want them to know that there's grandparents like me that care and love them dearly. And that no one outside should be raising them but their own blood relatives.*

Other GRG expressed similar sentiments but specifically used the term "culture" instead of "blood".

> *We take care of our grandchildren because they are our grandchildren. They should be raised in our culture. We take care because we love them of course, they are our grandkids.*

These comments reinforce what the literature says about the symbolic meaning of grandparenthood in Native Hawaiian culture. The Hawaiian language includes a phrase to describe grandchildren fortunate enough to live with their grandparents and learn tradition and lore from them. *Ka moʻopuna I ke alo* means "grandchildren in the presence" (Handy & Pukui, 1998, p. 179) and refers to grandchildren lucky enough to be hanaied by their grandparents' households.

The picture that emerges about the symbolic meaning of grandparenthood for many Native Hawaiians is one of stewardship and responsibility. As kūpuna, grandparents show love and responsibility for all children. It is apparent that they also feel a strong duty to guide the next generation, particularly in regards to culture and traditions. However it may be difficult for many Native Hawaiian grandparents to live up to these expectations, particularly those who are raising grandchildren without the supportive presence of the children's biological parents. In addition to traditional cultural notions of the symbolic meaning of grandparenthood, circumstances and events in the relatively recent history of the Native Hawaiian peoples have influenced the role of GRG.

Historical Context

Key Events

Any discussion of Native Hawaiian culture would be incomplete without inclusion of the social and historical circumstances of the Native Hawaiian people over the past two and a quarter centuries, since the arrival of Western visitors and settlers to the islands. Complete coverage of this time period is beyond the scope of this chapter, interested readers are referred to other sources for more information (Browne, Mokuau, & Braun, 2009; Duponte et al., 2010; Hope & Hope, 2003; McCubbin & Marsella, 2009). In order to understand the influence of this historical context on Native Hawaiian GRG, it is useful to divide this time into two periods: from 1778 to 1899, and the 20th century into the present. The period from 1778 to 1899 influenced Native Hawaiian culture because it laid the groundwork for assimilation into Western culture. The period from 1900 to the present has had a more direct effect on individual cohorts of GRG to whom the events have become personal histories (Browne et al., 2009).

In the 100 years following the arrival of Captain Cook, the population of Native Hawaiians in Hawai'i declined by over 90%, to a low of 40,000 individuals. This decline was due mostly to diseases, such as smallpox and syphilis, to which Native Hawaiian were exposed through contact with foreigners. Hawaiians had no immunity to these diseases (Browne et al., 2009; McCubbin & Marsella, 2009). Around 1820, American missionaries arrived in the islands to convert Native Hawaiians to Christianity. These missionaries condemned traditional Hawaiian worldviews, the result was a loss of religion and language for the remaining Native Hawaiians (Duponte et al., 2010). Because traditional Hawaiian culture did not have a concept of land ownership, another loss to the common Hawaiian people occurred in 1848 with a land division, the great *mahele* (division). This resulted in 30% of the Hawaiian people sharing only .8% of the land in what was later to become the state, the rest was granted to the Kingdom of Hawai'i and royalty. The last great loss occurred in 1898 when the Kingdom of Hawai'i was annexed as a territory by the United States, despite the fact that approximately half of the Native Hawaiian population at that time provided signatures in opposition of annexation (Hope & Hope, 2003).

Since 1900, many circumstances and events have impacted the lives of contemporary GRG, either through direct experience or through stories they were told by their parents and grandparents (Browne et al., 2009). The early 20th century saw the establishment of institutions formed to benefit Native Hawaiians. Between 1909 and 1911, Queen Liliuokalani established an organization to benefit destitute children in the State of Hawai'i that was later to become the Queen Lili'uokalani Children's Center (QLCC). To this day, QLCC has service units on the most populated Hawaiian Islands and works toward building "strong positive family attachment built on a cultural and spiritual foundation" (QLCC, 2011). In 1921, the U.S. Congress created the Department of Hawaiian Homelands to provide land and housing to Native Hawaiians. The mid 20th century saw military and political change. During the 1940s the U.S. military began to use the island of Koho'olawe off the coast of Maui as a bombing range; President Eisenhower officially commandeered the island for military use in 1953. The Island of O'ahu was a major center of operations for the United States military for two wars: World War I from the bombing of Pearl Harbor in 1941 until 1945, and the Vietnam War from 1964 until 1974. In between these wars, Hawaii became the 50th U.S. State in 1959.

The period from 1970 to the present has also brought rapid change to Native Hawaiian culture, including what some scholars have called "resilience events" (Browne et al., 2009), which center around links to traditional cultural practices, before Western settlers arrived on the islands. A Native Hawaiian cultural renaissance occurred in the mid-1970s. It included increased practice and interest in spirituality, healing traditions, hula, music, and language. The renaissance focused on restoring traditional meaning to these activities, in contrast to commercial stereotypes, which had been promoted by the tourist industry earlier in the century (Imada, 2004). Events during the 1970s also ushered in changes in political and social power leading to the establishment of the Office of Hawaiian Affairs, the teaching of the Native Hawaiian language in public and charter schools, and the eventual return of the island of Kaho'olawe to the State of Hawaii (Marsella & McCubin, 2009).

However, not all changes during this time were positive. Consistent increases in the costs of living and housing prices in Hawaii that began in the 1980s and continue through the present led to the outmigration of many Native Hawaiian families to the mainland United States (Browne et al., 2009). Native Hawaiian peoples continue to have disproportionally poor physical health. In addition to high rates of cancer and heart disease (Mokuau, 2011), rates of diabetes and asthma are twice that of the White population (CDC, 2011). Native Hawaiian peoples also face economic disparities, 18% of Native Hawaiian families live in poverty, compared to the U.S. average of 12% (WHIAAPI, 2011). The political identity of the Hawaiian People is also uncertain. Several versions of a Native Hawaiian Recognition Act, The Akaka Bill, have been introduced in the U.S. Senate over the past decade. These bills have been controversial due to problems with identifying individuals as Native Hawaiian, fair reparation for historical inequities, and equality of rights compared to other indigenous peoples in the United States.

Influence of Key Events on GRG

These events continue to influence the everyday lives of GRG in several ways and have prompted the need for resilience. Given the many losses discussed above, it becomes clear that Native Hawaiian people have not been well served by political and social systems over the past two centuries. They have also faced swift social, cultural, and political change. These two issues were evident in the comments from the GRG in our sample. Their comments indicated that many did not trust formal systems and most had a sense of rapidly changing circumstances.

Several of the comments made by the GRG indicated that they felt little protection from political and social systems, which some referred to as "the system." One grandparent's comments indicated that GRG, who often take in their grandchildren without formal legal arrangements, are at an unfair advantage compared to foster parents, who operate within the formal legal system.

> *I got very angry because the state should start changing their system. We as grandparents take care of our grandchildren because our children got into trouble. The Foster Parent gets more money than us and we do the same thing in caring for the children. If we the grandparents don't take care then the state has to find a foster parent and some of them are so mean to the children. Because I see it with my own eyes and love my grandchildren that's why I'm there for them.*

Many GRG referred to CPS, Child Protective Services, as a particularly untrustworthy system. The following comment expresses the common sentiment that the CPS system is not effective in protecting them and their grandchildren.

> *I would love to continue raising my grandchildren but with CPS involved, they always seem to focus on reunification, I really don't understand this system of ours. There should be a 3 strikes law regarding situations such as ours. My grandchildren have been through hell and back.*

A comment made by another grandparent expressed even greater mistrust, even hostility, toward CPS.

> *They took my grandson when he was 4 months old and gave me back the two older ones. They told me as soon as I got a place I was going to have him back, never did. I hate CPS, don't trust no one.*

These comments are even more meaningful when we consider that they were not prompted by a question asking what the GRG responding to our survey thought about CPS. We asked them to simply "share any comments." It is noteworthy that these grandparents felt that it was important to express their feelings about the system. When considered within historical and cultural contexts, some GRG appear to consider it important to shelter their grandchildren from the system.

The second way that the historical context was evident in the comments of these GRG was their sense of rapid historical change. Some comments made by the GRG responding to our survey conveyed their concern of the uncertain future of the Native Hawaiian culture. These comments appeared to express sadness that their grown children are dealing with the social problems such as economic disparities and substance abuse, which led to the abandonment of their grandchildren.

> *We take care of our grandchildren because their parents only think of themselves. My son was never raised the way he's raising his children. I'm very sad that he does things this way.*

A comment made by one grandfather indicated that he felt a generation gap between himself and his grandchildren and was looking for ways to connect with his grandchildren.

> *"Generational Gap" and our expectations for "our" children cause for concern (already future conflict apparent). Wife & I unable to maintain "new parental training techniques." We do the best we can, and we appreciate all the resources available to us.*

Another comment appeared to express consternation over the oddity of their having to assume the role of caregiving grandparents while they are still parenting their own children.

> *We have no choice. Today grandparents are working too. Children whose teenagers are parents and grandparents in their 30–40 and grandparents (adopted) are the ones to provide. Strange but that's the world today.*

These comments suggest that Native Hawaiian GRG are well aware of rapid historical change, which is understandable when one considers the many changes to the Native Hawaiian way of life that have occurred over the past century. This swiftly paced historical change might also explain why activities and practices emphasizing traditional values are a source of resilience for Native Hawaiian GRG.

Traditional Values as Sources of Resilience

Despite the hardships evident in the trauma and rapid change experienced by the Native Hawaiian culture, it was clear that the GRG responding to our survey were resilient. Their sources of their resilience appeared to be found in strength drawn from a sense of meaning derived from the caregiving role in line with the importance of kūpuna in traditional Native Hawaiian culture. One grandparent expressed the joy associated with taking care of grandchildren.

> *I take care of my grandson cause I love him like a son. He brings me love and joy and happiness!*

Other grandparents expressed their feelings toward their grandchildren simply and strongly.

> *My grandchildren and great grandchildren are my life. Mahalo* [Thank you].

Other grandparents acknowledged that raising grandchildren was a source of resilience in itself by bringing them joy to overcome other hardships in their lives. One grandmother noted that taking care of her granddaughter was a positive aspect in her life, and that it had helped her overcome the death of her husband.

> *I have not seek assistance since I returned to Hawaii. Been away in Maui for xx years and last xx years in California caring for my husband. He passed away .... and I haven't quite been able to come out of this mood that I am in. As for granddaughter, caring for her has given me some light in surviving.*

Given the symbolic and special meaning of kūpuna and grandparents in traditional Native Hawaiian culture, it becomes clear that the strength that these grandparents derive from taking care of their grandchildren derives from their cultural beliefs. One comment, in particular, supported the notion that cultural beliefs were a strong source of resilience for these GRG.

> *Although I mention cause of love, that had to be worked on because of not bonding from birth. It does take my family culture and religious belief to help me have thoughts to try to take on such a responsibility.*

Just as cultural practices have served as a source of resilience and strength in the history of the Native Hawaiian peoples, they may also be a great source of resilience for GRG. The following section describes implications for practitioners who work with GRG.

Implications for Professionals Working with Native Hawaiian Grandparents

Each of the Native Hawaiian cultural values discussed earlier may be used to foster resilience in clinical practice and service delivery to Native Hawaiian GRG. Incorporating these values into practice can help GRG trust service providers and feel comfortable expressing their needs. It can also help these GRG to focus on the opportunity to preserve a rapidly changing culture. The section below provides four recommendations for ensuring that Native Hawaiian values are included in interactions with GRG in both individual and support group settings. These recommendations are: maintaining harmonious relationships, incorporating rituals, keeping a light environmental footprint, and practicing integrity. They foster resilience because they stem from the traditional values previously discussed. Specific suggestions for implementing each recommendation in clinical and community practice are provided.

Emphasizing Positive and Harmonious Relationships

The most important recommendation for fostering resilience in work with Native Hawaiian GRG is maintaining harmonious relationships. This recommendation cultivates resilience by practicing the traditional values of laulima (cooperation) and lōkahi (unity).

Practitioners should keep in mind that the process of building unity and cooperation is more important than the execution of rules. Activities should be designed to create a unified and harmonious group. They should also encourage teamwork, focus on giving and receiving of support, and encourage feelings of inclusion. Specific suggestions for implementing this recommendation are: group planning, allowing plenty of time for "talk story" or informal conversation, including all members of the ʻohana in activities, potluck meals, and projects/exercises within which parties work together toward a common goal.

Incorporating Rituals

The second recommendation for using traditional values to foster resilience in Native Hawaiian GRG is to incorporate rituals into meetings and activities. Rituals contribute to resilience by evoking values of ho'omana (spirituality) and the practice of passing knowledge by an oral tradition, which includes music and chant. Rituals developed and led by kūpuna themselves are particularly effective in developing trust and collaboration between grandparents and professionals because they allow kūpuna to impart traditional knowledge as well as show humility on the part of the service provider by relinquishing a leadership position to become part of the group. Specific suggestions for implementing this recommendation are: beginning or ending each meeting with *pule* (prayer) led by a kūpuna, collectively choosing to sing a song or recite a poem to begin or end a meeting, incorporating music and singing into activities, beginning meetings with introductions that include location of origin as well as name (so kūpuna can place families with respect to location and genealogy), and beginning or ending meetings by sharing successes and words of wisdom or encouragement for others.

Keeping a Light Environmental Footprint

The third recommendation is keeping a light environmental footprint. This recommendation fosters resilience by reflecting the traditional value of aloha 'āina (caring for the land). Activities should be simple, casual, and inclusive of all family members. In our experience, Native Hawaiian GRG are more focused on the process of joining together as a group than the elaborateness of the setting. Specific suggestions for implementing this recommendation include: having meetings and activities outside or on a lanai (patio) whenever possible, centering projects and activities around nature, and having participants clean up and dispose of garbage after meetings and activities.

Practicing Integrity

The fourth recommendation is to ensure that work with Native Hawaiian GRG is characterized by integrity and focused on helping others. This recommendation reflects the traditional values of pono (uprightness) and kōkua (mutual assistance). All interactions should be in line with moral behavior and focus on positive outcomes for all parties involved.

Specific suggestions for implementing this recommendation include: ending activities by having participants share lessons learned from interactions, making sure to schedule meetings and activities at times that accommodate the greatest number of GRG, rotating meeting/activity schedules to accommodate all schedules, providing opportunities to assist others, and encouraging supportive projects, such as home yard cleanups, outside of regularly scheduled meetings.

Summary and Conclusions

This chapter has focused on aspects of Native Hawaiian culture that appear to be sources of strength and resilience in GRG. This is important because Native Hawaiian GRG are more likely than their White counterparts to face economic disparities and have poor physical health. The Native Hawaiian culture emphasizes spirituality, harmony with nature, respect for elders, and the importance of family and social relationships. Comments from contemporary GRG illustrate that these values remain salient. These GRG express responsibilities for ensuring the well-being of their families as well as safeguarding the spiritual and cultural development of future generations. However historical events also appear to have left their mark on the values of these GRG. Their comments also indicate that they feel let down by political and social systems and have faced a dizzying pace of social and cultural change. In light of these feelings of disenfranchisement and rapid change, traditional cultural beliefs and practices are an exceptionally important source of resilience for Native Hawaiian GRG.

Practitioners who work with Native Hawaiian GRG can incorporate traditional values into practice by working to maintain harmonious relationships, practicing rituals, keeping a light environmental footprint, and emphasizing integrity in both individual and group interactions. Emphasizing positive practices rooted in Native Hawaiian culture can help to offset the negative influence of historical events that led to suppression of Native Hawaiian peoples. Focusing on positive, culturally-centered, values can help Native Hawaiian GRG develop resilience to overcome challenges associated with raising grandchildren without assistance from the grandchildren's biological parents. Emphasizing these values can be an important resource for practitioners working with this population. As a people, the *Kanaka Maoli*, or Native Hawaiian peoples, have demonstrated an incredible capacity for resilience by drawing on many positive aspects of the Native Hawaiian culture. These same positive values can also be important sources of resilience for Native Hawaiian GRG.

Note

1 This research was supported in part by a grant from the State of Hawai'i Executive Office on Aging.

References

Ayers Counts, D. (2007). Introduction: The practice and prospects of grandparenting in the Pacific. *Pacific Studies, 30*(3), 4–16.

Browne, C. V., Mokuau, N., & Braun, K. L. (2009). Adversity and resiliency in the lives of Native Hawaiian elders. *Social Work, 54*(3), 253–261.

Cox, C. (2011). Ethnic, cultural, and gender issues in conducting caregiver educational and support groups. In R. W. W. Toseland, D. H. H. Haigler, & D. J. J. Monahan (Eds.), *Education and support programs for caregivers* (pp. 59–71). Springer: New York.

Cox, C. B. (2002). Empowering African American custodial grandparents. *Social Work, 47*(1), 45–54.

Centers for Disease Control (2011). Health disparities affecting minorities Native Hawaiian and other Pacific Islanders. Retrieved from http://www.cdc.gov/omhd/Brochures/PDFs/1PNHOPI.pdf.

Duponte, K., Martin, T., Mokuau, N., & Paglinawan, L. (2010). 'Ike Hawai'i—A training program for working with Native Hawaiians. *Journal of Indigenous Voices in Social Work, 1*(1).

Grieco, E. M. (2001). The Native Hawaiian and other Pacific Islander Population: 2000. Washington DC: US Census Bureau.

Handy, E. S. C., & Pukui, M. K. (1998). *The Polynesian family system in Kau'u, Hawai'i.* Mutual Publishing: Honolulu.

Hayslip, B., & Kaminski, P. L. (2005). Grandparents raising their grandchildren: A review of the literature and suggestions for practice. *The Gerontologist, 45*(2), 262.

Hope, B., & Hope, J. (2003). Native Hawaiian health in Hawaii: Historical highlights. *Californian Journal of Health Promotion, 1*(1), 1–9.

Ikels, C. (1998). Grandparenthood in cross-cultural perspective. In M. Szinovacz (Ed.), *Handbook on grandparenthood* (pp. 40–52): Westport, CT, US: Greenwood Press/Greenwood Publishing Group.

Imada, A. L. (2004). Hawaiians on tour: Hula circuits through the American empire. *American Quarterly, 56*(1), 111–149.

Ka'Opua, L. S. I., Mitschke, D. B., & Kloezeman, K. C. (2008). Coping with breast cancer at the nexus of religiosity and Hawaiian culture: Perspectives of Native Hawaiian survivors and family members. *Journal of Religion & Spirituality in Social Work: Social Thought, 27*(3), 275–295.

Kaomea, J. (2001). Dilemmas of an indigenous academic: A Native Hawaiian story. *Contemporary Issues in Early Childhood, 2*, pp. 67–82.

Kataoka-Yahiro, M., Yancura, L. A., Page, V., & Inouye, J. (2011). Advance care planning decision making among Asian Pacific islander family caregivers of stage 4 to 5 chronic kidney disease patients on hemodialysis. *Journal of Hospice and Palliative Nursing, 13*, 426–435.

McCubbin, L. D., & Marsella, A. (2009). Native Hawaiians and psychology: the cultural and historical context of indigenous ways of knowing. *Cultural Diversity and Ethnic Minority Psychology, 15*(4), 374–387.

McCubbin, L. D., Ishikawa, M. E., & McCubbin, H. I. (2008). The *Kanaka Maoli*: Native Hawaiians and their testimony of trauma and resilience. In A. J. Marsella, J. L. Johnson, P. Watson & J. Gryczynski (Eds.), *Ethnocultural Perspectives on disaster and trauma* (pp. 271–298). Springer: New York.

McCubbin, L. L. D. (2006). The role of Indigenous family ethnic schema on well-being among Native Hawaiian families. *Contemporary Nurse, 23*(2), 170–180.

Mokuau, N. (2011). Culturally based solutions to preserve the health of Native Hawaiians. [doi: 10.1080/15313204.2011.570119]. *Journal of Ethnic and Cultural Diversity in Social Work, 20*(2), 98–113.

Mokuau, N., Browne, C. V., & Braun, K. L. (1998). Na Kupuna in Hawai'i: A review of social and health status, service use and the importance of value-based interven. *Pacific Health Dialog, 5*(2), 282–289.

'Ohana Caregivers (2011). About us. Retrieved from http://www.ctahr.hawaii.edu/ohanacaregivers/about.asp.

QLCC (2011). Queen Lili'uokalani Children's Center. Retrieved from http://wwwqlcc.org.

Simmons, T., & Dye, J. L. (2003). *Grandparents living with grandchildren: 2000.* Washington, DC: U.S. Census Bureau.

U. S. Census Bureau (2011). *State and county quick facts.* [Online database]. Retrieved from http://quickfacts.census.gov/qfd/index.html.

Wood, J. H. (2007). Hanai tales. *Hana Hou! The Magazine of Hawaiian Airlines.* 10(4). Retrieved from http://www.hanahou.com/pages/magazine.asp?Action=DrawArticle&ArticleID=607&MagazineID=38&Page=1

(WHIAAPI, 2011). White House Initiative on Asian Americans & Pacific Islanders (WHIAAPI) Fact sheet: What you should know about Native Hawaiians and Pacific Islanders. Retrieved from http://www2.ed.gov/about/inits/list/asian-americans-initiative/what-you-should-know.pdf.

Yancura, L. A. (2010). Delivering culturally sensitive health messages: The process of adapting brochures for grandparents raising grandchildren in Hawai'i. *Health Promotion Practice, 11*(3), 400–407.

8 Mutual Exchange Within Skipped Generation Households

How Grandfamilies Support One Another

Stacey R. Kolomer, Sarah A. Himmelheber, and Cara V. Murray

Abstract

Social support networks of custodial grandparents are often fragile due to social isolation, lack of a peer cohort, and a multitude of family tribulations which plague skipped generation households. As a result, grandchildren and grandparents within these households become reliant on one another for support. The mutual exchange of instrumental and emotional support between the grandchildren and grandparents within skipped generation households may contribute to the positive adaptation to the demands of being custodial grandparents. One hundred and three custodial grandparents were asked a series of open-ended questions regarding their relationships with their grandchildren. Regardless of the age of the child(ren), over half of the custodial grandparents identified specific ways in which their grandchildren provided ongoing support to them. The mutual support between grandparents and grandchildren that occurs within skipped generation households is often not discussed and understudied. Gaining insight into how grandfamilies support one another within their households is critical to designing better programs that assist these families. Focusing on the adaptive means by which family members within skipped generation households cope will lead to the development of sustainable interventions that values and supports grandfamilies' interdependence.

Introduction

With approximately 4.5 million infants, children, and teens being raised in skipped generation households (Roberto & Qualls, 2003) it stands to reason that there is no single experience defining the "grandfamily." In an effort to understand this increasingly common familial structure, growing numbers of researchers are focusing on grandfamilies. Helping professionals recognize the unique circumstances of this population and the need to provide grandfamilies with targeted interventions and support. Research has helped to document and address some of the challenges faced by grandfamilies, such as health, custodial, education, and financial issues. Unfortunately with so much attention to the problems common to grandfamilies, little has been documented about how to help build upon their strengths and recognize the families' existing resources in the households.

Identification of risk factors has been the primary focus of intergenerational caregiving research. Grandparents raising their grandchildren have been characterized by increased risk for physical and mental health issues, legal obstacles, lack of social supports, and financial stressors and strains (Sands & Goldberg-Glen, 2000). Often relying upon fixed incomes, grandparent caregivers have named finances as the largest source of stress stemming from becoming the primary caregiver (Waldrop & Weber, 2001). Age-related changes have also been a source of stress for grandparent caregivers, as has the ambiguity felt when transitioning from grandparent to full-time parent (Landry-Meyer, Gerard, & Guzell, 2005).

Stress may also stem from the circumstances necessitating a child's transition to a skipped generation household. Often grandparents become primary caregivers as a result of substance abuse, incarceration, abuse, neglect, abandonment, HIV/AIDS, mental illness, military deployment, divorce, or death (Roe & Minkler, 1998). Consequently, children being raised by their grandparents are frequently dealing with some type of trauma that occurred prior to living with their grandparent. Caring for these children may require increased attention and emotional energy from their grandparents.

Social support networks of grandfamilies are often fragile due to social isolation, lack of a peer cohort, and a multitude of family tribulations which plague skipped generation households. One possible outcome of this is that grandchildren and grandparents within these households become reliant on one another for support. The mutual exchange of instrumental and emotional support between the grandchildren and grandparents within skipped generation households may contribute to the positive adaptation to the demands of being custodial grandparents.

Knowledge and understanding about the circumstances of grandfamilies and the negative consequences of caregiving have influenced the development of interventions and programming in many communities. Although research in this area needs to continue, using strengths perspective as the theoretical framework surrounding this research should be examined and its consequences fully explored. Focusing on the deficits and unmet needs in grandfamilies may systematically overlook the inherent strengths of these families.

Strengths Perspective

Increased stressors and risk factors have been well documented in grandfamilies (see, for example, Hayslip & Kaminiski, 2005; McCallion, Janicki, Grant-Griffin, & Kolomer, 2000; Sands & Goldberg-Glen, 2000). Many of the challenges associated with being a grandparent caregiver are fixed factors: physical health changes, unchanging financial means, and managing children who are often leaving chaotic or problematic environments. All of these circumstances are outside of the grandparents' control. It is imperative that interventions are designed to address these complicated and stressful circumstances. However, because many of these challenges may be understood as environmental constraints, it is also vital for social workers to focus on and advocate for interventions that build on the strengths inherent in grandfamilies.

The strengths perspective allows people to feel a sense of increased control and effectiveness in their lives. Social work research operating from this framework has been key in building understanding around resiliency in families. Strengths perspective research may be thought of as part of "a new paradigm, a new way of thinking about and working with human beings across the lifespan that focuses on assets instead of deficits and on working in partnership 'with' instead of doing 'to'" (Bernard, 2006, p. 197). Inclusion of the strengths perspective will enable helping professionals to build effective partnerships with grandfamilies, better responding to these families' needs.

Research has shown social support to be a protective factor for grandparents raising their grandchildren, and it has also shown that a lack of support correlates with higher stress levels (Sands & Goldberg-Glen, 2000). Validating the unavoidable stress involved in taking on primary parenting responsibility, Landry-Meyer, Gerrad, & Guzell (2005) describe social support as "an important component in determining the way in which a grandparent interprets the stress of raising a grandchild" (p. 73). The tremendous amount of day-to-day changes accompanying the main parenting role often results in grandparent caregivers having to abandon previous leisure activities and time for themselves (Myers, Kropf, & Robinson, 2002). This change in routine, which decreases peer support, is generally framed as an obstacle; however, when assessing the support needs and resources of grandparent caregivers, research needs to go beyond noticing what is lost with the arrival of full-time grandchildren. The contribution of grandchildren to the household needs to be included to fully understand how families can thrive on the internal mutual support of one another.

Caregiving Benefits and Mutual Support

Investigating the notion of mutual support is consistent with the strengths perspective. Most commonly associated with support groups (Heller, Hsieh, & Pickett, 1997), the idea of mutual support is also relevant to grandfamilies. Assessment of mutual support should include both instrumental and emotional supports. Instrumental support refers to provision of basic physical needs, such as those taken on by grandparents when they assume custody of their grandchildren. Emotional support is the act of family and friends helping one to feel better and improve quality of life. Consideration of the instrumental and emotional support provided by the grandchildren in the household, regardless of age, is important for understanding the household strengths overall.

Certain types of support may be simpler to notice than other types. For instance, the instrumental support provided for grandchildren by grandparents has clearly allowed for children with multiple risk factors to enjoy a modicum of stability and avoid placement in the foster care system (Bratteli, Bjelde, & Pigatti, 2008). Children have demonstrated their capacity to "flourish, even under adverse circumstances, if [they] encounter persons who provide them with the secure basis for the development of trust, autonomy, and initiative" (Werner & Smith, 1992, p. 209). Grandparents have stepped up and assumed this role. Although the benefits for the grandchildren may be more obvious, there may also be positive outcomes for the grandparent as well.

Studies examining the potential for caregiving relationships to be supportive and beneficial to both giver and recipient have been undertaken in other areas. For example, HIV/AIDS caregivers identified multiple benefits to their caregiving roles. In spite of the intense medical responsibility and the social stigma associated with the disease, caregivers articulated a more complicated caregiving relationship, characterized by "personal growth, a positive change in personality, an increased understanding of HIV/AIDS in the development of new relationships, [and] feelings of achievement and self-satisfaction" (McCausland & Pakenham, 2003).

Likewise, research in the developmental disabilities field has shown that caregivers benefit from certain aspects of their caregiving role (for example, Pakenham, Sofronoff, & Samios, 2004). A recent phenomenological investigation found that caregivers of autistic children had "a remarkable ability to refocus their energy and locate strengths and abilities largely untapped before autism came into their lives" (Phelps, Hodgson, McCammon, & Lamson, 2009, p. 29). This holistic analysis did not minimize the difficulties that accompany caregiving. However, the qualitative methodology, including analysis of 20 caregiver narratives, showed that positives and negatives were present in various spheres of life: psychological, social, familial, and spiritual (Phelps et al., 2009). This more complete understanding of strengths and challenges supports the development of interventions that build up families and remind them of their resilience.

The Multiple Sclerosis community has recently offered another example of mutual support being present in relationships typically discussed as caregiver-care recipient (Pakenham, 2005). In this repeated measures study, caregivers and care recipients completed questionnaires containing open-ended questions along with the Benefit Finding Scale (Mohr, Dick, Boudewyn, Likosky, & Goodkin, 1999). Results showed that "despite the 'chronic sorrow' often associated with caring for a person with MS . . . a wide range of benefits [were] associated with their loved one's illness" (Pakenham, 2005, p. 993). Responses to the questionnaire were grouped, and seven benefit-finding themes were constructed "including: greater insights into illness and hardship, caregiving gains, personal growth, the strengthening of relationships, increased appreciation of life, health gains, and a change in life priorities and personal goals" (ibid., p. 993). In this study, 20% of participants also named benefits related to their caregiving role not articulated in the Benefit Finding Scale.

Every family is different, and the challenges that accompany those dealing with HIV/AIDS, DD (developmental disorders), or MS may not parallel those experienced by grandfamilies. However, the common thread of closeness in relationships, mutual support, and mutual benefit does demonstrate the need to attend to these issues when investigating skipped generation households. How we approach knowledge development about the needs of grandparent caregivers matters. Inclusion of the strengths perspective in all levels of intervention, from direct service needs assessments to program planning and legislation, will allow for appropriate and effective supports so that grandfamilies may thrive.

Method

Sample

One hundred and three grandparents were interviewed about their relationships with the grandchildren in their care. The participants chose where the interview took place. Most participants preferred to be interviewed in their own home or local senior center. Most interviews took between one and two hours. Sometimes these interviews took longer because it was an opportunity for the grandparents to discuss their experiences with someone unfamiliar with their situation. All participants completed a consent form and received a $20 gift card to an area store as an honorarium.

Instrument

The interview instrument included questions regarding the demographics of the grandparent and grandchild(ren), diagnoses of grandparent, physical/developmental disability status of grandchild(ren), level of perceived stress, symptoms of depression of the caregiver, information about the informal and formal social support in their lives, medication and alcohol usage. This data was reported previously in Kolomer (2009). A representative from the Area Agency on Aging and the principal investigator developed the instrument with input from members of the local caregiving coalition. In addition, focus groups were conducted with grandparent caregiver support groups from two senior centers in the region; so as to better understand what information the caregivers themselves thought was of value to collect.

Questions asked of the grandparents included the following: What is your relationship like with your grandchild(ren) in your care, What kinds of help do these grandchildren provide to you? What do you do for fun with these grandchild(ren), How have your physical problems impacted your ability to play with your grandchild; what is your relationship with your grandchildren who do not live with you?

Results

Grandparents

Over 80% of the grandparents interviewed were grandmothers (see Table 8.1). Almost half the group identified as unmarried, divorced or widowed. The average age of the grandparents was 59.6 years old, s.d. 9.56 and ranged from ages 43 to 87 years old. Approximately 50% of the grandparents were white and approximately 48% were African-American. Nearly half were high school graduates and approximately 28% had attended college. Twenty-eight percent were retired and while nearly 46% were unemployed. In terms of financial stability Figure 8.1 illustrates that over one-quarter of the grandparents reported having a difficult time making ends meet and 43% reported having just enough to get by. Despite the financial challenges, 65% of the families lived in their own homes.

Caregiving

Nearly three quarters of the caregivers were caring for one to two children (see Figure 8.2). However, three of the grandparents in the sample were caring for

Table 8.1 Grandfamilies Demographics (n = 103)

	%
Grandmothers	83.5%
Grandfathers	16.5%
Race	
Black or African American	47.6%
Hispanic/Latino/Spanish Origin	1.9%
White	50.5%
Marital Status	
Married	51.1%
Separated	8.7%
Divorced	16.5%
Widowed	14.6%
Unmarried	8.6%
Education	
College graduate	12.6%
Some college	15.5%
High School graduate	21.4%
Some high school	40.8%
Junior high school	9.7%
Employment	
Working part time	12.6%
Working full time	11.7%
Retired	28.2%
Unemployed	45.6%

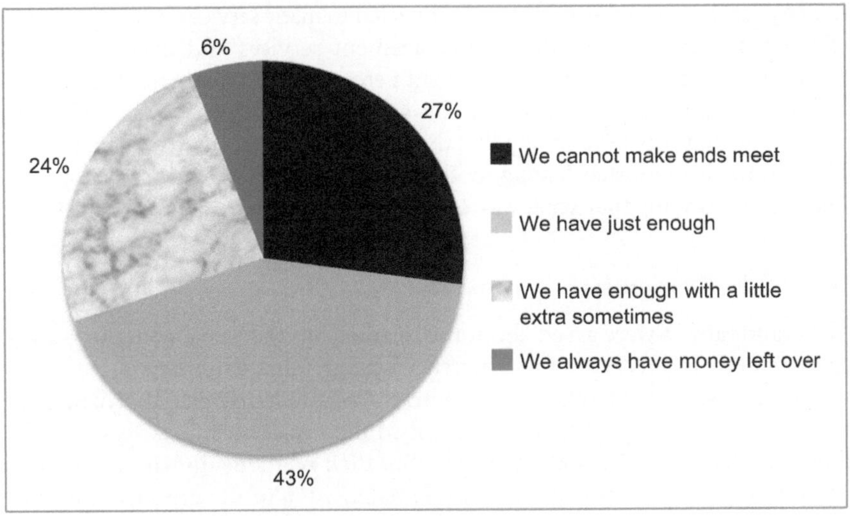

Figure 8.1 Financial Situation of Grandfamilies (n = 103)

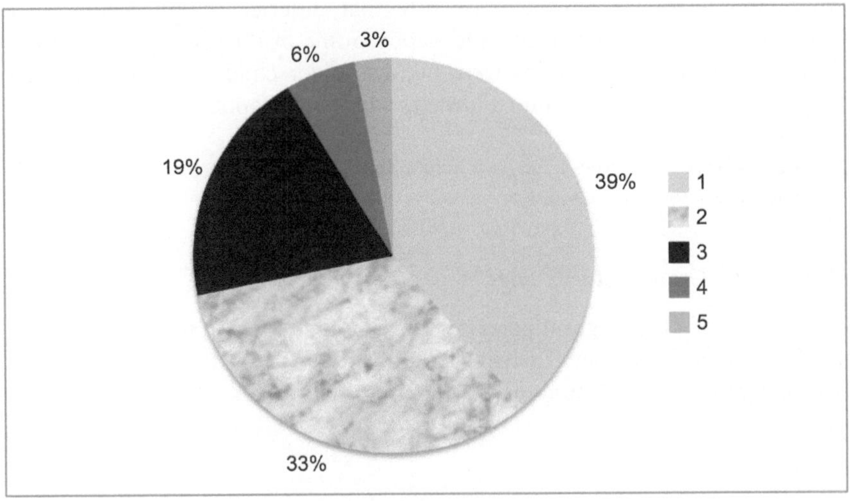

Figure 8.2 Number of Grandchildren being cared for in home

five grandchildren. The length of time for the most recent caregiving event ranged from one month to 16 years with the average length of time caregiving being four years and nine months, s.d. 3.8 years. The average age of the oldest child was 10.9 years old, s.d. 4.3 years with the age range being age three to 22 years old. Forty-five percent of the custodial grandparents reported that a child in their care had a disability or delay. The most common diagnosis of a grandchild as reported to the grandparent by a physician was Attention Deficit Disorder.

The participants in this study were connected to many services. Seventy percent of the participants received case management services and over 60% were involved in a support group. Twenty-eight percent of the grandparent caregivers had received individual counseling. This group was highly engaged in religious activities with nearly 69% stating that they were a part of religious organizations. This group also reported having moderate to strong informal social supports. The mean score for that scale was 15.57, s.d. 6.83, with a range of one-30.

State of the Relationship

The grandparents were asked about the relationship they have with the grandchildren in their care. Forty-three percent of the grandparents interviewed stated that they have a good relationship with their grandchildren. Approximately another 17% of the grandparents described their relationship as very close to their grandchildren. Only 8% reported that their relationship with the grandchildren in their care was poor. Approximately 31% of the grandparents had a blend of responses to the question. Those who talked about challenges in the relationships with their grandchildren said these changes to previously positive relationships occurred during the grandchildren's pre teen years and teen years. Words that were mentioned frequently that described relationships were caring, loving, close, wonderful, and happy. Some of the grandparents talked about how great relationships were because older children helped younger children, or because the grandchildren made A's in school.

> *I came into their lives at a time when they desperately needed someone and have been there ever since . . .*

How Do the Grandchildren Help

Nearly half of all the grandparents reported that their grandchildren were helpful to them. The ways in which grandchildren helped were divided into two categories, instrumental tasks and emotional tasks.

Instrumental

The instrumental ways that grandchildren helped included doing yard work, cleaning, cooking, washing clothes, sweeping, washing dishes, fixing cars, chopping and stacking wood, mowing the lawn, and taking out the trash. These activities are beneficial to the grandfamilies as the grandchildren were able to complete tasks that may be too physically demanding for their grandparents.

Emotional

Some ways in which grandchildren helped emotionally included keeping spirits high, providing company, support, improving mental health, and providing

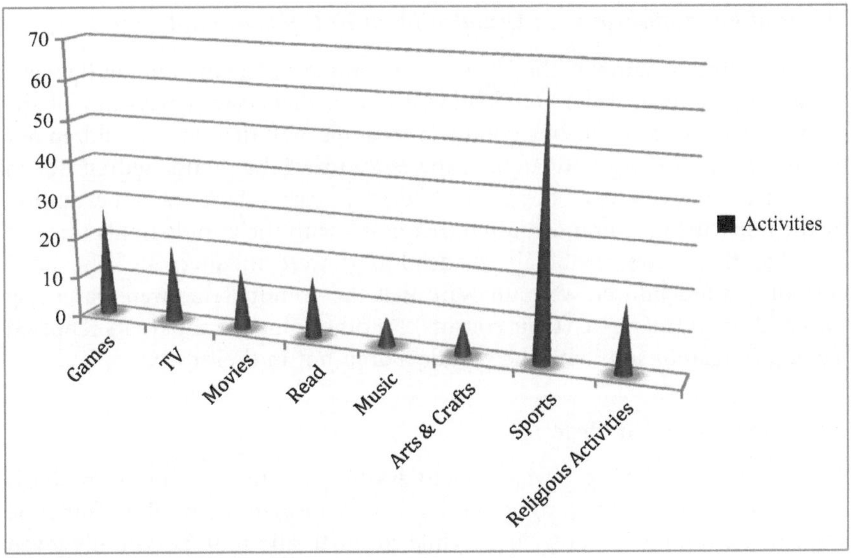

Figure 8.3 Activities Grandfamilies do together (n = 103)

personal attention. Just being able to laugh together greatly enhanced the mood of the grandparents. The grandchildren keep emotions high. One grandmother reported that she did not have time to get depressed when taking care of her grandchildren. *They make me laugh.*

Sharing activities and being together also provided positive aspects and emotional support to the caregiving relationship. As shown in Figure 8.3 many of the grandparents reported playing games, watching TV, arts and crafts, going to the movies, reading, playing music, and participating in sports, fishing, and religious activities as ways in which grandfamilies interacted together. However, nearly half of the grandparents said that their own physical limitations have impacted their ability to play with their grandchildren.

Physical Problems Impacting Play

A majority of the grandparents interviewed were struggling with significant health problems. Thirty-nine percent of the grandparents had one or two health problems. A fifth of the grandparents had five or more health problems. Over half reported diagnoses of hypertension, 42% had arthritis, and 27% had diabetes. Nearly one quarter of the grandparents reported having heart problems and nearly 12% reported having histories of cancer diagnoses. These numerous health problems impacted the grandparents and grandchildrens fun activities with one another.

> *I would like to do more active things like playing sports outside: bones are fragile and I am afraid I will fall.*

Status of Relationships with Grandchildren Not in Custodial Care

An interesting dynamic within these grandfamilies is the interaction between the grandparents and the grandchildren not in their care. Forty-four of the grandparents reported having good relationships with their grandchildren not in care. Nine of the grandparents experienced that the grandchildren not in their care were jealous of the grandchildren in care. There was a perception by the non-custodial grandchildren that living with the grandparents was fun and that they (non custodial grandchildren) were missing out. The non-custodial grandchildren were unaware that the grandparents were parenting the children in their care (their cousins). Another nine grandparents reported having no relationship with the grandchildren not in their care.

Considerations for Practice

As agencies are reducing services due to drastic economic cuts more emphasis should be placed on helping grandfamilies to insulate themselves from the stresses and strains of caregiving. While so much attention is typically given to either the grandparent or the grandchild, services that look at the strengths of the whole family will likely increase the support and resiliency within the family. Even very young grandchildren are capable of being supportive to adult caregivers. Families need to be given the tools to recognize their own strengths and resources within their families. Focusing on the adaptive means by which family members within skipped generation households cope will lead to the development of sustainable interventions that values and supports grand-families' interdependence. How can practitioners design interventions that build upon grandfamilies' interdependence on one another?

Building on Grandfamilies' Strengths and Resources

Awareness of one's own individual, family, and community protective factors is a beginning point for the development of strengths based interventions to support family resiliency (Benzies & Mychasiuk, 2009; Mendenhall & Mount, 2011). Skill building, education and informal and formal support all may help families accomplish long term goals, as well as address immediate crisis situations (Saint-Jacques, Turcotte, & Poulio, 2009). Considering what the grandparents in this study reported, grandfamilies already have a wealth of individual, family, and community protective factors, however, many times families are not in tune with their own strengths. It is up to helping professionals to assist grandfamilies with being able to recognize the existing strengths within the family unit. Often initial assessments identify negative factors and what is lacking rather than identifying the mutual exchange of instrumental tasks and emotional support between family members. Visual pictorials can go a long way in helping families be aware of their existing strengths. While individual assessments are important, family centered assessments for grand-families are critical for multidimensional interventions (see Figure 8.4).

Grandparent Strengths	Granchild(ren) Strengths	Family Strengths	Community Supports
•Belief system •Providing adequate housing •Being active	•Instrumental Tasks- help grandparents with chores in and out of the home •Emotional support	•Family cohesion •Supportive interactions •Emotional support	•Connection to mutiple community organizations •Identified strong informal support network •Active with religious organizations

Figure 8.4 Family Centered Assessment of Grandfamilies' Strengths

Helping grandchildren discover their contributions to the families' resiliency can build the children's self esteem and confidence (Lebya, 2004). For example, often grandchildren are not aware of how they provide emotional boosts to their grandparents and therefore have no knowledge of how they are contributing to the grandparents' emotional well-being. Knowing one's own positive contributions to the household may increase self-assurance and their own emotional health. Grandparents reported about how the grandchildren's contributions to the household contributed to good relationships. It is obvious from this study that grandparents recognize the support provided to them by the grandchildren but it is unclear whether the grandparents are sharing these reflections with the grandchildren in their care. The mutual exchange of support between grandparents and grandchildren leads to strengthening family ties and bonds, as well as increasing individual family members' well-being. Helping professionals can encourage grandparents to be open in their communication with the children about how the grandchildren contribute to the household.

Where Do We Go From Here?

There are several areas that could benefit from further exploration by helping professionals. For example, what do grandchildren think about their relationship with their custodial grandparents? Do they also feel close and happy about the relationships they share with their custodial grandparents? Are their perceptions congruent to custodial grandparents? How do the grandchildren perceive their grandparents' physical limitations? Are grandchildren even aware of the challenges grandparents have with their physical health problems and ability to participate in activities with the children? Another relationship to explore is perceptions of relationships with family members not living in the grandparent-headed households. How do these relationships strengthen grandfamilies' inherent resources? How do those relationships impact the support system in grandfamilies?

Further study is needed to evaluate whether grandparents who recognize their grandchildren as providing instrumental and emotional support are in fact less likely to experience the typical stressors and strains of skipped generation households as identified in the literature. It would seem that the grandparents who reported having good and very close relationships with their grandchildren may be less likely to have experienced emotional strain and symptoms of depression as so often documented in the literature. Another consideration is grandparents who are struggling with physical impairments that interfere with their interactions with their grandchildren may be more likely to experience emotional stress than grandparents who are not physically impaired. The mutual exchange of instrumental and emotional support between the grandchildren and grandparents within skipped generation households may contribute to the positive adaptation to the demands of being custodial grandparents but these interactions require closer examination.

For grandparents, stepping into a primary caregiver role often requires major adjustments in multiple aspects of life. Likewise, substantial changes in the lives of grandchildren also occur. Although transitioning into daily life together may disrupt the routines of both grandparents and grandchildren, the process for these two groups likely differs. Perhaps due to the divergent issues characterizing the experiences of these two ends of grandfamilies, research aimed at understanding the experiences of skipped generation households has primarily been framed either from the grandparents or the grandchildren. It is time for family-centered strengths-based approaches to become the model for assessing grandfamilies. Understanding the mutual exchange between family members will likely lead to improved self-esteem, self-assurance, and improved physical and emotional well-being for all members of grandfamilies.

References

Benard, B. (2006). Using strengths-based practice to tap the resilience of families. 197–221. In D. Saleebey (Ed.). *Strengths perspective in social work practice*, 4th ed. Allyn & Bacon/Longman.

Benzies, K., & Mychasiuk, R. (2009). Fostering family resiliency: a review of the key protective factors. *Child and Family Social Work, 14*, 103–114. doi:10.1111/j.1365-2206.2008.00586.x

Bratteli, M., Bjelde, K., & Pigatti, L. (2008). Grandparent and kinship foster care: implications of licensing and payment policies. *Journal of Gerontological Social Work, 51*(3/4), 228–246.

Evans, T. (2004). A multidimensional assessment of children with chronic physical conditions. *Health and Social Work, 29*(3), 245–248.

Hayslip, B., & Kaminski, P. L. (Eds). *Parenting the custodial grandchild.* New York: Spring Publishing.

Heller, T., Roccoforte, J. A., Hsieh, K., Cook, J. A., Susan A., & Pickett, S. A. (1997) Benefits of support groups for families of adults with severe mental illness. *American Journal of Orthopsychiatry, 67*(2), 187–198.

Kolomer, S. (2009). Grandparent caregivers' health and management of prescription medication. *Journal of Intergenerational Relationships, 1*, 243–258.

Landry-Meyer, L., Gerard, J. M., & Guzell, J. R. (2005). Caregiver stress among grandparents raising grandchildren: the functional role of social support. *Marriage & Family Review, 37*(1–2), 171–190. doi:10.1300/J002v37n01_11

Lebya, E. (2010). How school social workers integrate service opportunities into multiple elements of practice. *Children and Schools, 32*(1), 27–49.

McCallion, P., Janicki, M. P., Grant-Griffin, L., & Kolomer, S. R. (2000). Grandparent caregivers II: Service needs and service provision issues. *Journal of Gerontological Social Work, 33*(3), 57–84.

McCauseland, J., & Pakenham, K. I. (2010). Investigation of the benefits of HIV/AIDS caregiving and relations among caregiving adjustment, benefit finding, and stress and coping variables. *AIDS Care, 15*(6), 853–869.

Mendenhall, A., & Mount, K. (2011). Parents of children with mental illness: exploring the caregiver experience and caregiver-focused interventions, *Families in Society, 92*(2), 183–190. DOI: 10.1606/1044-3894.4097

Mohr, D. C., Dick, L. P., Russo, D., Pinn, J., Boudewyn, A. C., Likosky, W., & Goodkin, D. E. (1999). The psychosocial impact of multiple sclerosis: exploring the patient's perspective. *Health Psychology, 18*(4), 376–382.

Myers, L. L., Kropf, N. P., & Robinson, M. M. (2002). Grandparents raising grandchildren: Case management in a rural setting. *Journal of Human Behavior in the Social Environment, 5*(1), 53–71.

Pakenham, K., Sofronoff, K., & Samios, C. (2004). Finding meaning in parenting a child with Asperger's syndrome: Correlates of sense making and benefit finding. *Research in Developmental Disabilities, 25*, 245–264.

Pakenham, K. I. (2005). The positive impact of multiple sclerosis (MS) on carers: Associations between carer benefit finding and positive and negative adjustment domains. *Disability and Rehabilitation, 27*, 985–997.

Phelps, K., Hodgson, J., McCammon, S. L., & Lamson, A. (2009). Caring for an individual with autism disorder: A qualitative analysis. *Journal of Intellectual and Developmental Disability, 34*, 1–27.

Roberto, K. A., & Qualls, S. (2003). Intervention strategies for grandparents raising grandchildren: Lessons learned from the caregiving literature. In B. Hayslip & J. Patrick (Eds.). *Working with custodial grandparents* (pp. 13–26). New York, NY US: Springer Publishing Co. Retrieved from EBSCOhost.

Roe, K. M., & Minkler, M. (1998). Grandparents raising grandchildren: challenges and responses. *Generations, 22*(4), 25. Retrieved from EBSCOhost.

Saint-Jacques, M. C., Turcotte, D., & Poulio, E. (2009). Adopting a strengths perspective in social work practice with families in difficulty: from theory to practice, *Families in Society, 90*(4), 454–461.

Sands, R. G., & Goldberg-Glen, R. S. (2000). Factors associated with stress among grandparents raising their grandchildren. *Family Relations, 49*(1), 97–105.

Werner, E., & Smith, R. (1992). *Overcoming the odds: High risk children from birth to adulthood.* New York: Cornell University Press.

Waldrop, D. P., & Weber, J. A. (2001). From grandparent to caregiver: the stress and satisfaction of raising grandchildren. *Families in Society: The Journal of Contemporary Social Services, 82*(5), 461–472.

9 Formal Social Support

Promoting Resilience in Grandparents Parenting Grandchildren

Megan L. Dolbin-MacNab, Karen A. Roberto, and Jack W. Finney

Abstract

There is evidence that social support is associated with enhanced resilience among grandparents parenting their grandchildren. One type of social support frequently accessed by grandparents is formal social support delivered by professionals in a variety of service settings. Unfortunately, grandparents experience a number of barriers to accessing formal support. In this chapter, we draw on existing literature and examples from our own empirical research to provide an ecological (Bronfenbrenner, 1979) conceptualization of best practices for providing formal support to custodial grandparents. Our recommendations move from proximal environments such as the grandparents' attitudes and beliefs about formal supports to more distal elements of the formal service environment such as program accessibility and the training and education of program staff. We also provide recommendations for macro issues related to program structure and availability. Together, these recommendations can help practitioners create welcoming service environments that are positioned to meet grandparents' varied needs.

Formal Social Support: Promoting Resilience in Grandparents Parenting Grandchildren

With the recent growth in the number of grandparents who are parenting their grandchildren (Kreider & Ellis, 2011), grandparents' successes and challenges have come to the attention of a variety of practitioners and service providers. Custodial grandparents experience a number of stressors that can benefit from both formal and informal support including financial difficulties, legal problems, and physical and mental health concerns (Hughes, Waite, LaPierre, & Luo, 2007; Minkler & Fuller-Thomson, 1999; Minkler, Fuller-Thomson, Miller, & Driver, 1997). Grandparents may also need assistance obtaining housing and home modifications, finding services for their grandchildren, and meeting the family's nutritional needs. Additionally, as grandparents take on new roles and responsibilities with their custodial grandchildren, they may also struggle with social isolation, parenting stress, and grandchild behavior problems

(Hayslip & Kaminski, 2005; Hayslip, Shore, Henderson, & Lambert, 1998; Jendrek, 1993; Jendrek, 1994).

In response to these challenges and needs, there has been a substantial increase in the number of intervention programs and support services designed to promote resilience, or "positive adaptation in the context of significant risk or adversity" (Ong, Bergeman, & Boker, 2009, p. 1777), among grandparents and their custodial grandchildren. Building resilience is a worthy practice goal because, while grandparents may savor their close relationships with their grandchildren and feel a great sense of purpose related to parenting their grandchildren (Dolbin-MacNab & Keiley, 2006; Hayslip & Kaminski, 2005), they often need assistance adapting to their parenting responsibilities and managing those responsibilities in the face of limited resources and other stressors. Interventions that promote resilience by addressing grandparents' challenges can help enhance their quality of life, as well as that of their grandchildren.

One particular form of intervention shown to promote resilience among grandparents parenting grandchildren is seeking social support from existing and new social network members. Broadly, social support refers to "emotional, instrumental, and informational assistance from others"—whether through formal or informal channels (Gerard, Landry-Meyer, & Roe, 2006, p. 361). Despite evidence of the importance of both informal and formal support to the lives of custodial grandparents (e.g., Gerard et al., 2006; Kelley, Whitely, Sipe, & Yorker, 2000; Landry-Meyer, Gerard, & Guzell, 2005; Leder, Grinstead, & Torres, 2007), less attention has been given to how formal sources of social support, in particular, can help grandparents overcome the risks associated with parenting their grandchildren. To shed greater light on the value of formal support for promoting grandparent resilience, we draw on existing literature and examples from our own empirical research to provide an ecological (Bronfenbrenner, 1979) conceptualization of best practices for use by practitioners. We begin, however, with a brief discussion of the types of social support systems available to grandparents and the importance of these social support systems in helping grandparents successfully manage their unique family roles and relationships.

Social Support

Formal and Informal Social Support

Social support includes relationships with both informal and formal entities. Informal support is based on affiliation or norms of obligation and includes assistance and emotional support received from relatives, friends, and neighbors (Litwak, 1985). Emotional support, more so than actual assistance, acts as a buffer against the negative effects of stressful situations such as assuming responsibility for a grandchild. Thus, whereas grandparents may expect instrumental assistance from their relatives and friends, they value equally and perhaps benefit even more from the emotional support they receive from these relationships.

In contrast to informal support, formal social support is based on a contractual or paid arrangement (Litwak, 1985). Grandparents may turn to professional care providers and services to complement the support provided by their informal networks or when their informal networks are either unavailable or unable to assist them. Physicians, therapists, case managers, community service providers, and other professionals are examples of the types of individuals positioned to provide formal support to grandparents parenting their grandchildren. Such support may occur within the context of a variety of governmental assistance and support programs such as Temporary Assistance to Needy Families (TANF), the Supplemental Nutrition Assistance Program (SNAP, formerly known as Food Stamps), the foster care system, the Women Infants and Children (WIC) program, aging services, and community support groups.

Much of the existing research on social support among grandparents parenting grandchildren suggests that grandparents receive inadequate support from both their informal and formal networks (e.g., Burton, 1992; Jendrek, 1993; Minkler & Roe, 1993; Musil, 1998). Because they are assuming an off-time role and parenting grandchildren at a time when many of their peers are engaged in other activities, grandparents often experience less frequent contact with members of their informal support networks (Gerard et al., 2006; Minkler, Roe, & Robertson-Beckley, 1994). In the case of formal support, Gerard and colleagues (2006) argue that formal support may be more difficult for grandparents to access because seeking assistance from community organizations or other professionals requires motivation and autonomy. Grandparents may also experience a number of other significant barriers to accessing formal sources of support, which will be discussed in more detail in a later section of the chapter.

Dimensions of Social Support

Additional dimensions of social support address the size, availability, and responsiveness of grandparents' support networks. More specifically, grandparents' social support can be categorized into their social networks, perceived support, and enacted support (Landry-Meyer et al., 2005). The social network captures grandparents' level of social embeddedness or the number and types of people available to provide them with support (Barrera, 1986; Landry-Meyer et al., 2005). However, just because a grandparent has people available to provide support, it does not mean the grandparent is actually accessing this support or that the support is truly available. Thus, perceived support becomes an important consideration. Perceived social support reflects the degree to which a grandparent perceives that social support is available and adequate (Gerard et al., 2006; Landry-Meyer et al., 2005). Conversely, enacted support captures the actual support a grandparent receives (Landry-Meyer et al., 2005).

This could include support from friends and family as well as assistance received through formal assistance or support programs (Landry-Meyer et al., 2005; Vaux & Harrison, 1985).

The Intersection of Social Support and Resilience

Social support is influential in determining the degree to which grandparents are able to cope with and adjust to their caregiving responsibilities (Crowther & Rodriquez, 2003; Gerard et al., 2006; Landry-Meyer et al., 2005). In this sense, social support can be conceptualized as a protective factor that promotes grandparent resilience. Social support may encourage grandparent resilience by "compensating for or counteracting the negative influence of stressors on grandparents' well-being" (Gerard et al., 2006, p. 362). In this conceptualization, social support is thought to compensate for stressors by promoting positive outcomes and reducing negative outcomes (Gerard et al., 2006). For example, becoming friends with other custodial grandparents may prevent a grandfather from feeling isolated and becoming depressed. Alternatively, social support may buffer the influence of grandparents' stress on their well-being (Gerard et al., 2006). This conceptualization suggests that social support is most beneficial to grandparents experiencing high levels of stress. Grandparents experiencing lower levels of stress are hypothesized to be in less need of social support and, therefore, to benefit less from it (Gerard et al., 2006). In this case, a grandmother experiencing very high levels of parenting stress would benefit more from a supportive friend, relative, or practitioner than a grandmother who feels less stressed by her parenting responsibilities.

Though some contradictory findings exist, empirical research generally suggests that having strong informal and formal social support systems promotes positive outcomes for custodial grandparents. Enacted formal support has been shown to reduce the negative impact of specific stressors such as grandchild behavior problems and parenting hassles on grandparents' life satisfaction and caregiving stress (Gerard et al., 2006). It also has been found to be positively associated with grandparents' life satisfaction and generativity (Landry-Meyer et al., 2005). In other studies, perceived social support has been negatively associated with grandparent psychological distress and physical health (Kelley et al., 2000; Leder et al., 2007). Additionally, Muliira and Musil (2010) found that subjective and instrumental support was associated with greater use of preventative health care, gynecological exams, and blood pressure screenings. These authors suggested that addressing potential health problems ahead of time, through greater use of formal supports and preventative health care services, could have significant positive implications for grandparents' short- and long-term physical health.

Our own research findings lend further support to the conceptualization of social support as a factor that can promote resilience among grandparents parenting grandchildren. For example, in our study of 40 grandmothers parenting a grandchild aged 13 years or younger (Roberto, Dolbin-MacNab,

& Finney, 2008), higher perceived social support on the MOS Social Support Survey (Sherbourne & Stewart, 1991; example items include "someone to get together with for relaxation" and "someone you can count on to listen to you when you need to talk") was associated with better mental health (SF-36v2; Ware, Krosinski, & Keller, 2000; Ware & Sherbourne, 1992). Similarly, in a study of 95 grandmothers parenting grandchildren between the ages of 13 and 18 conducted by the first author, greater perceived social support, as measured by the MOS Social Support Survey (Sherbourne & Stewart, 1991), was associated with better mental health (SF-36v2; Ware et al., 2000; Ware & Sherbourne, 1992) and less parenting stress (Parental Stress Scale; Berry & Jones, 1995). Together, these and numerous other studies highlight the important role that social support plays in the lives of grandparents parenting grandchildren—especially in terms of promoting their health, well-being, and resilience.

Formal Social Support

When confronted with the challenges of parenting their grandchildren, many grandparents seek formal support from professionals including physicians, therapists, case workers, and teachers, among many others. It is generally thought that participating in formal systems of social support promotes grandparent resilience via decreasing isolation, developing skills and knowledge, meeting instrumental needs, and providing emotional support (Gladstone, Brown, & Fitzgerald, 2009; Hayslip, 2003; Kolomer, McCallion, & Janicki, 2002; Dannison & Smith, 2003). For example, Gerard and colleagues (2006) found that formal enacted support buffered "the negative impact of grandchild health problems and parent daily hassles on grandparents' general well-being" (p. 375). Similarly, in our study of 40 grandmothers raising young grandchildren (Roberto et al., 2008), we found that perceiving one's physician as being supportive (Self-Efficacy for Accessing Physician Assistance; Janicke & Finney, 2003) was positively associated with grandmothers' physical health (SF-36v2; Ware et al., 2000; Ware & Sherbourne, 1992). Others have also confirmed the value of formal support for grandparents' resilience, as part of grandparents' broader social support resources (Crowther & Rodriguez, 2003; Gerard et al., 2006; Kelley et al., 2000; Landry-Meyer et al., 2005; Leder et al., 2007).

Barriers to Accessing Formal Support

Despite evidence that accessing formal systems of support may promote grandparent resilience, studies by Hayslip and Shore (2000) and Gerard and colleagues (2006) suggest that many custodial grandparents fail to make use of a number of formal support systems including mental health counseling, kinship navigators, support groups, assistance programs, and medical services. This failure to access a potentially beneficial type of support is thought to reflect a number of personal, logistical, and structural barriers to service utilization. For grandparents, these barriers are likely to accumulate and prevent them from obtaining the support they need.

For grandparents parenting grandchildren, a significant barrier to seeking formal support is a lack of awareness of available services and support systems (Dolbin-MacNab, Johnson, Sudano, Serrano, & Roberto, 2011a; Gibson, 2002; Hayslip & Shore, 2000). Personal beliefs and stressors also serve as barriers to utilizing services. That is, grandparents may decide not to access formal support systems because they prefer informal sources of support, are in denial about the seriousness of their difficulties, feel ashamed about needing help, or believe that accessing formal assistance is an indicator of personal failure (Gibson, 2002; Henderson & Cook, 2005). Grandparents may also avoid utilizing formal supports in order to protect their privacy or because they are afraid of the consequences of government involvement in their lives (Gibson, 2002; Gladstone et al., 2009; Janicki, McCallion, Grant-Griffin, & Kolomer, 2000). There is also evidence that high levels of stress make it difficult for grandparents to access needed support (Sands & Goldberg-Glen, 2000), although others suggest that grandparents with the highest levels of adjustment might be the most likely to seek formal support (Hayslip & Shore, 2000).

Logistical difficulties also form barriers to grandparents' ability to access and utilize formal social support. Grandparent may not know whom to contact or where to go in order to obtain needed services or assistance. They may also lack transportation, childcare, or free time—all of which are needed in order to seek services (Gibson, 2002; Hayslip & Shore, 2000; Minkler, Driver, Roe, & Bedeian, 1993). Finally, grandparents often have childcare responsibilities, caregiving commitments, work duties, or health problems that make it difficult for them to find the time or energy to access formal systems of support (Dolbin-MacNab et al., 2011a).

Finally, in addition to personal and logistical barriers, structural barriers may prevent grandparents from accessing formal support systems. Structural barriers can include program staff who behave insensitively or policies and procedures that create an unwelcoming service environment (Dolbin-MacNab et al., 2011a). When accessing formal supports, grandparents may have difficulty establishing program eligibility, locating documentation, completing paperwork, and working their way through multiple service programs and providers (Gladstone et al., 2009; Gibson, 2002). For those grandparents who are able to make connections with formal support systems, many report that the program's policies and procedures are not sensitive to their family structure (Burnette, 1997; Gibbs & Muller, 2000; Gibson, 2002). These barriers may be further compounded by caseworkers and other program staff who lack an understanding of grandparents raising grandchildren or who hold negative stereotypes about grandparents' family situations (Dowdell, 1994; Gibson, 2002; Gladstone et al., 2009). Grandmothers may also express frustration with the differences in services available to custodial grandparents versus those available foster parents (Minkler & Roe, 1993).

Promoting Formal Social Support: An Ecological Framework for Practitioners

Given the multitude of barriers that prevent grandparents from accessing formal social support, practitioners interested in promoting resilience among grandparents parenting grandchildren must conceptualize and deliver services in ways that overcome as many of these barriers as possible. Ecological systems theory (Bronfenbrenner, 1979), which postulates that individuals and their environments are interdependent, provides a useful means for conceptualizing how practitioners and service programs can enhance grandparents' awareness of the formal support systems available to them (i.e., perceived formal support) as well as ensure that grandparents receive the assistance they need (i.e., enacted formal support). By taking steps to enhance grandparents' perceived and enacted formal support, practitioners can help promote grandparent resilience, despite the many challenges that grandparents are experiencing.

Based on ecological systems theory, a formal support system would consist of multiple nested environments ranging from the immediate elements of the formal support system that have a frequent, direct influence on grandparents (microsystem) to the broader sociocultural context in which the formal support system is located (macrosystem; Bronfenbrenner, 1979). Depending on the quality of the environments in which they are embedded, grandparents have various opportunities and limitations available to them (Bronfenbrenner, 1979). Those grandparents with more opportunities have more control over their situations and increased freedom in how they respond and adapt to stressors and other challenges in their lives. In the context of formal support, the quality of the micro (proximal) and macro (distal) elements of the formal support environment can vary greatly and, therefore, significantly impact the degree to which grandparents can obtain needed assistance and services.

To enhance formal support for grandparents parenting grandchildren, practitioners must address barriers at each level of the service environment and consider how these elements influence one another. In the following sections, we outline best practices for developing effective formal support systems for grandparents at four levels of the formal support environment—the grandparent, program accessibility, program staff, and program structure. Figure 9.1, which was developed for the purposes of this chapter, visually depicts our ecological conceptualization of best practices moving from grandparents' more proximal (i.e., the grandparent) to distal (i.e., program structure) environments. When implemented in concert, these best practices can improve the degree to which grandparents are able to access and utilize formal systems of social support. The arrows in this figure illustrate how each layer of the various formal support environments influences the others.

These best practices are derived from an integration of findings from several empirical projects. In the first project, 52 grandmothers raising adolescent grandchildren provided recommendations for practitioners delivering formal

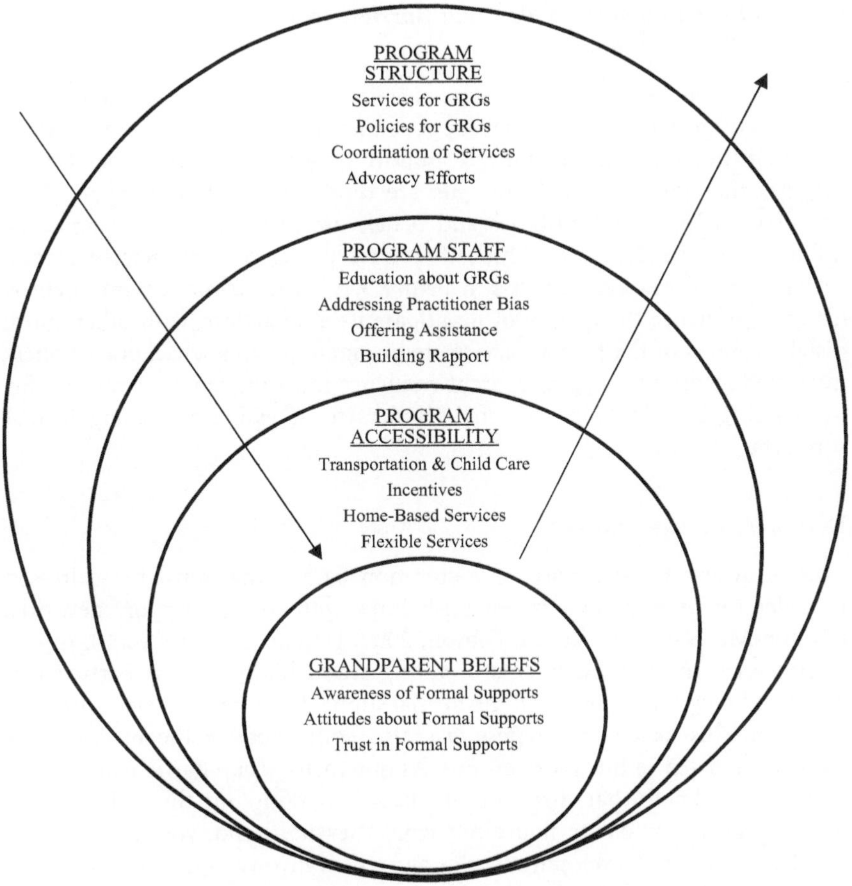

Figure 9.1 An ecological (Bronfenbrenner, 1979) conceptualization of strategies for the delivery of effective formal support to grandparents parenting grandchildren

support (Dolbin-MacNab & Keiley, 2006). Participants were recruited nationally and responded to a series of open-ended questions about their needs and the degree to which formal support services were able to meet those needs. In the second project, 59 professionals who work with grandparents and their custodial grandchildren participated in a series of focus groups (Dolbin-MacNab, Johnson, Sudano, Serrano, & Roberto, 2011a). Focus group participants provided suggestions for how best provide formal services to grandparents and grandchildren. Finally, we also draw from a series of qualitative interviews with 48 grandparents raising young grandchildren ages 5 and under (Dolbin-MacNab, Johnson, Sudano, Serrano, & Roberto, 2011b). During the interviews, grandparents were asked to make recommendations for how service programs could best meet their needs.

Overcoming Grandparents' Personal Barriers to Utilizing Formal Support

Although ecological systems theory suggests that both proximal and distal elements of grandparents' formal support environments determine the extent to which they make use of formal support systems, Bronfenbrenner (1979) suggests that proximal environments are often the most influential. Thus, grandparents' personal attitudes and beliefs are likely to have a significant influence on the degree to which they have perceived and enacted formal social support. And, as depicted in Figure 9.1, this proximal environment is likely to influence the quality of grandparents' interactions with other, more distal elements of the formal service environment. In this sense, practitioners interested in promoting grandparent resilience must implement strategies for overcoming grandparents' personal barriers to accessing and using formal supports.

Developing Service Awareness

Lack of awareness of services is a common barrier that must be addressed in order for grandparents to establish links with formal support networks (Dolbin-MacNab et al., 2011a; Gibson, 2002; Hayslip & Shore, 2000). In our interviews with 48 grandparents of young grandchildren, many participants reported being unfamiliar with the formal support services that were available to them. This lack of awareness was also confirmed by the professionals who participated in our focus groups. As one focus group participant shared, "They don't know that there are all these programs out there. They have to navigate the system to figure out what they need and, you know, what's worth their time." Developing service awareness involves spreading the word about potential sources of formal support in a variety of ways. Services should be advertised in locations that grandparents frequent, and should be delivered via multiple forms of media (e.g., television, radio, flyers). Because grandparents often experience barriers associated with eligibility, it is also important that efforts to promote service awareness be tailored to grandparents parenting grandchildren. That is, grandparents need to see themselves depicted in advertising materials and have it be clear that they may be eligible for services. Additionally, practitioners should actively work to develop word-of-mouth advertising among grandparents. One focus group participant shared how word-of-mouth among grandparents is a powerful way to overcome a lack of service awareness (and to build trust in formal support systems):

> I take somethin' over there to a neighbor, she gon' tell me a story, "Ms. Roberts bought me this. Look at this." So, they tell each other what they get . . . word-of-mouth to each other, you know, if they're in that type of community.

Addressing Helping-Seeking Attitudes

Even if practitioners are able to build awareness of sources of formal support, grandparents may still not make use of such services due to their personal beliefs about the acceptability of seeking assistance (Gibson, 2002; Henderson & Cook, 2005). In our focus groups, the professionals suggested that grandparents may not access formal services (despite their awareness and eligibility) because of a sense of pride or out of fear of not being self-sufficient. One participant shared how these beliefs could be both a strength and a limitation for grandparents in need of services: "So, that's [sense of pride and a desire to be self-sufficient] a strength, but it's kind of a weakness, too, because sometimes it holds you back from asking for things that you're—you and your children would be eligible for." To address these barriers, practitioners need to talk openly with grandparents about their feelings about seeking assistance, as well as any concerns that grandparents have about the process of utilizing formal systems of support. Practitioners can also normalize grandparents' feelings and assist them in accessing whatever forms of formal social support that they feel comfortable with and that will help meet their needs and those of their grandchildren.

Building Trust in Formal Support Systems

Even with these efforts, grandparents will not make use of formal systems of support if they do not believe that "the system" is looking out for their best interests (Gibson, 2002; Gladstone et al., 2009; Janicki et al., 2000). In our interviews with 52 grandparents raising adolescent grandchildren, many indicated that they did not trust formal support systems. Some of this distrust developed as a result of their experiences with practitioners they perceived as being judgmental or making too many assumptions about their families. One grandmother explained how her lack of trust in formal systems of social support stemmed from the fact that she did not feel understood by practitioners: "Unless you walk in our shoes, you really don't know what's going on. They can go by what they pick up and read, but unless they've truly walked in our shoes, they really don't know what's going on." To build grandparents' trust, practitioners must monitor their biases, build rapport, and provide excellent customer service. More detail about these recommendations is included in a later section of this chapter—however, the link between grandparents' attitudes and practitioners' behaviors highlight the interdependent nature of the environments surrounding formal systems of support and the need to intervene in both proximal and distal arenas larger formal support environments.

Additionally, because becoming involved in formal systems of support may bring grandparents to the attention of various sources of authority (e.g., Child Protective Services or the courts), practitioners must remain cognizant that some grandparents may be hesitant to seek formal social support (despite being eligible) out of fear of the consequences for themselves and their adult children. For instance, one focus group participant explained, "they [grandparents] want to get help, but they don't want to have to say that my child is a bad parent in order to get that type of help." To address this issue and assist grandparents in accessing needed formal support, practitioners should talk openly with grandparents about confidentiality and about their concerns associated with seeking services. When possible, practitioners should work with grandparents to devise a solution that provides them with the assistance they need—without compromising the well-being of their larger family system.

Enhancing the Accessibility of Formal Support Systems

In order for formal support systems to promote grandparent resilience, it is necessary for grandparents to be able to get to their doctor, case worker, therapist, support group, or government assistance program. Unfortunately, as discussed previously, grandparents experience a number of logistical barriers to accessing services (Gibson, 2002; Hayslip & Shore, 2000; Minkler et al., 1993). Whether they lack transportation, are experiencing health problems, or have difficulty using a computer, practitioners must actively work to remove as many logistical barriers to accessing services as possible. Removing these barriers would improve the quality of this layer of grandparents' environments (see Figure 9.1) and facilitate interactions among other more proximal and distal elements of the formal support environment. When this occurs, grandparents are more likely to benefit from services.

In our focus groups and in both sets of grandparent interviews, participants gave a number of useful ideas for removing logistical barriers that prevent grandparents from accessing formal supports. They recommended providing transportation and child care, and when possible and appropriate, offering meals and incentives for participation. One grandmother suggested,

> Feed the kids. Give them pizza and juice, and stuff like that. Give the kids help with their homework or play games. The grandparents can be in another place, and they can meet with experts who come in to talk about things.

Some participants even recommended providing home-based services to grandparents with health problems or who were otherwise homebound.

On a more macro level, part of removing logistical barriers to accessing formal support involves locating services in a comfortable and central part of the community—particularly in areas that are easily accessible via public transportation. To promote utilization by grandparents, programs should also offer flexible hours of service, including weekends and evenings, options for providing receiving services over the telephone, and services in multiple languages. While it is unlikely that any program will be able to remove all logistical barriers to accessing services, practitioners should still make attempts to address as many logistical barriers as possible.

Educating and Training Practitioners and Program Staff

Within the formal support environment, grandparents find themselves interacting with a variety of practitioners. As discussed previously, negative interactions with program staff can be a major barrier to grandparents' willingness to seek formal support and their satisfaction with that support (Dowdell, 1994; Gibson, 2002). Furthermore, as suggested by ecological systems theory (Bronfenbrenner, 1979), the quality of grandparents' interactions with program staff can impact other elements of their environments such as their attitudes about seeking services. Therefore, in order to enhance this aspect of formal support systems, practitioners must provide grandparents with a welcoming, non-judgmental service environment.

Providing Education About Grandparents Parenting Grandchildren

To create this type of environment, our grandparent participants recommended that program staff receive education about the challenges and needs of grandparent-headed families. Potential areas for education include reasons for the caregiving arrangement, the loss and trauma experienced by grandchildren, and grandparents' health challenges and sources of stress. For example, one grandmother raising an adolescent grandchild suggested that practitioners need to understand how the grandparent's age can impact his or her involvement with the grandchild:

> They need to take into consideration that my energy level at my age is far less than it was 10 years ago. People expect me to be available to go there, to do this. I think they [service providers] really must know that the grandparent raising a grandchild's energy level is going to be lower. It doesn't mean that they aren't capable, but if the energy level is low enough then they need to take this into consideration when expecting grandparents to attend or do for the grandchild.

Similarly, another grandmother recommended "making them [service providers] more aware of what these kids are going through. They go through loss and grief. They go through the unknown. Who's going to leave next? Is grandma going to die?"

Addressing Practitioner Biases

Beyond education about grandparents parenting grandchildren, to create a welcoming, non-judgmental environment, practitioners must also carefully examine their biases and assumptions and consider how these attitudes might consciously or unconsciously impact how they interact with grandparents and their grandchildren. Focus group participants highlighted two particularly problematic attitudes that are often held by practitioners—first, that grandparents are somehow at fault for their situations and, second, that custodial grandparents should be able to "take care of their own." As discussed previously, to combat these types of judgmental attitudes, practitioners need to be formally educated about the complexities of grandparent-headed households. As part of such professional development sessions, practitioners may also benefit from an open discussion about their previous experiences with grandparents raising grandchildren and an exploration of their attitudes and the potential impact of these attitudes on their delivery of formal support.

Offering Assistance and Building Rapport

In addition to monitoring biases and becoming more educated about grandparents parenting grandchildren, participants in both the focus groups and the interviews with grandparents indicated that, to be successful in supporting grandparents, program staff should develop a personal relationship and rapport with grandparents. Practitioners should also actively assist grandparents in meeting their service needs. The assumption was that, even if grandparents make use of one source of formal support, they may have other needs that are best met by other services or programs. As a result, a professional from the focus groups recommended that service providers should be willing to help grandparents access other formal supports by helping them complete paperwork, gather documentation, and make calls to other programs. She described how this has been helpful to her program in getting grandparents the formal support they need:

> [Grandparents need] someone who knows the kids, knows the situation, knows the family dynamics, who can walk them [grandparents] through the different systems, who can be the constant with all this change and chaos and stuff that goes on.

This level of intense assistance, coupled with a warm, supportive personal style was also valued by the grandparents we interviewed. As one grandmother of a young grandchild shared, "I feel like I know some of them [service providers] . . . personally, on a personal basis." Based on these observations, practitioners interested in promoting grandparent resilience should be familiar with the range of formal supports that are available to grandparents and ready to assist grandparents in accessing those services. Practitioners should also make an effort to form a personal connection with grandparents, and set aside some time for socializing and visiting.

Tailoring Programming for Grandparent-Headed Families

At the macro or most distal level of formal support systems, practitioners can promote grandparent resilience by improving the quality and availability of formal services available to custodial grandparents. As this element of formal support systems improves, in accordance with ecological systems theory

(Bronfenbrenner, 1979), it should also positively influence all other levels of the formal support environment depicted in Figure 9.1.

Developing Population-Specific Services

Given that formal systems of support cannot benefit grandparents if they do not exist, services tailored to the needs of grandparents parenting grandchildren should be developed. Grandparents in our two sets of interviews recommended needing interventions for grandchildren, programs that serve multiple needs in one location, and services that provide grandparents with respite care, among other suggestions. Practitioners could develop these grandparent-friendly services based on a community needs assessment that involves input from grandparents, grandchildren, a variety of professionals, and other significant community stakeholders.

Adopting Population-Sensitive Policies and Procedures

For existing services, practitioners must ensure that program policies and procedures are sensitive to grandparents' unique needs. For instance, in the focus groups, participants discussed how requiring that grandparents have custody of their grandchildren could result in many grandparents not being eligible for services. As one focus group participant shared, "If you don't have custody of the child . . . you are limited to whatever services you can receive." Another participant echoed the difficulty accessing services for grandchildren that can arise when grandparents do not have custody: "One of the issues that we see often—more than 50% of the time—is the grandparent doesn't necessarily have legal custody of the child and so navigating the system is really hard enough anyway, but throw that in there and it really makes it worse." Another issue that was described as making it difficult for grandparents to receive existing services was not having required documentation (e.g., grandchild birth certificates, immunization records). Finally, in the interviews with 48 grandmothers of young grandchildren, participants suggested that it was very helpful to them when programs were flexible and understood their busy schedules and multiple responsibilities. For example, one grandmother described how she appreciated how a government assistance program was responsive when she had to miss appointments: "I miss my appointments 50,000 times. Cause I'm so [busy] being a grandma . . . if I miss my appointment they try to set up appointment for me when like I'm off . . . You know, if somebody cancels they'll call me." Together, these empirical examples illustrate the importance of programs developing population-sensitive service eligibility, enrollment, and utilization policies.

Coordinating Services

Another strategy for enhancing grandparents' ability to access formal systems of support is to develop greater communication and coordination among the various formal support systems that grandparents already use. For instance, one focus group participant expressed her frustration in trying to help grandparents access multiple forms of formal support:

> Sometimes county to county it's not the same either. And I think that's the other thing, is that grandparents who live in different counties, we say, "You can apply for this and this." And then they go there and their local social services [manger] is saying, "You don't qualify for that." But we're saying, "Yes, you do and you would in our county." And so then that makes it further complicated . . . and does make it a lot more challenging.

For practitioners interested in enhancing grandparents' resilience via formal support systems, consideration should be given to providing grandparents with more centralized, one-stop services. To illustrate, one focus group participant described her vision for these services:

> What I would say is, because of the huge number of needs these families have, the more the services can be grouped together to reduce the amount of effort it takes to access them and the more there can be navigators to help work the way through the system to access the services, the better it will be.

Engaging in Advocacy

To promote the resilience of grandparents and their custodial grandchildren, practitioners must be willing to advocate for these families. Because grandparents lack power within formal support systems, practitioners must support grandparents who are being treated unfairly, bring their issues to the attention of funders and policymakers, and highlight the needs of this population for the general public. The grandmothers we interviewed explained that they could not bring about change in policies or the resources available to them on their own. In fact, they wanted practitioners to partner with them in advocating for more inclusive policies, greater grandparent rights, and better access to resources and services. For example, one grandmother explained, "They [practitioners] need to get involved with it [grandparents raising grandchildren]. And, maybe by getting involved, they can help these children too." Similarly, another grandmother shared that practitioners need to "network with us. We need to let the community know the numbers [of grandparent caregivers] because sometimes grandparents feel embarrassed. We want professionals to join our strength in numbers."

Summary and Conclusion

Despite evidence that adequate social support may be associated with greater grandparent resilience and well-being (Gerard et al., 2006; Kelley et al., 2000;

Landry-Meyer et al., 2005; Leder et al., 2007), many grandparents become isolated from their usual informal support networks due to their increased caregiving responsibilities (Jendrek, 1993; Minkler & Roe, 1993; Minkler et al., 1994; Musil, 1998). For this reason, formal systems of support can be central in developing grandparent resilience. As discussed in this chapter, grandparents parenting grandchildren experience a multitude of barriers to accessing and utilizing formal systems of social support. To promote resilience among grandparents parenting grandchildren, practitioners must assist grandparents in responding to and interacting with both proximal and distal elements of the formal service environment. Ideally, implementing the recommendations outlined in this chapter will allow practitioners to create a grandparent-friendly service environment that can promote greater grandparent adaptation and resilience.

References

Barrera, M. (1986). Distinctions between social support concepts, measures, and models. *American Journal of Community Psychology, 14*, 413–445. doi:10.1007/BF00922627

Berry, J. O., & Jones, W. H. (1995). The parental stress scale: Initial psychometric evidence. *Journal of Social and Personal Relationships, 12*, 463–472. doi:10.1177/0265407595123009

Bronfenbrenner, U. (1979). *The ecology of human development: Experiments by nature and design*. Cambridge, MA: Harvard University Press.

Burnette, D. (1997). Grandparents raising grandchildren in the inner city. *Families in Society, 78*, 489–501.

Burton, L. M. (1992). Black grandparents rearing children of drug-addicted parents: Stressors, outcomes, and social service needs. *The Gerontologist, 32*, 744–751.

Crowther, M., & Rodriguez, R. (2003). A stress and coping model of custodial grandparents among African Americans. In B.Hayslip, Jr. & J. H.Patrick (Eds.), *Working with custodial grandparents* (pp. 145–162). New York, NY: Springer.

Dannison, L. L., & Smith, A. B. (2003). Custodial grandparents community support program: Lessons learned. *Children and Schools, 25*(2), 87–95. doi:10.1093/cs/25.2.87

Dolbin-MacNab, M. L., Johnson, J., Sudano, L., Serrano, E., & Roberto, K. A. (2011a). *Focus groups: Professionals serving grandparent-headed families*. Blacksburg, VA: Virginia Tech.

Dolbin-MacNab, M. L., Johnson, J., Sudano, L., Serrano, E., & Roberto, K. A. (2011a). *Interviews: Grandparent raising WIC-enrolled grandchildren*. Blacksburg, VA: Virginia Tech.

Dolbin-MacNab, M. L., & Keiley, M. K. (2006). A systemic examination of grandparents' emotional closeness with their custodial grandchildren. *Research in Human Development, 3*, 59–71. doi:10.1207/s15427617rhd0301_6

Dowdell, E. B. (1994). A special population: Grandmother caregivers [Editorial: Views and Opinions]. *Psychological Nursing and Mental Health Services, 32*(11), 7.

Gerard, J. M., Landry-Meyer, L., & Roe, J. G. (2006). Grandparents raising grandchildren: The role of social support in coping with caregiving challenges. *International Journal of Aging and Human Development, 62*, 359–383. doi:10.2190/3796-DMB2-546Q-Y4AQ

Gibbs, P., & Muller, U. (2000). Kinship foster care moving to the mainstream: Controversy, policy, and outcome. *Adoption Quarterly, 4*, 57–87. doi:10.1300/J145v04n02_04

Gibson, P. (2002). Barriers, lessons learned, and helpful hints: Grandmother caregivers talk about service utilization. *Journal of Gerontological Social Work, 39*(4), 55–74. doi: 10.1300/J083v39n04_05

Gladstone, J. W., Brown, R. A., & Fitzgerald, K. J. (2009). Grandparents raising grandchildren: Tensions, service needs and involvement with child welfare agencies. *International Journal of Aging and Human Development, 69*, 55–78. doi:10.2190/AG.69.1.d

Hayslip, B. (2003). The impact of a psychosocial intervention on parental efficacy, grandchild relationship quality, and well being among grandparents raising grandchildren. In B. Hayslip, Jr. & J. Patrick (Eds.), *Working with custodial grandparents* (pp. 163–178). New York, NY: Springer.

Hayslip, B., & Kaminski, P. L. (2005). Grandparents raising their grandchildren. *Marriage and Family Review, 37*, 147–169. doi:10.1300/J002v37n01_10

Hayslip, B., & Shore, R. J. (2000). Custodial grandparenting and mental health services. *Journal of Mental Health and Aging, 6*, 367–383.

Hayslip, B., Shore, R. J., Henderson, C. E., & Lambert, P. L. (1998). Custodial grandparenting and the impact of grandchildren with problems on roles satisfaction and role meaning. *Journal of Gerontology: Social Sciences, 53B*, S164–S173. doi:10.1093/geronb/53B.3.S164

Henderson, T. L., & Cook, J. L. (2005). Grandma's hands: Black grandmothers speak about their experiences raising grandchildren on TANF. *International Journal of Aging and Human Development, 61*, 1–19. doi:10.2190/Q4A1-BG9G-XDXK-1VP0

Hughes, M. E., Waite, L. J., LaPierre, T. A., & Luo, Y. (2007). All in the family: The impact of caring for grandchildren on grandparents' health. *Journal of Gerontology: Social Sciences, 62B*, S108–S119. doi:10.1093/geronb/62.2.S108

Janicke, D. M., & Finney, J. W. (2003). Children's primary health care services: Social-cognitive factors related to utilization. *Journal of Pediatric Psychology, 28*, 547–558. doi: 10.1093/jpepsy/jsg045

Janicki, M. P., McCallion, P., Grant-Griffin, L., & Kolomer, S. R. (2000). Grandparent caregivers I: Characteristics of the grandparents and children with disabilities for whom they care. *Journal of Gerontological Social Work, 33*, 35–55. doi: 10.1300/J083v33n03_03

Jendrek, M. P. (1993). Grandparents who parent their grandchildren: Effects on lifestyle. *Journal of Marriage and the Family, 55*, 609–621. doi:10.1093/jpepsy/jsg045

Jendrek, M. P. (1994). Grandparents who parent their grandchildren: Circumstances and decisions. *The Gerontologist, 34*, 206–216. doi:10.1093/geront/34.2.206

Kelley, S. J., & Whitley, D., Sipe, T. A., & Yorker, B. C. (2000). Psychological distress in grandmother kinship care providers: The roles of resources, social support, and physical health. *Child Abuse & Neglect, 24*, 311–321. doi:10.1016/S0145-2134(99)00146-5

Kolomer, S., McCallion, P., & Janicki, M. (2002). African-American grandmother carers of children with disabilities: Predictors of depressive symptoms. *Journal of Gerontological Social Work, 37*(3/4), 45–64. doi:10.1300/J083v37n03_05

Kreider, R. M., & Ellis, R. (2011). *Living arrangements of children: 2009* (Current Population Reports, P70-126). Washington, DC: U. S. Census Bureau. Retrieved from http://www.census.gov/prod/2011pubs/p70-126.pdf

Landry-Meyer, L., Gerard, J. M., & Guzell, J. R. (2005). Caregiver stress among grandparents raising grandchildren: The functional role of social support. *Marriage and Family Review, 37*, 171–190. doi: 10.1300/J002v37n01_11

Leder, S., Grinstead, L. N., & Torres, E. (2007). Grandparents raising grandchildren: Stressors, social support, and health outcomes. *Journal of Family Nursing, 13*, 333–352. doi: 10.1177/1074840707303841

Litwak, E. (1985). *Helping the elderly: The complementary roles of informal networks and formal systems*: New York, NY: Guilford.

Minkler, M., Driver, D., Roe, K. M., & Bedeian, K. (1993). Community interventions to support grandparent caregivers. *The Gerontologist, 33*, 807–811.

Minkler, M., & Fuller-Thomson, E. (1999). The health of grandparents raising grandchildren: Results of a national study. *American Journal of Public Health, 89*, 1384–1392. doi: 10.2105/AJPH.89.9.1384

Minkler, M., Fuller-Thomson, E., Miller, D., & Driver, D. (1997). Depression in grandparents raising grandchildren: Results of a national longitudinal study. *Archives of Family Medicine, 6*, 445–452.

Minkler, M., & Roe, K. (1993). *Grandmothers as caregivers: Raising children of the crack cocaine epidemic.* Newbury Park, CA: Sage.

Minkler, M., Roe, K., & Robertson-Beckley, R. (1994). Raising grandchildren from crack-cocaine households: Effects on family and friendship ties of African American women. *American Journal of Orthopsychiatry, 64*, 20–29. doi: 10.1037/h0079493

Muliira, J. K., & Musil, C. M. (2010). Relationship between methods of coping, social support and receipt of preventive care procedures by primary grandmother caregivers. *Journal of Community Mental Health, 35*, 479–486. doi: 10.1007/s10900-009-9216-y

Musil, C. M. (1998). Health, stress, coping, and social support in grandmother caregivers. *Health Care for Women International, 19*, 441–455. doi: 10.1080/073993398246205

Ong, A. D., Bergeman, C. S., & Boker, S. M. (2009). Resilience comes of age: Defining features in later adulthood. *Journal of Personality, 77*, 1777–1804. doi: 10.1111/j.1467-6494.2009.00600.x

Roberto, K. A., Dolbin-MacNab, M. L., & Finney, J. W. (2008). Promoting the health of grandmothers parenting young grandchildren. In B. Hayslip & P. Kaminski (Eds.), *Parenting the custodial grandchild* (pp. 75–89). New York, NY: Springer.

Sands, R. G., & Goldberg-Glen, R. S. (2000). Factors associated with stress among grandparents raising their grandchildren. *Family Relations, 49*, 97–105. doi: 10.1111/j.1741-3729.2000.00097.x

Sherbourne, C. D., & Stewart, A. L. (1991). The MOS social support survey. *Social Science and Medicine, 32*, 705–714. doi: 10.1016/0277-9536(91)90150-B

Vaux, A., & Harrison, D. (1985). Support network characteristics associated with support satisfaction and perceived support. *American Journal of Community Psychology, 13*, 245–268. doi: 10.1007/BF00914932

Ware, J. E., Jr., Kosinski, M., & Keller, S. D. (1994). *SF-36: Physical and mental health summary scales: A user's manual.* Boston, MA: The Health Institute.

Ware, J. E., Jr., & Sherbourne, C. D. (1992). The MOS 36-item short-form health survey (SF-36): I. Conceptual framework and item selection. *Medical Care, 30*, 473–483. doi: 10.1097/00005650-199206000-00002

10 Social and Personal Resources of Grandmother Caregivers After Grandchildren Are Grown[1]

Catherine Goodman, Dolores Scorzo, Patricia Ernandez, and Araceli Alvarez-Nunez

Abstract

Grandparents have offered a stable source of parenting for grandchildren when parents are not able to provide for them. However, little is known about their well-being after their grandchildren have grown or their grandchild's assistance to these aging grandmothers in times of ill health. This pilot study of 50 grandmothers addressed the factors related to the well-being of grandmother caregivers who had raised grandchildren in terms of their personal and social resources. Considering personal resources, the grandmothers' resilience and their satisfaction with having raised their grandchildren were predictors of mental health and life satisfaction. In terms of social resources, closeness in the grandmother-grandchild relationship predicted mental health and lower depression; instrumental support from family and friends predicted lower depression; and subjective support from family and friends predicted life satisfaction. Grandmothers' poor health was marginally related to greater instrumental support from their grandchildren, possibly reflecting assistance mobilized in light of greater need. Interventions which enhance the essential grandmother-grandchild relationships are crucial, as well as interventions to foster other supportive relationships. Grandmothers can be encouraged to draw on the positives of their past caregiving experience and cultivate their own resilience in the face of adversity.

Introduction

Over the past three decades, researchers have described the issues facing grandparent caregivers (Hayslip & Kaminski, 2005) and risks to their well-being, such as depression and poor health (Bachman & Chase-Lansdale, 2005; Grinstead, Leder, Jensen, & Bond, 2003; Minkler, Fuller-Thomson, Miller, & Driver, 2000). Increases in numbers of grandchildren being raised by grandparents were substantial over the past 30 years, from almost 1 million grandchildren raised by their grandparents without a parent at home in 1980 (Saluter, 1996) to 1.8 million in 2009 (Kreider, 2011). These are skipped generation families, in which parents may be involved but do not live in the same household, leaving basic care to the grandparent.

To a considerable extent, grandparent caregivers are at risk for depression (Minkler, Fuller-Thomson, Miller, & Driver, 2000); poor health (Grinstead, Leder, Jensen, & Bond, 2003; Musil & Ahmed, 2002; Bachman & Chase-Lansdale, 2005); low income and poverty (Kelley, Whitley, Sipe, & Yorker, 2000; Fuller-Thomson & Minkler, 2003); social stresses, such as poor relations with adult children (Goodman & Silverstein, 2002; Waldrop, 2003); and struggles with parenting (Hayslip, Temple, Shore, & Henderson, 2006; Hayslip, King, & Jooste, 2008). In spite of the substantial knowledge about this population, little is known about the well-being and personal or resources of grandparents whose grandchildren have grown to maturity; or the types of relationships that exist between caregiving grandparents and their adult grandchildren.

Personal Resources

Grandparents raising a grandchild sustain their commitment, in spite of the risks and hardships that they experience. Personal resources, such as strength in adversity or resilience, may be related to the grandparents' well-being. Resilience is a concept applied to groups of people experiencing hardship, who have overcome their difficulties based on the observation that some individuals have good outcomes in spite of serious adversity (Rutter, 2007). Few studies have addressed resilience among caregivers, although literature is emerging on the resilience of grandchildren raised by grandparents (Downie, Hay, Horner, Wichmann, & Hislop, 2010; Sands, Goldberg-Glen, & Shin, 2009). In terms of grandparent resilience, Musil and colleagues (Musil, Warner, Zauszniewski, Jeanblanc, & Kercher, 2006) examined resourcefulness, one approach to resilience. They found self-regulatory efficacy and self-control—resourcefulness—to be related to family functioning, although resourcefulness did not differ by custodial caregiver, three-generational, or non-caregiver groups of grandmothers. Additionally, Waldrop (2003) identified a theme of strength in adversity through qualitative interviews with 37 grandmother caregivers and Fuller-Thomson (2005) described the strength and challenges of Canadian First Nations grandparents. Considering resilience in the family as a whole, adolescents in grandparent headed families were compared to those with parental caregivers. Those adolescents living with grandparents described an aspect of family resilience as seeking and accepted help from outside (Shin, Choi, Kim, & Kim, 2010). Resilience may be a personal characteristic of grandparent caregivers who have high morale and well-being as these grandparents typically must overcome difficult life circumstances, including the parents' circumstances, parenting a second time around, and seeing their grandchildren through to adulthood.

Satisfaction with raising grandchildren may also be considered a resource in that it verifies congruence and lack of inner-conflict with assuming an off time and long term second parenting commitment. Raising grandchildren offers benefits (Hayslip & Kaminski, 2005), a sense of purpose and the rewards of close relationships with grandchildren. Satisfaction with the parenting role has been found to be related to more emotional support from family (Hayslip, Temple, Shore, & Henderson, 2006); and conversely parenting stress was related to lower perceived social support from family and friends (Gerard, Landry-Meyer, & Roe, 2006). Lower parenting stress was also related to better physical and mental health (Leder, Grinstead, & Torres, 2007) and higher parenting self-efficacy (Ramaswamy, Bhavnagri, & Barron, 2008). In addition to satisfaction with parenting, parenting practices are integrally related to the grandparent's well-being: Negative parenting practices (e.g., harsh and inconsistent parenting) have been related to the grandmother's depression and anxiety, with positive practices related to lower distress (Smith & Richardson, 2008). Furthermore dysfunctional parenting practices (ineffective discipline and low nurturance) have been related to the grandchild's behavior problems, as well as to the grandparent's psychological distress (Smith & Hancock, 2010). Therefore, satisfaction with the parenting experience among older, experienced grandmother caregivers may be related to higher grandparent well-being as they look back and evaluate their lives. Satisfaction with parenting a second time around may have a cultural component: Pruchno (1999) determined that African-American grandmothers were more likely to view the role as an expectation of grandparenthood.

Social Support Resources

Generally, socially supportive relationships are reciprocal, with reciprocal give and take from family and friends related to greater life satisfaction among older adults. Factors that deter reciprocity are functional limitations and poor health, which have been documented in older adult parent-child relationships, as well as partner and other trusting relationships (Chandola, Marmot, & Siegrist, 2007). Reciprocity has been conceived as an internalized norm (Perugini, Gallucci, Presaghi, & Ercolani, 2003): According to the norm, returning help is the right thing to do, especially toward deserving others.

Thompkins (2007) has suggested that grandchildren will be the caregivers for aging grandparents who have raised them, returning care by providing for their grandparents in times of illness and frailty. And grandparent caregivers may expect more care from their grandchildren: Kaminski and Hayslip (2004) found that grandparent caregivers were more likely to turn to their grandchildren to meet their own social, emotional, and physical needs compared to looking to parents for need fulfillment (Hayslip & Kaminski, 2005). Indeed, grandchildren in general have joined the ranks of caregivers of older adults (Dellmann-Jenkins, Blankemeyer, & Pinkard, 2000).

One approach to social support, conceptualized by Barrera (1986) distinguishes between perceived and enacted support. Perceived support is often related to better mental health and well-being, whereas enacted support is often mobilized in times of special need and has been related to illness or crises. Another similar approach to classification of social support for older adults has been as instrumental versus subjective support (Musil & Ahmad, 2002), with subjective social support reflecting the appraisal or perception that support is available, satisfaction with support, or an evaluation of relationships as supportive. In contrast, instrumental social support is a description of specific ways that support has been provided, such as help with dressing, paying bills, and transportation. This help is often related to lower levels of physical and psychological well-being and could be consistent with support mobilized to handle stress and distress. Social support has also been conceived as social integration, such as social networks, although extensive social networks of middle age may decline in older adulthood (Rook, 2009).

Social support has been identified as important for the well-being of grandparent caregivers. Musil and colleagues (Musil et al., 2006) compared custodial grandmothers to grandmothers in multigenerational homes and those not involved in caregiving. Custodial grandmothers had less subjective support compared to non-caregivers; and less instrumental support than both other groups using subscales from the Duke Social Support Index. Musil and Ahmed (2002) also found subjective support to be related to lower depression and better health and to mediate the relationship between stress and depression/health in a sample of grandmothers who were primary, secondary, and non-caregivers. Other studies have found that less perceived social support is related to greater difficulties with grandchildren (Hayslip, King, & Jooste, 2008); and that greater social support from family and friends was related to less parenting stress, greater life satisfaction (Gerard, Landry-Meyer, & Roe, 2006), and less psychological distress (Smith & Hancock, 2010).

This study addresses circumstances in the lives of older grandmother caregivers who have raised their grandchildren. It looks at resilience and satisfaction with having raised a grandchild as personal self-appraisals that reflect the ability of grandmother caregivers to persevere and support their grandchildren over the years. It also addresses social factors, such as supportive relationships from family and friends. In particular, the study focuses on the quality of the grandmother's relationship with her grandchild; and assistance provided to her by her grandchild as enactment of intergenerational reciprocity.

Methods

Design

This is a cross sectional pilot study of grandmothers who had been involved in raising grandchildren 10 years earlier. One randomly selected grandchild was described in detail, the same one described 10 years before.

Sample and Data Collection

Fifty grandmother caregivers were recruited from grandmothers participating in a study 10 years earlier. A sample of 105 grandmothers (56 African-American and 49 White) was selected by drawing randomly for potential

African-American or White skipped generation respondents with a current address (no postal return). Of those we attempted to contact, the response rate was 32.1% for African-American, 65.3% for White grandmothers, and an overall response rate of 47.6%. Of those who were not interviewed 4.7% were deceased, 4.7% overtly declined, and 14.3% didn't respond to multiple calls. Other non-responders could not be reached due to lack of information or phone numbers. The previous sample had been broadly recruited through grandchildren in 223 schools in the Los Angeles Unified School District and through media announcements of the study (see Table 10.1).

The current pilot study of 50 African-American and White grandmothers offered a $20 incentive for the one-hour telephone interview. Telephone

Table 10.1 Demographic Description of Pilot Sample ($N = 50$)

Characteristic	n	%	m	*(sd)*
Grandmothers				
Age			67.26	(6.43)
Under 60	6	12		
60–69	29	58		
70–79	12	24		
80 or over	3	6		
Ethnicity				
African American	18	36		
White	32	64		
Married	18	36		
Family Income 2007				
$20,000 or less	6	12		
$20,001–40,000	16	32		
$40,001–60,000	10	20		
$60,001–80,000	7	14		
$80,001 and over	11	22		
Grandchildren				
Age			18.86	(3.54)
Under 18	20	40		
18 or over	30	60		
Gender				
Male	24	48		
Female	26	52		
Ethnicity				
African American	20	40		
White	30	60		
Currently Living with Grandmother	31	62		
Cumulative Years with Grandmother			14.37	(4.98)
Under 10	6	12		
10–19	37	74		
20 or over	7	14		

interviews were conducted by a team of three professional social workers and one master's level social work student.

Measures

Well-being for the grandmother was measured using the well-known SF-36 (Ware, 1993) to assess mental and physical health; the CES-D to assess depression (Radloff, 1977); and the Satisfaction with Life Scale (Diner, Emmons, Larson, & Griffin, 1985). The SF-36 consists of 36 items, producing eight subscales that are weighted and normed to result in mental and physical health indices. Coefficient alpha for subscales ranged from .76 for Role Emotional to .93 for Physical Functioning. The CES-D consists of 20 items, assessing frequency of symptoms, such as "You felt sad." Ratings were from 0 (never, rarely) to 3 (most all the time). Coefficient alpha in this sample was .89. Satisfaction with Life Scale was composed of five items, such as "I am satisfied with my life," rated from 7 (strongly agree) to 1 (strongly disagree), with a coefficient alpha in this sample of .87.

Personal resources consisted of resilience and satisfaction with having raised their grandchild. Resilience was measured using 25-item Connor-Davidson Resilience Scale (CD-RISC), with items such as "I am able to adapt to change," and "I tend to bounce back after illness or hardship." Items were rated on a 4-point scale from 1 (rarely) to 4 (nearly all the time; Vaishnavi, Connor, & Davidson, 2007) with coefficient alpha in this sample .90. Satisfaction with Grandparenting was measured by five items developed for this study to assess satisfaction with role performance and the choice to raise their grandchild. Examples are, "I feel satisfied with the way I parented my grandchild." Items were rated on a 5-point scale from 1 (strongly disagree) to 5 (strongly agree). For Satisfaction with Grandparenting, coefficient alpha was .78.

Support from family and friends was measured using the Duke Index for Social Support subscales for Subjective Social Support and Instrumental Social Support (Koenig, George, & Blazer, 1993). The Subjective Support Subscale consisted of seven items, such as "Does it seem that your friends and family understand you?" rated on a 3-point scale from 1 (hardly ever) to 3 (most of the time). Coefficient alpha in this sample was .73. The Instrumental Subscale was a list 12 specific yes-no items regarding ways that family and friends could help, including "shop or run errands for you?" and "help out when you are sick?" Coefficient alpha was .82 for this sample. To assess subjective support from the grandchild, the Bengtson (1991) affective solidarity scale was used to show close, presumably supportive relationships, consisting of five items rated on a 6-point scale from 1 (not at all) to 6 (extremely). Items addressed closeness, communication, getting along, understanding, and affection: coefficient alpha was .90 in this sample. To assess instrumental support from the grandchild, the Duke Instrumental Social Support Subscale was adapted to address help provided by the grandchild, using the same 12 items as for family and friends. Coefficient alpha for help provided by the grandchild was .75.

The sample consisted of older adult grandmothers (67 years old on average), African-American (36%) and White (64%), who were predominantly unmarried (64%) and living on family incomes of $60,000 or less (64%). Grandchildren were typically 19 years old, slightly more likely to be female (52%), and White (60%). Most grandchildren currently lived with their grandmothers (62%) and 88% had been living with their grandmothers 10 or more years (mean 14.4 years; see Table 10.1).

Results

Multiple regressions were used to look at well-being outcomes (mental health, physical health, life satisfaction, and depression) regressed on personal resources (Model 1: resilience and satisfaction with grandparenting) and social supports (Model 2: subjective and instrumental supports from family/friends and from grandchild) in separate analyses. With this small sample, the power to identify results was low; therefore the alpha $p \leq .10$ was discussed as a result to avoid false negatives or type 2 error. The dependent variables of life satisfaction and depression were transformed using square root transformation to improve their distributions. Four predictor variables were also transformed using square root (grandmother-grandchild closeness; instrumental social support from family and friends) or log transformations (grandmother satisfaction; subjective social support from family and friends).

Mutivariate analysis showed that personal resources predictors in Model 1 (resilience and grandparent satisfaction) were related to mental health (accounting for 28% of the variance) and life satisfaction (accounting for 39% of the variance). Both resilience and grandparent satisfaction were significant predictors for the grandmother's mental health and life satisfaction. This model trended for depression (but accounted for only 11% of the variance) and was not significant for physical health (see Table 10.2 and 10.3).

Social support predictors in Model 2 showed significance for mental health, depression, and life satisfaction and trended for physical health. Mental health was strongly predicted by closeness of the grandmother-grandchild relationship, with this model accounting for 35% of the variance. Depression was also predicted by a less close relationship between grandmother-grandchild; and by fewer instrumental supports from family and friends, the model accounting for 24% of the variance. Life satisfaction was predicted by close grandmother-grandchild relationships (trend) and by greater subjective social support from family and friends, with this model predicting 23% of the variance. Although the physical health analysis only trended, greater instrumental support from the grandchild was significantly related to lower levels of physical health (the model accounting for 17% of the variance; see Table 10.2 and 10.3).

Table 10.2 Personal and Social Resource Predictors of Mental Health, Depression, and Life Satisfaction: Standardized Regression Coefficients ($N = 50$)

Predictors	*Mental Health*		*Physical Health*	
	Model 1	*Model 2*	*Model 1*	*Model 2*
Resilience	.309*		.088	
Grandparenting Satisfaction	.388**		–.284*	
Instrumental SS		.156		.015
Subjective SS		.153		.119
Instrumental SS-GC		.025		–.445*
Emotionally Close GM-GC		.534**		.057
R^2 =	.276***	.350***	.082	.168†
Adjusted R^2 =	.245***	.292***	.043	.094†
F =	8.958***	6.063***	2.103	2.275†
Df =	2, 47	4, 45	2, 47	4, 45

Note: SS = Social Support; GC = Grandchild; GM = Grandmother.
†$p \leq .10$, *$p \leq .05$, **$p \leq .01$, ***$p \leq .001$.

Table 10.3 Personal and Social Resource Predictors of Mental Health, Depression, and Life Satisfaction: Standardized Regression Coefficients ($N = 50$)

Predictors	*Depression*		*Life Satisfaction*	
	Model 1	*Model 2*	*Model 1*	*Model 2*
Resilience	–.260†		.348**	
Grandparenting Satisfaction	–.171		.472***	
Instrumental SS		–.305*		–.107
Subjective SS		–.169		.327*
Instrumental SS-GC		–.149		–.007
Emotionally Close GM-GC		–.368*		.322†
R^2 =	.108†	.244*	.386***	.229*
Adjusted R^2 =	.070†	.177*	.360***	.160*
F =	2.848†	3.637*	14.765***	3.332*
Df =	2, 47	4, 45	2, 47	4, 45

Note: SS = Social Support; GC = Grandchild; GM = Grandmother.
†$p \leq .10$, *$p \leq .05$, **$p \leq .01$, ***$p \leq .001$.

Discussion

Summary

This study has identified resilience and satisfaction with raising a grandchild as robust predictors of mental health and life satisfaction after the grandchildren are raised. Closeness of the grandmother-grandchild relationship was a key factor in the current well-being of these older grandmothers, predicting mental health and lower depression (and marginally life satisfaction). Furthermore, instrumental support from the grandchild was higher amongst grandmothers in less good health, although the model only trended. Results suggest that grandchildren step in when their grandmothers were ill or need assistance with basic tasks. On the other hand, subjective support from family and friends was related to higher life satisfaction; and instrumental support from family and friends was related to lower depression, demonstrating that other support relationships are also important after years of raising grandchildren.

Personal Resources

Resilience, the ability to show strength in adversity and bounce back after difficult times (Rutter, 2007), was related to self-ratings of high mental health and life satisfaction in this pilot study. Musil and colleagues (2006) found qualities related to resilience (self-regulatory efficacy and self-control) to be important for family functioning amongst grandparents in varying circumstances (caregiving, co-parenting, traditional). As researchers turn to the construct of resilience using self-ratings, more evidence will emerge that resilience is part of the self-image of grandparent caregivers with high morale. The challenge of raising children in later middle age involves flexibility and persistence: Strong grandmothers who had the high levels of well-being endorsed resilience as part of their self-image. Indeed, raising grandchildren is often born of adversity and involves persistence, making unpopular decisions, and coping with unexpected stresses in order to keep the family together—all aspects of resilience (Vaishnavi et al., 2007).

Satisfaction with having raised their grandchildren was related to mental health and life satisfaction, demonstrating the centrality of this choice, and the importance of self-appraisal of success. Studies of coping with stress have demonstrated that positive reappraisals are used to cope by older adults more often compared to young adults. Furthermore, this type of coping has been related to higher subjective well-being in older adults (Wrosch, Heckhausen, & Lachman, 2000). Older adults evaluate their lives, referred to as life review, which involves coming to terms with choices they have made over the life span, a process related to self-esteem (Chiang, Lu, Chu, Chang, & Chou, 2008). Raising grandchildren is a long-term commitment, which sometimes involves sacrifices with spouses (14% found it caused problems in marriage; Pruchno, 1999) and adjustments in the workplace (45% changed hours worked, 15% changed employers; Pruchno). At best, raising grandchildren involves lifestyle shifts that often lead to financial shortages, role overload, and lack of privacy. This study demonstrates that in spite of the struggles, many grandmothers look back at their caregiving lives with pride in themselves and in their choice to raise grandchildren.

Social Support Resources

In terms of support in times of need, the relationship with the grandchild is central. A close relationship to their grandchild is related to mental health, lower depression, and marginally to life satisfaction. High quality grandparent-grandchild relationships could be the caregiving relationships of the future as older adult grandparent caregivers need assistance due to illness and find their adult children may be unavailable (Thompkins, 2007). The marginal health finding in this small pilot suggests that indeed, as grandmothers' health declines, grandchildren provide greater assistance with instrumental tasks.

In terms of support from family and friends, ratings show the importance of instrumental types of assistance in deterring depression. Instrumental support in particular is a needed resource for skipped generation grandparent caregivers, who have been found to have lower instrumental support than grandparents in multigenerational families or non-caregivers (Musil et al., 2006). Apparently, the benefits of practical assistance from others can provide protection to grandmother caregivers against the common risk of depression experienced by many caregivers.

On the other hand, the subjective appraisal that family and friends are supportive is related to positive life satisfaction. This result echoes findings of other researchers who also identified perceived/subjective social support to be related to life satisfaction and lower parenting stress (Gerard, Landry-Meyer, & Roe, 2006); lower depression, greater health (Musil & Ahmed, 2002); and lower psychological distress (Smith & Hancock, 2010).

Implications for Research

This pilot study provided insights into potential benefits of strong relationships with grandchildren; and self-perception as resilient and satisfied with parenting a second time. A larger study could address these issues with greater power to identify subtle contributors to well-being. Additionally, grandmothers in the study were typically 67 years old, and many were in good health: More advanced age and greater frailty would demonstrate more surely the possible involvement of grandchildren as caregivers, providing reciprocally to their grandmothers who raised them. Another research approach to resilience might be to identify successful and satisfied grandmother caregivers in high risk circumstances, such as poverty, or broken and conflicted families. Researchers could assume these grandmothers were resilient and search for factors that may have enabled their success. This is consonant with Rutter's (2007) definition of resilience as persons who succeed in spite of high risks.

Implications for Practice

This study focuses on the importance of the grandmother-grandchild relationship over time, as the grandmother ages and may become ill or frail. Grandchildren have become caregivers for grandparents in other circumstances (Dellmann-Jenkins, Blankemeyer, & Pinkard, 2000) and the potential of close bonds and reciprocal obligations generated from caregiving enhance this likelihood. Social workers and other mental health professionals should look toward grandchildren as a personal resource for grandparents in confronting illness and frailty in older years. Although the age gap may be a deterrent to providing assistance because grandchildren are establishing families and raising their own children, this type of sandwich generation may still provide a resource for aging grandparent caregivers. Other family and friends may also be supporters, and grandparent caregivers should be encouraged to cultivate relationships that enrich their lives and offer support. Lastly, social workers should support the grandmother's self-image as resilient and assist her to resolve regrets and reevaluate her caregiving efforts to emphasize the positives.

Grandparent caregivers provide for young children when these children are vulnerable and in need. They often struggle with serious challenges and their flexibility, generosity, and strength enable them to persevere through the years until their grandchildren are grown. The well-being of grandmothers across the life-span is important as society becomes more aware and supportive of their efforts.

Note

1 This study was supported in part by a Scholarly and Creative Activities Award, California State University, Long Beach.

References

Bachman, H. J., & Chase-Lansdale, P. L. (2005). Custodial grandmothers' physical, mental, and economic well-being: Comparisons of primary caregivers from low-income neighborhoods. *Family Relations, 54*, 475–487.

Barrera, M., Jr. (1986). Distinctions betweens social support concepts, measures, and models. *American Journal of Community Psychology, 14*, 413–445.

Bengtson, V. L. (1991). *The longitudinal study of three-generation families: 1991 Survey*: Unpublished survey instrument, Andrus Gerontology Center, University of Southern California.

Chandola, T., Marmot, M., & Siegrist, J. (2007). Failed reciprocity in close social relationships and health: Findings from the Whitehall II study. *Journal of Psychosomatic Research, 63*, 403–411.

Chiang, K., Lu, R., Chu, H., Chang, Y., & Chou, K. (2008). Evalution of the effect of a life review group program on self-esteem and life satisfaction in the elderly. *International Journal of Geriatric Psychiatry, 23*, 7–10.

Dellmann-Jenkins, M., Blankemeyer, M., & Pinkard, O. (2000). Young adult children and grandchildren in primary caregiver roles to older relatives and their service needs. *Family Relations, 49*, 177–186.

Diener, C., Emmons, R. A., Larson, R. J., & Griffin, S. (1985). The Satisfaction With Life Scale. *Journal of Personality Assessment, 49*, 71–75.

Downie, J. M., Hay, D. A., Horner, B. J., Wichmann, H., & Hislop, A. L. (2010). Children living with their grandparents: resilience and wellbeing. *International Journal of Social Welfare, 19*, 8–22.

Fuller-Thomson, E. (2005). Canadian First Nations grandparents raising grandchildren: A portrait in resilience. *International Journal of Aging and Human Development, 60*, 331–342.

Fuller-Thomson, E., & Minkler, M. (2003). Housing issues and realities facing grandparent caregivers who are renters. *The Gerontologist, 43*, 92–98.

Gerard, J. M., Landry-Meyer, L., & Roe, J. G. (2006). Grandparents raising grandchildren: The role of social support in coping with caregiving challenges. *International Journal of Aging and Human Development, 62*, 359–383.

Goodman, C., & Silverstein, M. (2002). Grandmothers raising grandchildren: Family structure and well-being in culturally diverse families. *The Gerontologist, 42*, 676–689.

Grinstead, L. N., Leder, S., Jensen, S., & Bond, L. (2003). Review of research on the health of caregiving grandparents. *Journal of Advanced Nursing, 44*, 318–326.

Hayslip, B., Jr., & Kaminski, P. L. (2005). Grandparents raising their grandchildren: A review of the literature and suggestions for practice. *The Gerontologist, 45*, 262–269.

Hayslip, B., Jr., King, J. K., & Jooste, J. L. (2008). Grandchildren's difficulties and strengths impact the mental health of their grandparents. In B. Hayslip, Jr., & P. L. Kaminski (Ed.), *Parenting the custodial grandchild: Implications for clinical practice* (pp. 53–73). New York: Springer.

Hayslip, B., Jr., Temple, J. R., Shore, R. J., & Henderson, C. E. (2006). Determinants of role satisfaction among traditional and custodial grandparents. In J. B. Hayslip, & J. H. Patrick (Ed.), *Custodial grandparenting: Individual, cultural, and ethnic diversity* (pp. 21–35).

Kaminski, P. L., & Hayslip, B. (2004, August). *Parenting attitudes of custodial grandparents.* Paper presented at the annual meeting of the American Psychological Association, Honolulu, HI.

Kelley, S. J., Whitley, D., Sipe, T. A., & Yorker, B. C. (2000). Psychological distress in grandmother kinship care providers: The role of resources, social support, and physical health. *Child Abuse and Neglect, 24*, 311–321.

Koenig, H. G., George, L. K., & Blazer, D. G. (1993). Abbreviating the Duke Social Support Index for use in chronically ill elderly individuals. *Psychosomatics, 34*, 61–69.

Kreider, R. M., & Ellis, R. (2011). Living arrangements of children: 2009 *Current Population Reports* (P70–126). Washington DC: U.S. Census Bureau. Retrieved 12-28-11 from http://www.census.gov/prod/2011pubs/p70-126.pdf

Leder, S., Grinstead, L. N., & Torres, E. (2007). Grandparents raising grandchildren: Stressors, social support, and health outcomes. *Journal of Family Nursing, 13*, 333–352.

Minkler, M., Fuller-Thomson, E., Miller, D., & Driver, D. (2000). Grandparent caregiving and depression. In B. Hayslip, Jr., & R. Goldberg-Glen, (Ed.), *Grandparents raising grandchildren: Theoretical, empirical, and clinical perspectives* (pp. 207–220). New York: Springer.

Musil, C. M., & Ahmad, M. (2002). Health of grandmothers: A comparison by caregiver status. *Journal of Aging and Health, 14*(1), 96–121.

Musil, C. M., Warner, C. B., Zauszniewski, J. A., Jeanblanc, A. B., & Kercher, K. (2006). Grandmothers, caregiving, and family functioning. *Journal of Gerontology: Social Sciences, 61B*, S89–S98.

Perugini, M., Gallucci, M., Presaghi, F., & Ercolani, P. (2003). The personal norm of reciprocity. *European Journal of Personality, 117*, 251–283.

Pruchno, R. (1999). Raising grandchildren: The experiences of Black and White grandmothers. *The Gerontologist, 39*, 209–221.

Radloff, L. S. (1977). The CES-D scale: A self-report depression scale for research in the general population. *Applied Psychological Measurement, 1*, 385–401.

Ramaswamy, V., Bhavnagri, N., & Barton, E. (2008). Social support and parenting behaviors influence grandchildren's social competence. In B. Hayslip, Jr., & P. L.

Kaminski (Ed.), *Parenting the custodial grandchild: Implications for clinical practice* (pp. 165–178). New York: Springer.

Rook, K. S. (2009). Gaps in social support resources in later life: An adaptational challenge in need of further research. *Journal of Social and Personal Relationships, 26*(1), 103–112.

Rutter, M. (2007). Resilience, competence, and coping. *Child Abuse & Neglect, 31*, 205–209.

Saluter, A. F. (1996). Marital status and living arrangements: March 1994, Current Population Reports (Series P20–484). Washington, DC: U.S. Government Printing Office.

Sands, R. G., Goldberg-Glen, R. S., & Shin, H. (2009). The voices of grandchildren of grandparent caregivers: A strengths-resilience perspective. *Child Welfare, 88*(2), 25–45.

Shin, S. H., Choi, H., Kim, M. J., & Kim, Y. H. (2010). Comparing adolescents' adjustment and family resilience in divorced families depending on the types of primary caregiver. *Journal of Clinical Nursing, 19*, 1695–1706.

Smith, G. C., & Hancock, G. R. (2010). Custodial grandmother-grandfather dyads: Pathways among marital distress, grandparent dysphoria, parenting practice, and grandchild adjustment. *Family Relations, 59*, 45–59.

Smith, G. C., & Richardson, R. A. (2008). Understanding the parenting practices of custodial grandmothers: Overcompensating, underserving, or overwhelmed? In B. Hayslip, Jr., & P. L. Kaminski (Ed.), *Parenting the custodial grandchild: Implications for clinical practice* (pp. 131–147). New York: Springer.

Tompkins, C. J. (2007). Who will care for the grandparents? *Journal of Psychosocial Nursing, 45*, 19–22.

Vaishnavi, S., Connor, K., & Davidson, J. R. T. (2007). An abbreviated version of the Connor-Davidson Resilience Scale (CD-RISC), the CD-RISC2: Psychometric properties and application in psychopharmacological trials. *Psychiatry Research, 152*, 293–297.

Waldrop, D. P. (2003). Caregiving issues for grandmothers raising their grandchildren. *Journal of Human Behavior in the Social Environment, 7*, 201–223.

Ware, J. E., Jr. (1993). *SF-36 health survey: Manual and interpretation guide.* Boston, MA: The Health Institute, New England Medical Center.

Wrosch, C., Heckhausen, J., & Lachman, M. E. (2000). Primary and secondary control strategies for managing health and financial stress across adulthood. *Psychology and Aging, 15*, 387–399.

Part III

Strength-Based Interventions with Grandparent Caregivers

11 Orienting to the Positive

A Practice Framework for Grandparent Caregiving

Francine Conway and Nathan S. Consedine

Abstract

The increasing numbers of grandparents providing primary care for their grandchildren in the United States continues to pose an enormous challenge for clinicians. Ongoing research suggests that grandparent caregivers (GPCs) are confronted with a large number of practical and psychological difficulties in caring for their grandchildren—age-congruent life tasks are interfered with, fulfilling aspects of the grandparenting role are obstructed, and GPCs report greater levels of stress, physical illness, alcoholism, smoking, anxiety, and depression. However, not all individuals suffer as greatly and some report deriving meaningful benefits from their grandparenting experience. In an exploratory study of 85 grandmothers raising their grandchildren, grandparents engaged in benefit finding with resulting benefits for their psychological and physical health. Consequently, while research documenting the problems confronting GPCs is important, an exclusive emphasis on the negative obscures an understanding of the benefits that may inhere. Because the literature on GPCs has focused on negative outcomes, we know little about who benefits, how they benefit, why they benefit, or implications for these potential differences. This chapter examined several bodies of literature germane to the GPCs' experience, offers evidence of both positive and negative valance experiences of GPCs and advances a practice framework for a positive and at least balanced orientation towards clinical practice with GPCs.

Adversity, no less than prosperity, can change us for better as well as for worse
(Affleck & Tennen, 1996)

Introduction

The number of grandparents who are currently providing primary care for their grandchildren has been on the rise. At one time, relatively few grandparents had primary responsibility for raising their grandchildren; however in the early 1980s grandparenthood arrived as a research focus for developmental researchers, and the resulting literature indicates that there has been a massive increase in this phenomenon to the extent that approximately 5% of contemporary American children live with grandparents, and in about one third of these cases neither biological parent is in the home (Conway, 1999). Additional data (Casper & Bryson, 1998) corroborate this trend and show that 3.9 million children were living with grandparents in 1997. According to the 2000 US Census, 4 million grandparent caregivers are caring for their grandchildren (Simmons & Dye, 2003). Although the US population has also grown since the 1980s, the intervening 30 years has nonetheless seen a relative increase from 3% to over 5% of all children. Increases have occurred in situations where the parent remains present as well as in those where the grandparent is the primary caregiver. Some combined households may reflect economic pressures, but situations where grandparents act as primary caregivers to their grandchildren represent the single greatest growth category between 1992 and 1997 (Casper & Bryson, 1998).

Both demographic patterns and public health considerations are contributing factors in this phenomenon. The increase of social problems that impact family structure is a major contributing factor to the unavailability of parents, while longer life spans and increased activity among the older populations, along with increasing rates of parental divorce, teen pregnancy, single parenting, and increases in the number of orphans are all thought to have a bearing on this trend. In addition, substance abuse, death due to AIDS, documented cases of child abuse and neglect, mental and physical illness and the incarceration of parents with a consequent court sanctioned termination of parental rights have all been cited as factors precipitating the grandparent caregiving situation (see Burton, 1992; Casper & Bryson, 1998; Hayslip & Kaminski, 2005; Kelly, 1993; Minkler, et al., 1992; Minkler, Roe, & Price, 1994; Poe, 1992). Consistent with these putative social-causative factors, Casper and Bryson's (1998) demographic analysis shows that a greater proportion of co-resident grandparents (i.e., those who live with their grandchildren but may or may not provide primary care) are female, perhaps because of greater male mortality and a lower likelihood of female remarriage following spousal death. In contrast, grandparent caregivers (i.e. those grandparents providing primary care) tended to be younger than the typical co-resident grandparent, although their health status tends to be similar. They are more likely to work and be educated than grandparents living in parent maintained households.

One must consider that, for previous studies, conclusions drawn may only emphasize the cost or burden associated with the grandparent caregiving experience. Undoubtedly, for the grandparent caregiver, the task of caring for one's grandchild may seem emotionally overwhelming and at times physically daunting. The stresses associated with caregiving tend to exacerbate existing medical conditions and allow grandparents little private time. However, despite these problems associated with caregiving, the parenting experience could prove gratifying and maybe even pleasurable for some grandparents. Therefore, it is our objective to present a broader view of the grandparenting experience by focusing on the benefits of caregiving as well as the cost in relation to traditional expectations (or sacrifices) made in assuming the grandparent caregiving relationship.

Role Conflict in Grandparent Caregiving

Grandparents parenting their grandchildren experience a grandparenting role that is markedly different from that which is more common in Western society. Grandparent caregivers are not as likely to experience grandparenting as only an opportunity to enjoy their grandchildren void of parental responsibilities. Rather, they become fully responsible for the child and are positioned to re-enter the parenting role. For grandparent caregivers, a Western perspective of grandparenting is unattainable because their circumstances dictate otherwise.

Unlike grandparents who develop traditional relationships with their grandchildren, grandparents who parent have the added responsibilities that accompany the parental role. Grandparent caregivers not only attend to the child's daily care, but also are responsible for their intellectual and emotional growth and development. Often, the child's needs require grandparents to accompany the child to weekly appointments with medical, mental health, and school professionals. In other words, attending to the child's well-being is an active, rather than passive, endeavor for grandparents. More compelling are the reasons grandparents offer for assuming caregiving responsibilities for their grandchildren. Grandparents assume primary caregiving roles that often stem from problems or deficits in the birth parent's relationship with the child; this pattern may, in part, explain the generally problem-focused portrayal of the grandparent caregiver phenomenon. Given that grandparent caregiving typically occurs in the context of negative circumstances, it seems unsurprising that the quality of life of grandparent caregivers has begun to suffer as they are increasingly drawn into the task of providing primary care for their grandchildren.

In order to appreciate the impact of parenting one's grandchild on grandparents, it is imperative that this examination occurs in the context of role expectations of grandparenting in general. A traditional classification of the grandparent role includes three dimensions: formal, fun seeking, and distant (Neugarten & Weinstein, 1964). Grandparents often opt for a fun seeking (pleasurable) relationship with their grandchild, one that is largely devoid of responsibility (Albrecht, 1954; Apple, 1956; Conway & Stricker, 2003), or one in which they function as mentors and role models (Conway & Stricker, 2003; Kornhaber & Woodward, 1981). A study by Kivnick (1982) found that grandparents derive meaning from their relationships with their grandchildren on several dimensions including: (a) centrality (role of grandparent is central in the grandparent's life); (b) valued elder (grandparent is the prized holder of tradition); (c) immortality through clan (grandparent's identification with grandchild as well as feelings of responsibility for family members); and (d) re-involvement with personal past (reliving their own lives through their grandchildren).

Sociological analyses stress the problems that arise due to conflicts between the necessary roles of the grandparent caregiver and the "expected" or traditional grandparenting roles. Jendrek (1993) suggests that grandparenting impacts four main areas of life: lifestyle, as well as relationships with friends, families and spouses. Conway (1999) likewise suggests that grandparent caregivers may well be deprived of the enjoyment of anticipated leisure and social life, a discrepancy referred to by Seltzer (1976) as "time disordered role desynchronization". Mui's (1992) conceptualization of role strain is similar in suggesting that there is an emotional cost to caregiving, particularly in circumstances characterized by major role changes (as in grandparent caregiving).

Empirical data are consistent with this view. Bongaarts, Menken, and Watkins (1984) have found that "parental" responsibilities adversely affected developmental milestones like retirement and leisure. Minkler et al. (1994) found that despite the supportive attitude of the spouse, female grandparents' relationships were negatively affected by the assumption of the caregiver role. Again, these authors ascribe this consequence to the infringement of caregiving on expected leisure time. In an intensive interview of 14 grandparent caregivers, Poe (1992) found that guilt characterized most grandparents' experience of caregiving, particularly where their role stemmed from their birth child's drug use. There were also feelings of self-blame, obligations, and a sense of betrayal. Although indirect, this latter finding, the "sense of betrayal", is likewise consistent with a view in which expectations have been violated.

Negative Impact of Grandparent Caregiving

Given such demands and pervasive role conflict, the fact that research generally offers a bleak picture of the mental and physical health of grandparent caregivers is perhaps not surprising. Roe, Minkler, Saunders, and Thompson (1996) report grandparent caregivers have poorer self-reported health and greater depression and anxiety compared to non-caregiving grandparents. Burton (1992) reported increases in physical illness, alcoholism, smoking, depression, and anxiety (see also Force, Botsford, Pisano, & Hobert, 2000), although she notes that stresses were not limited to the grandparenting situation, but were also related to family members and the neighborhood. However, compared to non-caregiving grandparents, depression and anxiety were more prevalent among younger grandparent caregivers and among those caregivers with lower educational backgrounds (Kolomer, McCallion, & Janicki, 2002; Sands & Goldberg Glen, 2000). The caregiver is often confined to the home and ties to other people may be compromised (e.g. Pietromonaco, Manis, & Frohardt-Lane, 1986). Kelly (1993) reported heightened stress and negative impact on relationships with friends, family, and spouses (see also Jendrek, 1993). Overall, researchers have found grandparent caregivers report more impaired health compared to their non-caregiving peers (Grinstead, Leder, Jensen, & Bond, 2003; Whitley, Pipe, & Crofts Yorker, 2000).

The extent to which these concerns are relevant is presumably influenced by the extent of the grandparent's involvement in parenting, legal status, and day care responsibilities. Minkler, et al. (1994) found that the stress of grandparenting children born with *in utero* exposure to drugs was moderated by informal support from friends and family. This support may be both instrumental and emotional. Kelly (1993) found that stress, social isolation, and role restriction were good predictors of stress in caregivers. In contrast, however, Conway (1999) found that assistance from others did little to alleviate the impact of caregiving on grandmothers. She suggests that while assistance is helpful, it does not reduce strain, but rather makes the grandmother feel better about having adopted caregiver responsibilities. Additionally, grandmothers who were married experienced less strain, and it may be that the support offered by a spouse is more regularly and directly practical or emotionally supportive than that offered by other individuals in the social network.

According to Thomas, Sperry, and Yarbrough (2000) an understanding of adult outcomes must be explicated in relation to the characteristics of the children involved, and these children are typically troubled (see e.g. Dubowitz & Sawyer, 1994). The rationale underlying this assertion stems from the fact that custodial grandparenting nearly always emerges in response to a crisis in the family of origin. Indeed, while most grandparent caregiving experiences seem to be characterized by some level of financial, physical or psychological difficulty, the difficulties increase in circumstances where grandparents assume custody of grandchildren because their own children are abusive, incarcerated, or too ill to care for their children (Thomas et al., 2000). Conway (1999), for example, reports that the number of behavioral problems the child was having was an important predictor of whether grandmothers reported strain (see also Daly & Glenwick, 2000). Schwartz (1994) suggests that the discrepancy between the age of the caregiver and the child may make it difficult for the grandparent to negotiate issues relating to the child's development, academic life, and peer interactions.

The Conceptual and Philosophical Problems

Orienting to the Negative

> "Psychology is not just the study of pathology, weakness, and damage; it is also the study of strength and virtue"
>
> Seligman & Csikszentmihalyi (2000)

Inherent in the "problem" of grandparent caregiving are a number of conceptual and methodological issues. Below, we consider a conceptual problem evident in the literature on grandparent caregiving; the distorted picture engendered by near-singular emphasis on negative outcomes and adjustment difficulties. As is quickly evident in a consideration of the literature on the social, psychological, and physical consequences of grandparent caregiving described above, we know vastly more about the problems caregiving grandparents experience than we do about how successfully they adapt to their circumstances, or any positive outcomes that might accrue. In part, this jaundiced view may simply represent a specific instantiation of psychology's historical orientation to investigating the negative aspects of human functioning. As Seligman and Csikszentmihalyi (2000) have noted, post World War II psychology has been predominantly a science of healing that concentrates on repairing damage within a disease model of human functioning. Given this legacy, we have comptively scant knowledge regarding what makes life worth living or how and why people flourish.

However, recent developments in preventative and emerging positive psychology traditions naturally lend themselves to the understanding of human strength and successful adaptation under adversity. Concepts and personal attributes like faith, optimism, courage, and the ability to find benefits in adversity now represent major research areas, and several researchers are beginning to document how positive human attributes can prevent dysfunction (see e.g. Taylor, 1983, 1989; Taylor & Brown, 1988, 1994). Saleeby's (1996, 1997) "strengths perspective" is similar in that it provides a more inclusive view of the individual's situation, focusing not only on deficits, but also on the individual, family, and community's capacities, talents, competencies, possibilities, visions, values, and hopes (Saleeby, 1996). Attributes such as humor, loyalty, insight, and management skills can be enlisted to overcome adversities (Valliant, 1993).

Although this approach has yet to be systematically applied in the context of grandparent caregiver research, theory provides sound grounds for expecting that these individuals may gain meaningful benefits from their experience. The view offered by Whitley, White, Kelley, and Yorke (1999) emphasizes concepts such as empowerment and resilience and their use in coping among grandparent caregivers. Below, we continue to develop this alternative to the predominantly palliative, negative, or deficit-based approach that dominates contemporary grandparent caregiver research. We suggest that a substantial proportion of grandparent caregivers may obtain meaningful benefits from their experiences and outline an applied practice considerations for positive approaches to grandparent caregiving.

Orienting to the Positive

Saleeby (1996) offered a supplementary view of the client's presenting problem that we advance as applicable to work involving grandparents parenting their grandchildren. The strengths perspective offers a holistic view of the client's situation, focusing not only on deficits, but on the individual, family, or community's intellectual, emotional, and physical capabilities however distorted these may have become through circumstance (Saleeby, 1996).

In making an argument for the strengths perspective, Saleeby's approach is in stark contrast with the more conventional pathology-based view of clients' circumstances. The strengths perspective offers a unique view that supports the accomplishments of individuals who may be experiencing difficulty in their lives. Although the difficulties are very salient for the client, a strengths approach dictates that practitioners and helping agents empower the client through identifying, acknowledging, and making use of the client's internal and external resources (Pinderhughes, 1995). Internal resources incorporate personal attributes of the individual that could be used as coping/survival tools. For example, humor, loyalty, insight, and management skills could be enlisted to help overcome present adversities (Vaillant, 1993). However, external resources are more exemplified by one's membership in a community that offers informal social and intergenerational networks, and fosters friendships and supportive relationships, which serve a protective function and minimize risks (Saleeby, 1996). Consideration of the grandparent caregiving situation from a strengths perspective offers a supplementary view of the experience that serves to empower grandmothers, emphasize their personal attributes, and help them to view community memberships as a source of support.

Benefit Finding in Grandparent Caregivers

There is very little research on benefit finding in grandparent caregivers. Research by Neugarten and Weinstein (1978) shows that grandmothers often view grandparenting as an opportunity for "biological renewal" while grandfathers view it as an opportunity for emotional fulfillment, although whether these same experiences remain for grandparents of the current birth cohorts, or those who provide primary care for their grandchildren remains unclear. Although a less documented view, grandparent caregiving, while stressful, is not entirely a negative experience. A few studies have considered the benefits of grandparent caregiving.

Grandparent caregiving has been found to be physically beneficial to grandparent caregivers in providing grandparents with increased opportunities to have active lifestyles and in preparing healthier meals (Hayslip & Kaminski, 2005). Also, psychological gains in relationship closeness with grandchildren enhance grandparent caregiver's sense of purpose gained from carrying out caregiving tasks (Hayslip & Kaminski, 2005; Kropf & Yoon, 2006). Moreover, among African-American grandparent caregivers, for approximately 10% of the caregivers, assumption of the caregiving role reinforces a tradition of surrogate and extended family care which is valued in the culture (Goodman & Silverstein, 2006; Hunter & Tayler, 1998). In addition, African-American grandmothers obtain a sense of pride from caregiving particularly in situations where caregiving leads to enabling young mothers to pursue and accomplish their career goals (Minkler & Fuller-Thomson, 2005).

It is decidedly the point of this chapter to advance a more positive and empowering perspective of a most challenging life situation that grandparents experience as primary caregivers. In order to apply the strengths perspective to the grandparent caregiver situation, a description of both aspects (costs vs. benefits) of the grandparent caregiving experience should be made salient. Moreover, consistent with Saleeby's conceptualization of the strengths perspective, it is imperative that grandparents' needs are explored in the context of existing sources of supports. This contrast between need and support is important in demonstrating the shift in perspective from a problem-focused orientation to a strengths perspective. A unique aspect of this study is the formulation of an intervention model that can be used to empower grandparents who parent.

Aims

1. To present a balanced view of the grandparent's experience of their caregiving role by describing the differential nature of their experience.
2. To identify and present grandparent caregivers' needs in the context of external resources available to grandparent caregivers.
3. To formulate a model of intervention with grandparent caregivers based on the strengths perspective.

Method

Participants

Eighty-five grandmothers who were recruited to participate in this study cared for at least one grandchild (18 years or younger) at least five days/week. The participants were recruited from grandparent support programs, schools, doctors' offices, parenting classes, gerontology, and aging organizations, and foster care agencies in the New York metropolitan area. Grandmothers participated voluntarily and without remuneration.

Procedure

Grandmothers who expressed interest in the study were contacted by phone, introduced to the study, and a telephone interview was conducted. Of those interviewed 82.4% were primary caretakers in parent-absent households; 96.5% cared for their grandchild seven days per week while the remaining 3.5% cared for their grandchild at least five days per week.

A brief screening interview established the grandmother's eligibility for the study as follows: (1) grandmothers who were primarily responsible for their grandchild's care five or more days per week and (2) grandmothers parenting grandchildren who were under 18 years old. Demographic information was obtained using a questionnaire that was piloted for clarity of language. Grandmothers were then asked open ended questions about the following: (a) what sacrifices they make for their grandchild; (b) what they liked least and liked best about the grandchild; (c) benefits obtained from the caregiving relationship; (d) assistance the grandmother receives; and (e) what the grandmother needs to help in her parenting role. An initial sample was used to develop qualitative categories and train coders. Independent raters were used to code the test data and to establish inter-rater reliability ($r = .85$).

Demographic Characteristics of Grandmothers

The mean age of grandmothers and their grandchildren was 59.6 years and 7.9 years respectively. The ages of the children ranged from newborn to 18 years old. The mean age of the grandchildren when they first came to live with their grandmother was 2.9 years. Forty-six percent of the grandmothers cared for one grandchild; 25% of the grandmothers cared for two grandchildren; and 24.7% of the grandmothers cared for 3–5 grandchildren. Sixty-six percent of the participants were maternal grandmothers. The mean age for the grandchild's biological parent was 32.6 years, ranging from 16 to 50 years. Sixty-two percent of the parenting arrangements were permanent ones, and 51.8% of all grandparent-grandchild relationships were legally mandated.

Results

In order to apply the strengths perspective to the grandparent caregiver situation, it is necessary to understand the types of benefits associated with caregiving. The study considers the grandmothers' parenting experience in terms of sacrifices made for her grandchildren, benefits received from the relationship, and aspects of the relationship reported as most and least favorable. Consideration of grandmothers' needs in the context of external resources is also a key component of the strengths model that requires exploration of not only grandmother's needs, but also assistance received with regard to caregiving.

Eighty-five percent of the grandmothers reported making sacrifices for their grandchildren, including time, money, infringement on personal needs, privacy/home, work/professional goals, and favorite activities, and others report they gave up having a "life" for their grandchildren (Table 11.1). However, only 58.8% of grandmothers could identify what those sacrifices were.

In spite of the difficulties, 83.5% of the grandmothers also reported that they benefit from the caregiving relationship. Of the grandmothers, 36.5%

Table 11.1 Sacrifices Experienced in the Grandparent Caregiving Experience

Types of Sacrifices	*Percentage of Grandmothers reporting sacrifice (N = 85)*
Cannot identify	23.5
Money	16.5
Personal needs	14.1
I've given up having a life	8.2
Time	7.1
Favorite activities	4.7
Profession	3.5
Various other	3.5
Privacy/home	1.2
None	15.3

Table 11.2 Benefits of the Grandparent Caregiving Experience

Types of Benefits	*Percentage of Grandmothers reporting benefits (N = 85)*
Enhanced psychological well-being	36.5
Companionship	14.1
Inspirational	12.9
Positive [observed] voyeuristic experiences	11.8
Caring for the child	10.6
Education	9.4
Various other	7.1
Assistance with chores and other duties	4.7
Qualities of the child	1.2
None reported	15.3

reported that the relationship enhanced their psychological well-being. Some grandmothers who benefited from the relationship offered more varied and individual reasons such as companionship, assistance with chores and other duties, educational enhancement, inspiration/motivation, caring for the child, qualities of the child, and various other benefits (Table 11.2).

Furthermore, 96% of the grandmothers identified something they liked best about the caregiving role. Twenty-five percent (25.9%) enjoyed the psychological aspects of the relationship, 22.4% liked the qualities of the grandchild best, and other grandmothers offered a variety of experiences they liked best about the parenting experience.

Grandmothers also identified an aspect of the relationship they liked least (75.3%). Disciplining (21.2%) and some behavioral characteristics of the grandchild (16.5%) were aspects of the relationship grandmothers liked the least. Other reasons such as the chores, time commitment, financial demands, and emotional strain were also offered to a lesser extent.

Most grandmothers (55.3%) received some help in parenting their grandchildren. Grandparents were helped by a relative (32.9%); and various friends, churches, social service agencies, legal agencies, schools, jobs, and grandparent support services (Table 11.3). Nevertheless, 71% of the grandmothers expressed need of more assistance. Grandmothers' needs included financial assistance, respite care, psychological/emotional support for themselves and their grandchildren, help negotiating with various agencies on behalf of their grandchild, and various other needs (Table 11.4).

Discussion

The grandparenting experience for grandmothers who serve as caregivers for their grandchildren is admittedly a strenuous and difficult one. However, consideration of this unusual parenting arrangement from a strengths perspective offers a broader model for understanding this complex relationship and has

Table 11.3 External Resources Available to Help Grandmothers Parent Grandchildren

Type of Assistance	*Percentage of grandmothers receiving assistance (N = 85)*
Relative	32.9
Friends	9.4
Churches	7.1
Grandparent support services	5.9
Social service agencies	3.5
Legal agencies	3.5
Other	3.5
Schools	2.4
Jobs	2.4
None	43.5

Table 11.4 Areas in Which Grandmothers Need Assistance in Parenting Their Grandchildren

Areas of need	*Percentage of grandmothers reporting areas of needed assistance (N = 85)*
Financial assistance	12.9
Respite care	10.6
Assistance in negotiating various agencies	10.6
Psychological support for self and grandchild	3.5
Various others	9.4
None	28.2

the potential to empower grandmothers seeking assistance with the emotional adjustment to parenting a second time. Perhaps most importantly, this report found that grandmothers' identification of sacrifices made in the relationship did not preclude them from identifying benefits associated with caregiving; grandmothers presented a balanced view of the parenting experience by reporting favorable as well as unfavorable aspects of the caregiving experience. Finally, although grandmothers' caregiving needs were pervasive, participants reported that their ability to obtain help was limited.

Grandmothers' ability to identify benefits as well as sacrifices in their caregiving suggests that grandparent caregiving is experienced in a highly differentiated manner. Firstly, grandmothers' acknowledgment of sacrifices associated with the caregiving experience suggests they are not simply denying the difficulties that arise from caregiving. Some of the sacrifices grandmothers reported affected their ability to provide self-care. For example, grandmothers often sacrificed personal time and attention to personal needs. In addition, other sacrifices interrupted grandmothers' professional development. Some grandmothers reported quitting their jobs or not pursuing advancements in their profession because it would take away from the time needed to meet the child's needs. Often grandmothers' available time was limited by the child's school schedule and grandmothers arrange their days around drop-off and pick-up times for school. Grandmothers spoke at length about the sacrifice of their homes. Grandmothers find housekeeping a challenge due to the enormity of the chores, and some grandmothers even gave up their sleeping accommodations to make a comfortable habitat for their grandchildren.

Secondly, however, and in spite of the many sacrifices, grandmothers were able to identify benefits associated with the caregiving experience. Grandmothers' described concrete rewards such as help with the chores and enjoying the companionship the child offered. Some grandmothers took very real pleasure in the actual caring for the child such as dressing them, giving a bath, and the like. Other grandmothers felt inspired by the child and derived a sense of vicarious pleasure from observing the child learn. Grandmothers' optimism may bode well for their psychological well-being. Moreover, the identification of benefits associated with parenting their grandchild suggests some mutual exchange between grandparent and grandchild. Awareness of what the child offers may serve to strengthen the relationship in the grandparent-grandchild dyad. The child's awareness of what he/she brings to the relationship may also serve to build self-esteem and feelings of being important in the face of having been abandoned.

Further support of grandmothers' balanced view of the parenting experience is evident in grandmothers' report of favorable as well as unfavorable aspects of the parenting experience. This finding is consistent with earlier research demonstrating that grandmothers have some ability to consider both aspects of the parenting experience (Burton, 1995; Jendrek, 1993). Grandmothers experienced disciplining their grandchildren as an unpleasant task and did not enjoy the demands of time and money. Nevertheless, they were able to enjoy personal characteristics of their grandchild such as their sense of humor.

Finally, the prevalence of grandmothers' reported need for assistance with parenting (71%) is in stark contrast to grandmothers' perception of identifiable resources available to them to assist in caregiving (only 56% reported receiving any help). Grandmothers reported that some of their needs included financial assistance, a respite from the caregiving, help negotiating the various bureaucratic systems to obtain services for their grandchild, and emotional support for themselves and their grandchild. Grandmothers who received assistance identified informal sources (such as friends and families) as well as more formal ones (such as legal aid, churches, places of employment, and schools). Grandmothers' identification of others who are emotionally invested in their grandchildren is an invaluable source of support, along with those who may offer concrete support such as finances and childcare.

Strengths Intervention Model

The results of this study support the adoption of a strengths perspective when working with grandparents who are raising their grandchildren. A strengths perspective offers a viable means of a therapist's intervention with grandmother caregivers. The identification of positive aspects of the experience constitutes the first level of intervention that can be achieved through interviewing grandparents about their experiences. Therapeutic efforts to help grandparents integrate both positive and negative aspects of the caregiving experience are necessary. Grandmothers who deny the realistic hardships as well as grandmothers who only view the experience negatively may have difficulty in adjusting to their parenting role.

The second stage of intervention with grandmother caregivers might benefit from focusing on identification of resources within their community and providing grandparents with skills to help them better utilize available resources. Grandmothers, with the help of a worker, can identify and enlist support of others and learn how to make use of problem solving skills when faced with difficult child rearing circumstances. Some grandmothers may need further assistance in constructing a formal support network of institutional resources. Helping agents should be aware of the areas in which grandmothers may require assistance. Grandmothers' needs ranged from concrete support such as finances and childcare to emotional support for themselves and their grandchildren.

Grandmothers would benefit from a therapeutic relationship with the clearly defined goal of helping them to identify personal attributes they may utilize in the parenting experience as well as to identify any skills, abilities, knowledge, and insight they have gained as a result of this challenging parenting experience. Often, grandmothers are burdened under the myriad tasks the parenting role demands. They tend to feel overwhelmed and may have little available time for introspection and consideration of their situation. Exploration of personal attributes serves to empower grandmothers whose resources may be depleted as a result of the caregiving situation. In addition, insight gained from the caregiving experience points to grandparents' adaptive and coping abilities in the long run.

Benefit Finding in Grandparent Caregivers: A Practice Framework

Having outlined several major bodies of literature germane to the consideration of benefit finding in grandparent caregivers, we conclude by offering some preliminary guidelines, clinical practice and devote some consideration to two key questions, the answers to which we feel will stimulate theory and practice approaches in the field.

Question 1: What Is the Source of Benefit Finding in Grandparent Caregivers?

Of the questions considered here, the one with the greatest practical potential relates to the nature of benefit finding. Both among grandparents and more generally, it remains unclear whether benefit finding is a trait-like personality variable or whether it is a coping ability that can be learned. In considering the former possibility, authors have linked benefit finding to dispositional optimism (Tennen, Affleck, Urrows, & Higgins, 1992), as well as to Extraversion and Openness to Experience. Several studies using the Life Orientation Test (LOT; Scheier & Carver, 1985) have shown that certain types of belief and perceptions closely related to benefit finding are related to optimistic expectations. In a study of grandmothers raising their grandchildren, Conway and colleagues found less adverse health outcomes among those grandmothers rating high on dispositional optimism (Conway, Magai, Springer, & Jones, 2008). Benefit finding may represent a specific instantiation of dispositional optimism (Scheier & Carver, 1985) insofar as optimists are more likely to perceive benefits (e.g. Tedeschi & Calhoun, 1996) and be less distressed by adversity (Scheier, Carver, & Bridges, 1994).

Question 2: How Does Age Impact on the Ability for Grandparent Caregivers to Find Benefits?

Perhaps because people are led to expect that old age will be a time of loss, older people often see themselves as faring better than most other people or as surpassing their expectations of age (Carstensen, Gross, & Fung, 1998). There is empirical evidence that older people engage in relatively more downward and less upward social comparison than younger people (Heckhausen & Krueger, 1993). There is also some suggestion that benefit finding may be a developmental trend. More generally, age is generally thought to be associated with improved emotion regulatory capacities (Gross, Carstensen, Pasupathi, Tsai, Gotestam-Skorpen, & Hsu, 1997). It is quite possible that developmentally older grandparents are more likely to value social relations, preserving the grandparent-grandchild relationship takes precedence over the demands of caregiving.

Concluding Remarks

This chapter demonstrates that having participants identify costs or sacrifices in a caregiving relationship did not preclude them also reporting substantial benefits, and indeed, most individuals reported a balance of benefits and costs. In terms of specific benefits, the data presented here suggest that grandmothers derive a great deal of pleasure directly through the relationship itself. Future research and case presentations are needed to support this strengths approach of working with grandparents and its impact on their ability to adjust to the caregiving role.

Although grandparent caregivers are confronted with a large number of practical and psychological difficulties in caring for their grandchildren, we have argued that an exclusively negative practice orientation to grandparent caregiving may overshadow a more positive outlook and the potential benefits to the grandparents and grandchildren. We have outlined a number of difficulties within current conceptualizations of grandparent caregiving, and offer an approach based on the notion that many grandparents find significant meaning and positive benefits in their experience.

References

Affleck, G., & Tennen, H. (1996). Construing benefits from adversity: Adaptational significance and dispositional underpinnings. *Journal of Personality, 64*, 899–922.

Albrecht, R. (1954). "The parental responsibility of grandparents," *Marriage and Family Living, 16*, 201–204.

Apple, D. (1956). "The social structure of grandparenthood," *American Anthropologist, 58*, 656–663.

Bryson, K., & Casper, L. (1998). "Co-resident grandparents and their grandchildren: Grandparent maintained families," U.S. Census Bureau, Population Division.

Bowers, B. F., & Myers, B. J. (1999). Grandmothers providing care for grandchildren: Consequences of various levels of caregiving. *Family Relations: Interdisciplinary Journal of Applied Family Studies, 48*(3), 303–311.

Boyer, N. C., & Poindexter, C. C. (2005). Barriers to permanency planning for older HIV affected caregivers. *Journal of Gerontological Social Work, 44*(3/4), 59–74.

Burton, L. M. (1992). "Black grandparents rearing children of drug-addicted parents: stressors, outcomes and the social service needs." *The Gerontologist*, v32 n6, 744–751.

Burton, L. M., Dilworth-Anderson, P., & Merriwether-de-Vries, C. (1995). "Context and surrogate parenting among contemporary grandparents." *Marriage-and-Family-Review, 20*(3–4), 349–366.

Carstensen, L. L., Gross, J. J., & Fung, H. H. (1998). The social context of emotional experience. In. K. W. Schaie & M. P. Lawton (Eds.), *Annual review of gerontology and geriatrics, vol. 17: Focus on emotion and adult development* (pp. 325–352). New York, NY: Springer.

Carver, C. S., Pozo, C., Harris, S. D., Noriega, V., Scheier, M. F., Robinson, D. S., Ketcham, A. S., Moffatt, F. L., & Clark, K. C. (1993). How coping mediates the effect of optimism on distress: A study of women with early stage breast cancer, *Journal of Personality and Social Psychology, 65*, 375–390.

Cherlin, A. J., & Furstenberg, F., Jr. (1986). "Grandparents and family crisis." *Generations, 10*(4), 26–28.

Consedine, N. S., & Fiori, K. L. (2009). Gender moderates the associations between attachment and discrete emotions in middle age and later life. *Aging and Mental Health, 13*(6), 847–862.

Conway, F. (1999). *A role theory perspective of grandmothers' emotional cost of caregiving to their grandchildren: Its significance on developmental stages in their life cycle.* Adelphi University.

Conway, F., Magai, C., Springer, C., & Jones, S. (2008). Optimism and pessimism as predictors of physical and psychological health among grandmothers raising their grandchildren. *Journal of Research in Personality, 42*(5), 1352–1357.

Conway, F., & Stricker, G. (2003). An integrative assessment model as a means of intervention with grandparent caregivers. In Hayslip, B. & Hicks Patrick, J. (Eds.), *Working with custodial grandparents* (pp. 45–57). New York, NY, US: Springer Publishing Co.

Curbow, B., Somerfield, M., Baker, F., Wingard, J., & Legro, M. (1993). Personal changes, dispositional optimism, and psychological adjustment to bone marrow transplantation. *Journal of Behavioral Medicine, 16*, 423–443.

Fiori, K. L., Consedine, N. S., & Magai, C. (2009). Patterns of relating among men and women from seven ethnic groups. *Journal of Cross-Cultural Gerontology, 24*(2), 121–141.

Fontaine, K. R., Manstead, A. S., & Wagner, H. (1993). Optimism, perceived control over stress, and coping. *European Journal of Personality, 7*, 267–281.

Garmezy, N. (1993) "Children in poverty: Resilience despite risk." *Psychiatry: Interpersonal and Biological Processes, 56*(1), 127–136.

Grinstead, L. N., Leder, S., Jensen, S., & Bond, L. (2003). Review of research on the health of caregiving grandparents. *Journal of Advance Nursing, 44*(3), 318–326.

Gross, J. J., Carstensen, L. L., Pasupathi, M., Tsai, J., Goestestam Skorpen, C., & Hsu, A. Y. C. (1997). Emotion and aging: Experience, expression, and control. *Psychology and Aging, 12*, 590–599.

Hayslip, B. J., & Kaminski, P. L. (2005). Grandparents raising their grandchildren: A review of the literature and suggestions for practice. *The Gerontologist, 45*(2), 262–269.

Heckhausen, J., & Krueger, J. (1993). Developmental expectations for the self and most other people: Age grading in three functions of social comparison. *Developmental Psychology, 29*, 539–548.

Heckhausen, J., & Schulz, R. (1995). A life-span theory of control. *Psychological Review, 102*, 284–304.

Janicki, M. P., McCallion, P., Grant-Griffin, L., & Kolomer, S. R. (2000). Grandparent caregivers I: Characteristics of the grandparents and the children with disabilities for whom they care. *Journal of Gerontological Social Work, 33*(3), 35–55.

Jendrek, M. (1993). "Grandparents who parent their grandchildren: effects on lifestyle." *Journal of Marriage and the Family, 55*, 609–621.

Johnson, C. L. (1983). "A cultural analysis of the grandmother." *Research-on-Aging, 5*(4), 547–567.

Kelly, S. (1993). "Caregiver stress in grandparents raising grandchildren." *Image: Journal of Nursing Scholarship, 25*(4).

Kelley, S. J., Whitley, D., Sipe, T. A., & Crofts Yorker, B. (2000). Psychological distress in grandmother kinship care providers: The role of resources, social support, and physical health. *Child Abuse & Neglect, 24*(3), 311–321.

Kivnick, H. Q. (1982). Grandparenthood: An overview of meaning and mental health. *The Gerontologist, 22*, 59–66.

Kolomer, S. R., McCallion, P., & Janicki, M. P. (2002). African American grandmother carers of children with disabilities: predictors of depressive symptoms. *Journal of Gerontological Social Work, 37*(3/4), 45–63.

Kornhaber, A., & Woodward, K. L. (1981). Grandparents/Grandchildren: The vital connection. Garden City New York: Anchor Press/Doubleday.

Kropf, N. P., & Yoon, E. (2006). Grandparents raising grandchildren: Who are they? In B. Berkman (Ed.), *Handbook of social work in health and aging* (pp. 355–362). New York: Oxford.

Lazarus, R. S., & Folkman, S. (1984). *Stress, appraisal and coping*. New York. Springer.

Lee, R. D., Ensminger, M. E., & LaVeist, T. A. (2005). The responsibility continuum: Never primary, coresident and caregiver: Heterogeneity in the African-American grandmother experience. *International Journal of Aging and Human Development, 60*(4), 295–304.

Lehman, D. R., Davis, C. G., DeLongis, A., Wortman, C. B., Bluck, S., Mandel, D. R., & Ellard, H. (1993). Positive and negative life changes following bereavement and their relations to adjustment. *Journal of Social and Clinical Psychology, 12*, 90–112.

McCrae, R. R., & Costa, P. T. (1986). Personality, coping and coping effectiveness in an adult sample. *Journal of Personality, 54*, 385–405.

Merz, E.-M., & Consedine, N. S. (2009). Attachment security moderates the links between emotional and instrumental family support and wellbeing in later life. *Attachment and Human Development, 11*(2), 203–221.

Minkler, M., Roe, K. M., & Price, M. (1992). "The physical and emotional health of grandmothers raising grandchildren in the crack cocaine epidemic," *The Gerontologist, 32*, 752–761.

Neugarten, B., & Weinstein, K. (1964). "The changing American grandparents," *Journal of Marriage and Family, 26*, 199–204.

Pinderhughes, E. (1995). "Empowering diverse populations: Family practice in the 21st Century," *Families in Society, 76*(3), 131–140.

Poe, L. M. (1992). Black Grandparents as Parents. Library of Congress.

Roe, K. M., Minkler, M., & Barnwell, R. (1994). "The assumption of caregiving: grandmothers raising the children of the crack cocaine epidemic." *Qualitative-Health-Research, 4*(3), 281–303.

Rutter, M. (1985). "Resilience in the face of adversity: Protective factors and resistance psychiatric disorder," *British Journal of Psychiatry, 147*, 598–611.

Saleebey, D. (1996). "The strengths perspective in social work practice: Extensions and cautions." *Social Work, 41*(3), 296–305.

Sands, R. G., & Goldberg-Glen, R. S. (2000). Factors associated with stress among grandparents raising their grandchildren. *Family Relations, 49*, 97–195.

Sands, R. G., Goldberg-Glen, R. S., & Thornton, P. L. (2005). Factors associated with the positive well-being of grandparents caring for their grandchildren. *Journal of Gerontological Social Work, 45*(4), 65–82.

Scheier, M. F., & Carver, C. S. (1985). Optimism, coping, and health: Assessment and implications of generalized outcome expectancies. *Health Psychology, 4*, 219–247.

Simmons, T., & Dye, J. L. (2003). *Grandparents living with grandchildren: 2000.* Washington, DC: U.S. Dept of Commerce. Retrieved July 20, 2008, from http://www.census.gov.

Tedeschi, R. G., & Calhoun, L. G. (1996). The posttraumatic growth inventory: Measuring the positive legacy of trauma. *Journal of Traumatic Stress, 9*, 455–472.

Tennen, H., Affleck, G., Urrows, S., & Higgins, P. (1992). Perceived control, construing benefits, and daily processes in rheumatoid arthritis. *Canadian Journal of Behavioral Science, 24*, 186–203.

U.S. Census Bureau 2000 Special Report (2004, March). Children and the households they live in: 2000. Retrieved from: www.census.gov/prod/2004pubs/censr-14.pdf.

Vaillant, G., & Koury, S. (1993). Late midlife development. In Pollock, George H. & Greenspan, Stanley I. (Eds.), *The course of life, Vol. 6: Late adulthood* (rev. and exp. ed.) (pp. 1–22). Madison, CT, US: International Universities Press, Inc. x, 550 pp.

Waldrop, D. P., & Weber, J. A. (2001). From grandparent to caregiver: The stress and satisfaction of raising grandchildren. *Families in Society, 82*(5), 461–472.

Winston, C. A. (2006). African American grandmothers parenting AIDS orphans: grieving and coping. *Qualitative Social Work, 5*(1), 33–43.

12 Skip Generations

A Strength-Based Mentoring Program for Resilient Grandparent Caregivers

Linda C. James and Christopher R. Ferrante

Abstract

Skip Generations, a program of Family Resource Centers of Crestwood, located in Rochester, NY, offers a unique and empowering mentoring program to grandparents and other kin who are the primary caregivers for children. A pair of two kinship caregivers—primarily grandmothers raising their grandchildren—provides support and mentorship to other kinship caregivers in the community through home visits twice a month. The hope is that, after ayear of support from their mentors, the mentees will join one of the support groups that *Skip Generations* offers and eventually become mentors themselves. This program is driven by a philosophy of empowerment, and the immeasurable experience that these mentors have not only ensures they will be empathetic, but also makes certain they will become a valuable resource to their mentees. In the process of rearing their grandchildren, the grandparents in this program have endured a wide range of feelings and emotions. Through the home visits, participants in *Skip Generations* learn how to express—and work through—these emotions. They realize that they are not alone, and that they must be healthy themselves in order to adequately provide care and support to the children they are raising.

Isolated, shocked, uncertain, hopeless. These are some of the words that *attempt* to describe what Linda James was feeling when her life took a drastic turn in 1987, when she was just 40 years old. Linda shares her story with as much passion as she has when she cares for her beloved grandchildren:

> *My story, like those of so many grandparents who are raising their grandchildren, began many years ago. In 1987, when my granddaughter was born, she weighed 1 lb. 4 oz. at birth. She was born in a drug house and later transported to Children's Hospital in Washington, D.C. I was notified by the hospital that my granddaughter needed surgery and that the hospital couldn't find her mother. I gave consent for the surgery and asked the hospital to stay in contact with me because I would take responsibility for my granddaughter when it was time for her to be released. I knew that my daughter would not*

be located because she was back on the streets. When the hospital notified me that she could be released, I had to find a way to bring her here to Rochester. She was hooked-up with a heart monitor and breathing machine that would require a private plane with a medical staff. After many attempts to find an agency to help me, a local radio station (WVOR) arranged a flight to Washington, D.C. for me and also helped to arrange a Mercy flight from Washington to Rochester with a nurse aboard.

This was a journey that would dramatically change my life. I was forced to quit my job at Strong Memorial Hospital in order to take care of her and apply for assistance through our local Department of Human Services.

Two years later, I was making that same journey to pick up her brother who also was born prematurely. His weight was 1 lb. 4 oz.; my daughter, at the time of his birth, was still using drugs.

In 1990, I was able to bring my daughter to Rochester, hoping that the change would give her the desire to change her lifestyle. She stayed clean for six months, and then returned to her patterns of drug abuse. A year later, her body was found in an abandoned field; she was strangled two days before her 26th birthday. After the death of my daughter, I received, along with my grandchildren, counseling to help us deal with loss and grief.

In time, I found a job at Family Resource Centers of Crestwood, and eventually my experience and passion for supporting my grandchildren carried over to what is now my professional career. For the past fourteen years, my full-time work continues as the Community-Based Supervisor for Skip Generations, providing education and support for grandparents who are raising their grandchildren.

Families comprised of grandparents and other relatives raising children are not new. In many of these kinship care families, the grandparent becomes the child's custodian for many reasons, including, but not limited to: parental drug abuse, incarceration, military duties, child abuse, and neglect. In a high number of these cases, the children have special needs. Grandparents and relatives often choose not to refer the children to the foster care system because of their desire to keep the children in the family, in the neighborhood, close to their relatives and siblings. In more collectivist, group-oriented cultures, this is a value highly regarded. The result, however, is a financially-burdened family with fewer resources for both the aging grandparent and the children in his or her care. Grandparents and relatives providing kinship care have cited their own need for support, with the following goals: reducing their isolation, gaining valuable information and sources of referral, receiving assistance in working with the children's parents, learning to navigate the education system for children with special needs, receiving respite care and emergency clothing and food, reducing stress, finding social activities for the family, finding adequate housing, gaining access to community resources, a supportive network, and financial assistance—and this is not an exhaustive list by any means.

Linda James is not alone in parenting a second time around. Nationwide, the 2010 Census data shows a 7% increase in children under the age of 18 living in grandparent-headed households (4.9 million, up from 4.5 million 10 years ago). Grandparents taking on the sole responsibility of providing a stable home for their grandchildren are steadily increasing in numbers. Approximately 11,500 grandchildren in Monroe County alone are being raised by their grandparents. The custodial grandparent role is often overlooked in the community, yet there is a cohort of committed individuals who care for their grandchildren as they did for their own children years earlier.

With questions such as: Will I have enough money to feed my household, or to make sure everyone has clean clothes for school? Is there anyone else in my situation? Is there support for me in my new role as a custodial grandparent? These grandparent caregivers are coping with situations they had not anticipated. Nonetheless, an underlying motivation of love for their grandchildren has allowed them to prevail despite the many challenges they have faced. They raise their grandchildren not because they are forced to—but rather, because they love their grandchildren—and soon grow committed to every aspect of raising them.

In Rochester, NY, there is support for kinship caregivers via the Skip Generations program, offered in the context of Family Resource Centers. The Skip Generations program is a gathering of highly motivated and committed individuals who, rather than running from the challenge of parenting for a second time, have stepped up to the plate and found their inner strength—their resilience. By forming a support group, they have empowered each other, and eventually other grandparents, to become advocates for themselves and for their grandchildren.

History of Skip Generations

It all began in 1989 with one woman, a pioneer if you will, who sought not only to receive support, but also to offer her support to others. Raising three of her grandchildren by herself, Shirley Wilmoth realized that there was no support in the community to help her and others in their new roles. Shirley not only found strength within herself, but was able to empower others to find their inner strength. This sense of empowerment is the element that turned a small support group, a gathering, into what is now viewed as a replicable model by the National Council on Aging (NCOA)—that others across the U.S. are using as an exemplary strength-based program.

When Shirley took it upon herself to start a support group for others like herself, who were faced with the many challenges that raising grandchildren brings, she decided to call it, very fittingly, "Skip Generations." The program was originally a part of the grassroots efforts of Family Resource Centers of Crestwood, which focused on parenting and early childhood education. Shirley, an advocate herself, led the support group in its early stages. The original group consisted of only three members, and Shirley facilitated the group until her health began failing in 1995. In 1997, due to its past experience in offering grandparent support groups, Family Resource Centers (FRC) of Crestwood was approached by the Monroe County Office for the Aging (MCOFA) to apply for a grant through the Brookdale Foundation. FRC applied for, and received, the grant, but then was faced with another challenge: the program needed a facilitator. Ms. Linda James, an Administrative Assistant at FRC, was approached to become facilitator of the Skip Generations program.

Although she had no previous experience running groups, Linda agreed to take on the challenge. Thus, a resilient coordinator was hired to lead a resilient group of individuals who would soon be working together to enrich one another through the sharing of personal stories and experiences and their desire to learn.

When Ms. James began, she did not have much of a participant-base from which to work, other than lists of former Skip participants. She kick-started her recruitment efforts by making phone calls to previous participants, writing letters to those she knew were interested, and providing home visits to those who needed mentorship. She ran the program from her car with her carry-on case (which, very much like her grandchildren, never left her side) as she traveled to these other grandparents' homes. Her home visits were very much a snapshot of what eventually evolved into the current mentoring program.

Later in 1997, Ms. James was able to start an evening group as a result of a grant Skip received from The Brookdale Foundation. The group hosted speakers who shared information about community resources and spent the rest of the time providing support to one another. They talked about important, relevant issues that were going on in their lives at the time in a family-like atmosphere at the center. No longer were grandparents alone; they had each other, and this was the bud of a flower that would soon be in full-bloom. Funding support grew through the Monroe County Office for the Aging and fell under the targeted services to special populations in Family Resource Centers' Empowerment grant through the New York State Children and Family Trust Fund.

Linda began her advocacy efforts for kinship caregivers by approaching legislators and promoting the Skip Generations program by sharing her personal story and representing the needs of some of the grandparents in the group. She soon realized that one support group simply was not enough to meet the needs of grandparents in the Rochester community. In time, she started a second support group, which was vital to the program. This new group was a daytime group; the evening group continued, but took a different focus. The day group was an educational and support group, while the evening group became known as "A Gathering of Women," this was a result of The Brookdale Foundation's pilot mental health program. In partnership with the University of Rochester's HRSA-funded Geropsychology Fellowship Program, Skip Generations provided a focus on the mental health of the grandparents and the children in their care. This was in keeping with the program's basic premise of "you must be healthy yourself before you can raise your grandchildren."

Now there was a group on Tuesday mornings and A Gathering of Women met on Tuesday evenings. The evening group's name was chosen in an effort to avoid the social stigma associated with such labels as "counseling" or "therapeutic" and the negative connotation such words might have had for the participants.

A Gathering of Women was a group of ten grandmothers who met weekly with a Psychology Fellow from the University of Rochester (UR), with whom Skip Generations had closely collaborated since 2000. The Psychology Fellow helped facilitate the group and introduced topics such as stress reduction and recognizing depression in order to support the mental health of the grandmothers. A Clinical Psychologist from the UR would provide therapeutic sessions with the children while their grandmothers met in their own group. This weekly program was provided for one year. It allowed the grandparents to have individual counseling to complement the group sessions. The UR also held depression screenings for all of the grandparents that were conducted by the Psychology Fellow, and some individuals were seen by the Fellow for individual counseling that complemented the group sessions. The group talked about anger, guilt, and shame—issues that were very relevant to them at that time. It was a time of soul-searching, looking within themselves and realizing that some things in their lives had to change in order for them to become better-suited to take on the responsibility of raising their grandchildren. On Saturday mornings, the UR Child Psychologist taught the children specific techniques to control and manage their anger. Skip Generations became a family of individuals with one focus: to enrich one another in order to more effectively parent their grandchildren.

A Gathering of Women was the precursor to the Skip Generations Mentoring Program. At the conclusion of one of the group sessions, Linda James and her UR partners posed the question: "What can these women—who are now well-equipped to tackle this challenge and also who are healthy and more empowered—do to give back to others in the community like themselves?" From this idea the Mentoring Program emerged. Ms. James and her UR colleagues began putting together a training curriculum that is still in use. The training manual and curriculum have been tested, revised, and supplemented over the years so that the information is up-to-date and accurate. The first training of 10 mentors took place in 2006, then another eight mentors were trained in 2009, and finally 10 more were trained in 2010. Each year, a UR Psychology Fellow co-facilitates the training, and these caregivers are then prepared to provide home visits to others in the community.

A Closer Look at the Mentoring Program

The mentors are trained in a 15-week curriculum facilitated by Linda James and a Psychology Fellow from the University of Rochester's Department of

Psychiatry. This curriculum works to equip the mentors with a solid knowledge-base that is integral to their roles as kinship caregivers on the following topics: child development, child mental health, adult physical health, adult depression, legal, legislative, financial, educational, and mandated reporting. Pre- and post-session assessments are conducted at each session. Completion of this curriculum is followed by a celebratory graduation ceremony, after which the mentors are ready to serve in their community. The mentors also participate in training on safety in home visits provided by Hillside Family of Agencies (HFA), and are required to be fingerprinted and receive child abuse clearance prior to embarking on their first home visit.

During the home visits, the mentors provide the support kinship caregivers need: they listen, provide encouragement and resources, and are empathic and understanding to their mentees' needs because at one point or another, the mentors have walked in their shoes. Through the sharing of personal stories, mentors can easily relate to, and help with, anything that may be needed. They also provide linkage to community resources that are available to the mentees. The mentors empower the other grandparents or relative caregivers to get out of deficit mode and into empowerment mode in order to become strong advocates for themselves and the children in their care. The mentors guide their fellow kinship caregivers through the many challenges involved in getting public services for their grandchildren.

Simply knowing that there is someone to say "I have been there" and "I am here for you" surely provides much more than reassurance: it inherently reduces isolation. The mentoring program also aims to decrease the incidence of depression among this population, to reduce grandparents' (or relative caregivers') stress by providing a solid base of knowledge, and to educate them on topics such as financial literacy, parenting skills, and help them with required paperwork. Additional evaluation measures were put in place for both the mentors and the mentees in order to track the program's effectiveness and impact on all of its participants.

The Structure of Skip Generations

The Skip Generations support group sessions provide a warm and supportive atmosphere for those in the custodial grandparent role living in Rochester, NY. They include various topics regarding outreach and advocacy. Along with the support group sessions, Skip Generations offers a mentoring program, where experienced grandparent caregivers can visit other kinship caregiver homes in the community in order to bring resources and serve as a sounding board to them. Some of those grandparents and relatives are pursuing custody and include those who are denied visitation rights.

There are three levels of participation in the Skip Generations Program. Level I is the educational support group for new participants (kinship caregivers) who have never been part of Skip before. In Level I, members also have the option of receiving in-home visits by the trained (Level III) mentors as well as linkage to Parents As Teachers (PAT) a program of Family Resource Centers for parents or grandparents who have children in their care from ages zero to 5. In this program, the parents or grandparents are taught how to play with their children using simple items readily available in their home. The age-appropriate activities of play offer a lens into the child's early development. Also in this level, a curriculum called Parenting A Second Time Around (PASTA) is offered to participants.

Level II is for those members whom are referred to as "veterans" of the program. These grandparents have been in the program the longest, some have even been participants since the program started, and have not yet been trained to be mentors, or simply express a need for ongoing support in the weekly support groups. The Level II support group also provides an opportunity for outside agencies to inform the grandparents about resources that they can offer in order to assist them or the children in their care. This provides a good interface between the participants and available resources in the community. The Community-Based Supervisor is also trained to provide two evidence-based parenting skills curricula in this level: the Effective Black Parenting Program and The Incredible Years.

Level III is the Mentoring Program, including the 15-week training course and then a twice-a-month commitment to providing home visits to other caregivers in their homes for the duration of one year.

Finding Inner Strength: Skip Generation's Impact on Its Participants

The mentors will tell you that they have become resourceful, and while this has certainly helped them to more effectively raise their grandchildren, it has also been a crucial part of their mentorship. Mentees often do not have access to many of the resources they may need. The structure of this program facilitates resourcefulness: the mentors receive, in their weekly meetings, resources and other valuable information that they can use for themselves and also to empower other grandparents.

One might think mentees would be hesitant at first to allow other people in their homes, especially someone who is going to help them with parenting their grandchildren. Though this hesitancy may exist, the common ground they share with the mentors trumps any hesitancy, and in nearly every case, the mentees look forward to their bi-weekly visits from the mentors. In a typical home visit, two mentors go into the home of a grandmother who may be unfamiliar with how to fill out an application for services. The grandmother has dinner cooking, laundry going, and is struggling to keep up with her children who are running around the house. She is overwhelmed. This grandmother struggles to get ahead because she is alone. She seldom gets the space to fill out an application for a service; the time is always occupied with the most immediate tasks, for example, getting the kids' clothes ready for school tomorrow. This situation is common when the mentors enter a grandmother's home; a stress-filled life is temporarily calmed by the presence of two people who were in the very same position not long before this visit. In an effort to empower, the mentors help their mentees find their own strength so that they can then do what is necessary to most effectively raise their grandchildren. The mentors do not directly do the work for the mentees, but rather empower them to do everything themselves. This empowerment, first and foremost, comes from their example. The mentors' lives are exemplary of how, when people face a seemingly impossible situation, there is a certain inner strength that can be accessed. For many, this cannot be accessed without the guidance and example of someone who has endured a similar hardship.

Perhaps the most remarkable fact about Skip Generations is that many mentees proceed through the various levels of the program and eventually become mentors. A mentor who was at one time a mentee, visits a mentee, knows exactly what the grandparent is going through and what he or she might need, because the mentor has needed similar services at one point. This type of mentor has endured; she has gone from needing twice monthly home visits in order to find resilience to finding it within herself to parent again, and then share her empowerment with others.

Ms. Rosena Addison shares her personal experience with the Skip Generations Mentoring Program:

> *My oldest daughter went into the military overseas and there was a problem with an abusive babysitter, so I said, "Bring the kids to me." I eventually took in grandchildren from my son and younger daughter, and have been raising them for 24 years. I had seven at one time in my house—six of them went to school and I was home with the little one. I fell into a depression. Skip Generations, thankfully, sent a mentor to the house. I was so enthused, I started coming to meetings and I brought the little one with me. At the support group meetings, I learned about Head Start and other programs available to me and my grandchildren. One of my grandchildren had lead poisoning, and I found out about the symptoms and treatments at a Skip Generations meeting. The meetings were a time to talk about our problems and I saw that my problems weren't so bad after all. We became one big family. I learned how to deal with the teen years. It's just been great—I can help the kids with any problem. If I don't know how to handle it, I know where to turn. Skip Generations has empowered me. There are so many people who don't know where to turn. You just don't realize how much Skip Generations is needed.*

Program Evaluation: Measuring Impact and Effectiveness

The kinship caregivers in Skip Generations have endured many changes in their lives when they took on the care of their grandchildren. In the process of raising their grandchildren, they experienced a wide range of emotions, including guilt, shame, and anger, to name just a few. By attending these educational support groups, or by receiving home visits, participants have learned how to express, and work through, these feelings. There is a lot of power and validation in realizing that others share the same feelings. They grow to realize that they have to be healthy themselves in order to raise healthy children.

Beyond providing information and support to alleviate isolation and decrease the incidence of depression among this population, Skip Generations also provides a source of empathy, information, counsel, education, and support so grandparents can properly care for the children in their care. Outcomes for this program include: reducing caregivers' stress; increasing parenting skills of kinship caregivers; improving financial literacy skills of kinship caregivers; and increasing the ability of kinship caregivers to advocate for their children and for themselves. The degree to which this program meets or exceeds these named outcomes is measured in various ways by means of surveys and other assessments.

Participants in Skip Generations report that:

- They feel less isolated as kinship care providers through the supportive groups and home visits.
- They see the program as a source of empathy, information, counsel, education and support, empowering them to care for their grandchildren.
- They have learned parenting skills, greater financial literacy, and how to reduce their stress as primary caregivers to their grandchildren.
- They are better able to advocate for their grandchildren and for themselves.

With a three-year Multi-Generational Civic Engagement grant through the National Council on Aging, Skip Generations staff developed strategies to strengthen and expand the capacity of Skip Generations. With increased volunteer resources, the program is focusing on enhancing its outreach in the community and developing a process of evaluation to clearly show its effectiveness.

In 2010, we realized, through our community outreach, that we needed to reach more of the males who are raising their relatives. So we developed a grandfathers group called Skip Generations II, which meets every second and fourth Friday of the month.

Evaluating the mentoring program involves the use of various measures to track effectiveness, including recruitment and training, change in knowledge-base, and level of satisfaction.

The Pre- and Post-training Efficacy Surveys are completed by every mentor-in-training at the beginning of the first training session and at the end of the final week of training. In order to assess participants' understanding of each domain in the mentor training, and to ensure the effectiveness of the implementation of each topic, everyone takes a Pre- and Post-training Knowledge Assessment each week. The assessment is the same before and after the training session, and the results are tracked to check the effective facilitation of these trainings. The Pre- and Post-training Knowledge Assessments are completed by every mentor-in-training at the beginning and end of each training session. There is a different assessment for each week, specific to the subject and focus of each session.

The Protective Factors Survey is completed by every mentee at the first visit, three months later, and every six months thereafter. The Crestwood Children's Center Customer Satisfaction Survey is completed by every mentor and mentee every six months. A Training Satisfaction Survey is also administered to every mentor at the end of the final training session. The Mentoring Survey is completed by every mentee on the first home visit, every three months, and again on the final home visit.

The overall results of the Pre- and Post-training Knowledge Assessments from the 2010 mentor training are as follows: Pre: 52.5% correct; Post: 77.2% correct. Results of participant surveys in the mentoring program showed the program's benefits. Participants consistently reported they have: received the empathy and support of a primary caregiver; gained knowledge of advocacy skills; learned ways to relieve stress; and gained access to information about available resources in the community.

Results from the Customer Satisfaction Survey are as follows. One hundred percent responded that: the program is scheduled at a time that is convenient for me; the program builds on my strengths as a parent; my understanding of child development has improved my relationship with my child. Ninety-five percent responded that: I have an opportunity to offer my input on the program; the Family Resource Center staff listens and understands my concerns; the Family Resource Center staff respects my family's cultural values and customs; I am kept informed about issues that affect my family/child; I have learned ways of responding positively to my child's behavior; overall, I am satisfied with my service experience. Ninety percent responded that: the Family Resource Center staff members are available to me when I need them; I have learned skills to advocate for my child.

These outcome measures speak powerfully to the impact that Skip Generations has had on the many kinship caregivers who have participated over the history of this program. Their personal stories now include a new message of hope and celebration of resiliency, growth, and family well-being.

FRC is a service of Crestwood Children's Center, which is one of seven affiliates of Hillside Family of Agencies, a nonprofit system of human services for youth and families across Western and Central New York and in Prince George's County, Maryland. Crestwood Children's Center provides an array of behavioral, child welfare, mental health, education and family development services to children ages birth to 21 and their families.

We are indebted to the continuing support of the Monroe County Office for the Aging as well as the Children and Family Trust Fund in the NYS Office of Children and Family Services and the generous contributions of our Rochester community. We also recognize the importance of our Multi-Generational Civic Engagement grant from the U.S. Administration on Aging to the National Council on Aging, with support from The Atlantic Philanthropies and the MetLife Foundation.

The evolution of Skip Generations has been greatly enhanced through our collaboration with the University of Rochester. This work was supported in part by a grant from the Health Resources Services Administration (HRSA) T06HP01830: "The University of Rochester Geropsychology Education Program."

13 Challenges in Translating an Evidence-Based Health Self-Management Intervention for Grandparent Caregivers[1]

Philip McCallion, Lisa A. Ferretti, and Jwakym Kim

Abstract

It is well established that there are concerns that grandparent caregivers rarely take good care of their own health. A focus on the well-being of their grandchildren rather than self, high levels of physical and psychosocial health concerns for all grandparents, and low levels of health insurance access for younger primary caregiver grandparents combine to increase their health risks. This is a population that would benefit from evidence based health promotion and self-management strategies but time, respite, and transportation constraints further isolate grandparent caregivers from such resources. This chapter will illustrate that grandparent caregivers do benefit from evidence based programs, in this case the Chronic Disease Self Management Program, but acknowledges that self-reported benefits for grandparent completers of the program were not as robust when compared with those reported by an age matched sample of other older persons. Insights on why such programs should and could become more accessible to grandparent caregivers.

Introduction

Perspectives on family caregiving generally begin with the care of children by parents but given reports of 29% of the U.S. population providing such care for an average of 20 hours per week (NCA/AARP, 2009; NCA/Evercare, 2009), in many ways caregiving discussions are increasingly focused on family caregivers as the mainstay of both long term care and of the management of care for people with chronic illness and disability. With values of as much as $375 billion being placed upon this unpaid care (NCA/Evercare, 2009), there have been long standing policy level concerns that public support of caregivers may result in families giving over this responsibility to "the state" (McCallion & Kolomer, 2003). However, there has been recognition of the need to support family caregivers most particularly embodied in the National Family Caregiver Support Program which supports assistance in locating services, counseling and training and respite care services throughout the country (http://www.aoa.gov/AoARoot/AoA_Programs/HCLTC/Caregiver/index.aspx). Growing recognition of the increasing size of the aging and infirm population, the decline in birth rates and in family size and (if caregivers are not available) the challenge to locate sufficient levels public replacement care resources (Jackson, Howe, & Nakashima, 2010) has brought into focus:

- The demands being placed on family networks.
- The absolute reliance of states on families to divert people from nursing home placement and to support quality lives in the community.

A critical concern that has emerged is the health of this caregiver resource.

Data increasingly points to caregivers providing intensive levels of care despite their own ill-health (Navaie-Waliser et al., 2002), high levels of depression and other mental health concerns (Marks, Lambert, & Choi, 2002), stress (Grunfeld, 2004), cognitive decline (Vitaliano, et al., 2005), poorly managed chronic health conditions of their own (Pinquart & Sorensen, 2003) and poor self-care (Lee et al., 2003). Such findings have encouraged the development of caregiver focused interventions (for reviews see Cook et al., 2001; Toseland, Smith, & McCallion, 2001).

Into this increasing complex caregiving picture have emerged grandparent or kin caregivers of children, on the one hand fulfilling a more traditional caregiving role of child care but on the other assuming this responsibility at ages and stages of life more similar to adult caregiver populations. Latest data from the 2008 American Community Survey suggests that 6.4 million grandparents of all ethnicities, a range of ages and in all locations have children under 18 living with them <http://www.census.gov/acs/www/guidance_for_data_users/guidance_main/>); and for many grandparents are the primary caregiver. Here too there is growing evidence of health care needs and concerns among these caregivers given the stress of what may be a new caregiving role and their own aging related health concerns (Baker & Silverman, 2008; Musel et al., 2009). Similar to other caregiving populations, this may manifest in poor self-care, depression, not managing their own chronic illnesses and reliance on wishful thinking as a health care strategy (Kolomer, 2008).

Faced with these challenges researchers have developed and tested a number of interventions targeted specifically at grandparent caregivers and offering case management (Kelley, Yorker, Whitley, & Sipe, 2001; Robinson, Kropf, & Myers, 2000; McCallion, Janicki, Grant-Griffin, & Kolomer, 2000; Cohon et al., 2003), support groups (McCallion et al., 2000; Robinson et al., 2000; Burnette, 1998), school-based medical, service and counseling (Grant, Gordon, & Cohen, 1997; Smith & Dannison, 2002); empowerment training and support (Cox, 2002; McCallion et al., 2000) and computer training to increase skills and support (Strozier et al., 2004). In reviewing these interventions Kolomer (2008) concluded that their successful delivery and dissemination is hampered by a lack of effectiveness evidence. Reviewing the same data, such interventions are further challenged by (1) their inability to be broadly adopted by the range of agencies with which grandparent caregivers come in contact; (2) not including sufficient attention to the support the grandparents themselves and/or their health management, and (3) being bound to specific funding sources such as time limited grants which means their reach to date has been quite limited. These are challenges equally faced by other caregiver interventions.

Hoagwood and Johnson (2003) argue that the research processes that enhance credibility of research findings around the development and testing of interventions also reduce the interventions' applicability to every day practice; randomized control trials by definition seek to control the environment in which a practice intervention is implemented and tested:

- Controlled trials benefit from protocols, practitioner training and supervision, and researcher oversight to ensure fidelity.
- Participants are screened and selected to be likely to benefit from the intervention, which also increases research control.

However, implementation in real world settings is less controlled and multiple challenges derail many new interventions. The interventions for grandparent caregivers are further stymied by the rarity of additional randomized control studies testing the interventions with new populations and settings.

Fortune, McCallion and Briar-Lawson (2010) have refined Hoagwood and Johnson's (2003) conceptualization of why evidence based interventions often do not work in the real world supporting that (a) implementation may not be supported within reimbursement and regulatory requirements (extra-organizational context); (b) implementation is difficult if the intervention conflicts with the organizational culture or with the manner in which services are delivered (organizational fit); and (c) practitioners often do not adopt interventions if their underpinnings are seen as conflicting with practitioner practice philosophies and training, or supervisory staff ability to provide the intensity of supervision needed (intervention processes). Additionally, in this case, (d) grandparent caregivers may not be as ready for the challenges and opportunities of these interventions as were the volunteer participants in the research studies (grandparent choice and control).

These concerns are not unique to grandparent caregiver interventions. Wilson and Fridinger (2008) argue that there are three phases in developing and implementing an intervention: research, translation, and institutionalization. The research phase is focused upon:

- Discovery (the underpinnings of the intervention).
- Efficacy (will desired benefits emerge).
- Implementation (effective implementation in real world settings).

For available grandparent caregiver interventions, even the research phase is incomplete, largely ending with the assessment of efficacy. There remains the need to demonstrate in an implementation research phase that controlled evaluation findings can be repeated in real world settings followed by attention to translation tasks:

(1) Dissemination—active participation and collaboration of stakeholders to change systems, policies, programs, and practices.
(2) Adoption by local agencies and providers.
(3) Practice implementation at the individual, organization, community and policy levels (Wilson & Fridinger, 2008).

The final phase of embedding intervention programs within regulatory and reimbursement schemes (institutionalization) is also absent for grandparent caregiver interventions.

Perhaps, these tasks are too much to ask of the grandparent caregiver intervention field, that we are at too early a phase in its development. Also, although the unique needs of grandparent caregivers are well documented (Musil et al., 2009), there is also much commonality with other caregivers and indeed older adults, particularly in terms of health needs, health care utilization and self-management of care. Rather than the development of unique interventions there should be an implementation and translation focus instead on the usefulness and accessibility for grandparent caregivers of more widely available and tested interventions, particularly interventions where implementation, translation, and institutionalization efforts are more advanced. For these reasons, within a larger implementation of the Chronic Disease Self-management Program (http://patienteducation.stanford.edu/programs/cdsmp.html) in New York State targeted at adults age 60+ with at least one chronic condition (and/or the caregivers of individuals with such conditions), it was decided to examine the usefulness of CDSMP for grandparent caregivers.

Intervention

The Chronic Disease Self-management Program (CDSMP) consists of workshops given in two and a half hours, once a week, for six weeks in community settings such as senior centers, churches, libraries, clinics, and hospitals. CDSMP was developed for people with chronic health problems and their significant others (often caregivers) and people with different problems attend the same workshop together. Workshops are facilitated by two trained workshop leaders, one or both of whom are non-health professionals with at least one chronic condition and groups usually consist of 12–16 participants. These trained workshop leaders follow a scripted Workshop Leaders Manual each time they facilitate the program. To support fidelity in delivery the course developers have scripted every minute of the course for content as well as the management of interactions involving the workshop leaders and workshop participants.

The program content includes:

- Developing decision-making and problem-solving skills.
- Developing and maintaining a safe and long-term physical activity program.
- Fatigue management.
- Dealing with anger, depression, and other difficult emotions.
- Cognitive management of pain and stress.
- Communicating effectively with family, friends, and health professionals.
- Using prescribed medication appropriately.
- Healthy eating.
- Making informed treatment decisions.
- Planning for future health care.

There is considerable randomized control-based evidence for the efficacy of CDSMP from studies completed by both the developer and by other research teams. Most of these studies assume that a completer of the program has attended four of six sessions in the belief that such a level of participation is required to adequately experience and benefit from CDSMP. A recent meta-analysis (Brady et al., 2011) has supported positive effects for completers across studies for self-efficacy, psychological health, health behaviors, and self-rated health.

The most systematic and longitudinal data includes an Agency for Healthcare Research and Quality (AHRQ)-funded investigation that compared health behaviors, health status, and health services use in patients age 40 to 90 years (average age 65) who had completed the CDSMP (Lorig et al., 1999). When 6 month post-test findings were compared to baseline measures researchers found (as compared to controls) that CDSMP participants had:

- Increased exercise.
- Better coping strategies and symptom management.
- Better communication with their physicians.
- Improvement in their self-rated health, disability, social and role activities, and health distress.
- More energy and less fatigue.
- Decreased disability.
- Fewer physician visits and hospitalizations.

In further follow-ups, Lorig et al. (2001a) found that after one year, CDSMP participants had:

- Significant improvements in energy, health status, social and role activities, and self-efficacy.
- Less fatigue or health distress.
- Fewer visits to the emergency room.
- No decline in activity or role functions, even though there was a slight increase in disability after one year.

After two years, for the same CDSMP participants, Lorig et al. (2001a) found:

- No further increase in disability.
- Reduced health distress.
- Fewer visits to physicians and emergency rooms.
- Increased self-efficacy.

The increase in patients' perceptions of their self-efficacy was also found to be associated with reduced health care use (Lorig et al., 2001a). Specifically, CDSMP participants were found to have used less hospital and physician services than they had used before participating in the program, and less than those in the CDSMP control group (Lorig et al., 1999; Lorig et al., 2001a). Savings found ranged from $390 to $520 per patient over a two-year study period (Lorig et al., 2001a). In a further study 12 months post-intervention, Kaiser Permanente CDSMP participants were found to have fewer visits to the emergency room and fewer hospital days compared to the year prior to completing the CDSMP. Kaiser Permanente paid approximately $200 per participant for CDSMP training, materials, and administration. With 489 participants, Kaiser's total cost was $97,800. Given that the cost to care for each participant was found to have decreased approximately $990 (fewer health services used), this yielded net savings of nearly $400,000 (Lorig, Sobel, Ritter, Laurent, & Hobbs, 2001b).

Supported by this evidence, implementation and translation demonstrations of CDSMP have been supported by a range of Foundations and by programs funded by the Centers for Disease Control and Prevention, the Center for Medicaid and Medicare Services and by the U.S. Administration on Aging. These demonstrations have included technical assistance supports to build infrastructure, fidelity monitoring, expansion of reach to diverse populations and sustainable delivery planning. CDSMP therefore represents an intervention that has transitioned from research to translation and institutionalization efforts (including beginning efforts at reimbursement) and its value for grandparent caregivers should be considered.

Research Design

Glasgow and colleagues (2001) have proposed the RE-AIM Framework which focuses on individual and institutional outcomes along five dimensions (see Figure 13.1) as a useful design for assessing the implementation, translation, and institutionalization of interventions. RE-AIM supports the investigation of Reach, Efficacy, Adoption, Implementation and Maintenance for an intervention through consideration of related guiding questions and use of diverse data sources.

In the contextual framework of Re-AIM, the focus is not simply on participant outcomes but also on reach, adoption, implementation, and maintenance issues that are influenced by the extra-organizational outcomes, organizational fit, intervention processes, and participant choice and control issues outlined earlier. The RE-AIM Framework provided the basis for the evaluation here.

- Reach into the target population especially to those who can most benefit.
  Guiding Questions
  -What percentage of the target population will be reached by the intervention?
  -Does the intervention reach those most in need?
  -Will participants be representative of persons served by the provider?
- Efficacy or effectiveness
  Guiding Questions
  -Does program achieve greater key targeted outcomes compared with other interventions?
  -Does it produce unintended adverse consequences?
  -How will or did it impact quality of life (QoL)?
- Adoption widely by a range of settings, particularly agencies working with populations most likely to benefit
  Guiding Questions
  -Will organizations have underserved or high-risk populations use the intervention?
  -Does the intervention help the organization address its primary mission?
- Implementation—consistency of delivery of intervention by staff members with moderate levels of training and expertise
  Guiding Questions
  -How many staff within a setting will try the intervention?
  -Can different levels of staff implement the program successfully?
  -Are the different components of the intervention delivered as intended?
- Maintenance of positive intervention effects (and minimal negative impacts) in individuals and populations over time at reasonable cost
  Guiding Questions
  -Does the program produce lasting effects at individual level?
  -Can organizations sustain the program over time?
  -Are those persons and settings that show intervention maintenance those most in need?

Figure 13.1 The RE-AIM Framework and Associated Research Questions (adapted from Glasgow et al., 2001)

Sample

From a larger dataset of 509 completers, first the grandparent caregivers were identified. Other completers in the dataset were then matched to this group on age, gender, ethnicity, and health status using a propensity score approach that found the best match for each randomly selected grandparent caregiver from the larger pool of comparison cases, with the comparison case then removed and not reconsidered for subsequent matches. A matched sample of 62 completers was identified: 31 grandparent caregivers and 31 non-grandparent caregivers. Baseline demographics of the sample may be found in Table 13.1.

Table 13.1 Baseline Demographics and Measure Scores

	Grandparent Caregiver (n = 31)	*Non-Grandparent Caregiver (n = 31)*
Age range	60–84 years old	60–84 years old
Mean age (years)	71	71
Gender	26 female; 5 male	26 female; 5 male
Health status (mean)	**3.10**	**3.03**
Fatigue (mean)	4.13	4.40
Pain (mean)	4.42	4.50
Shortness of Breath (mean)	2.97	2.10
Physician visits (mean)	3.85	3.39

Measures

Specifically to address stability in efficacy, secondary analysis of three measures contained in the demonstration dataset were utilized:

1. Self-rated health: 1 = excellent, 2 = very good, 3 = good, 4 = fair, 5 = poor
2. Self-reported fatigue, pain, and breathing difficulty were measured using visual numeric: 0 = no symptoms ~ 10 = severe symptoms
3. Physician visit: The self-report number of visits was collected (in the past six months, how many times did you visit a physician?)

Measures were all drawn from the original data tools. The data was collected as a pre-test before the class began and again at six months.

To address reach, adoption, implementation, and maintenance, quality assurance data gathered under the larger project was examined using a structured data collection protocol targeting information on host (organizations responsible for the management of recruitment, delivery and leaders) and implementation (organizations providing locations for delivery of the intervention and offering some help with recruitment) sites, fidelity, and intention to continue delivery.

Analysis

When an intervention is established as evidence-based, as is CDSMP, and the interest is the pursuit of translation and institutionalization, the analysis strategy is to examine stability in findings as compared to randomized control data rather than a replication of randomized trials. In pursuit of understanding whether stability was present, pre to post change scores were developed for the efficacy measures and percentages of those who experienced change in each group were generated. Descriptive findings were generated for the other RE-AIM dimensions.

Results

Findings for each of the RE-AIM dimensions included:

Reach

None of the host or implementation sites operated grandparent specific programs and all acknowledged that they made no specific outreach efforts to grandparent caregivers. It was acknowledged that the programs have reached only a small percentage of eligible grandparent caregivers, with the need for respite and transportation cited as the biggest barriers to a more extended reach. The sites with the most success on reaching such caregivers were faith communities, programs with associated food pantries and community based health clinics. Here grandparent caregivers were recognized as being an important but not exclusive component of the populations served. Because the target for the overall project was persons over age 60 there were no under 60 grandparents in the dataset. All the host and implementation sites that recruited grandparent caregivers also served persons under 60 so CDSMP participants were not completely representative of their persons served. Because grandparents in CDSMP at baseline, on average had two additional chronic conditions and scored lower on health self report measures when compared to all other participants, regardless of caregiver status, and were also a more ethnically diverse group, host and implementation sites felt strongly that their success in reaching grandparent caregivers meant that they were reaching people most in need.

Efficacy

For all five outcome measures, at six months, self-reported health, fatigue, pain, and breathing difficulty and physician visits, there was a higher level of improvement in the non-grandparent caregivers than in the grandparent caregivers (see Table 13.2) and the non-grandparent outcomes were similar to what has been reported in the randomized control studies. There was, however, some improvement for the grandparent caregivers. No adverse effects were noted and anecdotal reports from grandparents indicated that quality of life was improved through participation. Although participation levels were low,

Table 13.2 Percentage with Improved Scores Six Months Post-intervention

Condition	*GP (%)*	*Non-GP (%)*	*All (%)*
Health Status	13.8	13.3	13.6
Fatigue	27.6	40.0	33.9
Pain	22.6	53.3	37.7
Shortness of Breath	21.4	13.8	17.5
Physician Visits	28.0	44.0	36.0

host and implementation sites indicated that this program was more successful than other efforts to include grandparents in other non-grandparent specific programming.

Adoption

For the host and implementation sites the utility of serving grandparent caregivers per se was not reported as being of influence in their decision to adopt the program. Decisions to adopt were reported to be much more driven by low cost, encouragement from champions/community leaders/funders, availability of training and fidelity support, and utility for clients/consumers/patients/parishioners with chronic conditions. However, there were reports that grandparent caregivers were among the underserved and high health risk populations and that finding a program where they also participated helped sites better meet their mission. This further encouraged adoption of the program.

Implementation

Leaders were a combination of staff at sites and recruited volunteer peer leaders, all of whom completed leader training. There were no reports that there were unique difficulties in implementing the program with grandparent caregivers. A number of challenges were identified in the implementation of the program with grandparent caregivers: attendance challenges, requests for service information and supports for grandchildren, younger age compared to other participants, difficulties with attendance and with completion of action plans, and scheduling leaders/classes at times that suit grandparents. Despite these challenges there was consistent evidence that the different components of the intervention were delivered as intended.

Maintenance

At the individual level effects (percentage of participants who report pre to post improvements) at six months for grandparent caregivers were lower than for other participants and as compared to the reported randomized control data. Nevertheless, at the organizational level the host and implementation sites where grandparents attended indicated their intention to continue to make the opportunity to attend available to grandparent caregivers. Again host and implementation sites identified grandparent caregivers as among the most in need and that their impressions of positive effects for participating grandparent caregivers were higher than the self-report data.

Discussion

Translation and institutionalization of interventions requires an expanded research agenda and a repertoire of additional research methods. For this reason application of the RE-AIM Framework as has been undertaken here is an important expansion in the approach to intervention development and implementation for grandparent caregivers. The Framework's use also reflects that translation and institutionalization require much more attention to measures beyond efficacy. Finally, translation and institutionalization require that interventions be at a much more advanced stage of development than is true for most, if not all grandparent focused interventions. This concern is all the more pressing in environments where resources are strained and where grandparent caregivers are one of a number of populations that a provider or community organization is engaged with. It was noted in this study that none of the host and implementation sites saw themselves as primarily serving grandparent caregivers but did see grandparents as one of their most at risk subpopulations.

Many of the interventions previously found to be successful with grandparent caregivers have emphasized better health self management and empowerment approaches (see for example Cox, 2002; McCallion et al., 2000; Robinson et al., 2000) suggesting a proven health self management program for adults, including older adults and adults who are caregivers, may be useful for grandparent caregivers. Further, adoption and maintenance of programs is probably more likely if other caregivers or other older adults may also be included in the groups. Again, because none of the host and implementation sites exclusively served grandparent caregivers, the ability to serve multiple groups was highly valued and increased the likelihood that there would be sufficient attendees to successfully mount and deliver programs.

There were some grandparent-specific challenges identified in delivery: attendance challenges, requests for service information and supports for grandchildren, younger age compared to other participants, difficulties with attendance and with completion of action plans, and scheduling leaders/classes at times that suit grandparents. These challenges often reflected the different lives of grandparent caregivers driven by school, vacation and appointment schedules for their grandchildren which often meant a more varied schedule over the six week period of the class than was true for other participants. Also, the completion of between class action plans was at times more difficult and even among the 60+ group targeted, grandparents were more likely (but not always) to be at the lower end of the ages within a particular group.

Leaders found these issues to be difficult but not impossible to manage and host and implementation sites reported that they were probably a barrier to the decision by a grandparent to participate rather than to one's ability to remain in the class. If CDSMP is to be a more viable and widespread resource for grandparent caregivers there is a need to consider these challenges and identify responsive modifications in marketing and delivery that do not compromise the integrity required to ensure that the evidence based program is still delivered as intended. One strategy already underway is the training of grandparent caregivers who have completed the class as peer leaders to lead future classes. Another would be to recognize that the press of responsibilities is greater for many grandparent caregivers compared to their age and even health status peers and that more supports (e.g., respite, transportation, service assistance) are likely to be needed if they are to experience similar levels of or improved intervention outcomes. This suggestion is borne out in other grandparent caregiver research (McCallion et al., 2004).

To date, no grandparent specific programs have been participating in the delivery of CDSMP in New York State. It is likely that reach will be extended if such programs were included in the network of participating host and implementation sites. There is therefore a challenge to be met by CDSMP providers to seek to include grandparent specific programs but also to those programs to be open to the value of participation in a program that deals more generically with self-management of health concerns.

The review undertaken here of grandparent caregivers who have participated in CDSMP suggests that this is a program that is useful for at least some grandparent caregivers with chronic illnesses. The efficacy findings were not as strong as for other groups of participants and appear less robust than those found for interventions designed specifically for grandparents (see for example Burnette, 1998; McCallion et al., 2000; Robinson et al., 2000). However, if the concern is that there be a low cost, proven health focused or inclusive intervention that can be sustained as a service option, available through a wide range of agencies, and easily accessed by and welcoming of grandparents, then perhaps an option like CDSMP should be advanced over a grandparent specific intervention. Demonstrated better individual outcomes will not influence health and health habits for a population if the intervention is grant dependent, suffers from low attendance, is not widely available and fails to connect with those who need it most. The widespread infrastructure, fidelity approaches and value for multiple population of CDSMP make it more ideal to effect changes for large numbers of people even if those changes are small.

Note

1 The activities reported on here have been supported through a cooperative agreement with the U.S. Administration on Aging, the New York State Office for the Aging and the New York State Department of Health.

References

Baker, L. A., & Silverstein, M. (2008). Depressive symptoms among grandparents raising grandchildren. *Journal of Intergenerational Relations*, *6*(3), 285–304.

Burnette, D. (1998). Grandparents raising grandchildren: A school-based small group intervention. *Research on Social Work Practice*, *8*(1), 10–27.

Cohon, D., Hines, L., Cooper, B. A., Packman, W., & Siggins, E. (2003). Preliminary study of an intervention with kin caregivers. *Journal of Intergenerational Relationships*, *1*(3), 49–72.

Cooke, D., McNally, L., Mulligan, K., Harrison, M., & Newman, P. (2001). Psychosocial interventions for caregivers of people with dementia: A systematic review. *Aging & Mental Health*, *5*(2), 120–135.

Cox, C. B. (2002). Empowering African American grandparents. *Social Work, 47*(1), 45–54.

Fortune, A. E., McCallion, P., & Briar-Lawson, K. (2010). Building evidence-based intervention models. In A. E. Fortune, P. McCallion & K. Briar-Lawson (Eds.). *Social work practice research in the 21st century*. (pp. 279–295). New York: Columbia University Press.

Glasgow, R., McKay, H. G., Piette, J. D., & Reynolds, K. D. (2001). The RE-AIM framework for evaluating interventions: What can it tell us about approaches to chronic illness management? *Patient Education and Counseling, 44*, 119–127.

Grant, R., Gordon, S. G., & Cohen, S. T. (1997). An innovative school-based intergenerational model to serve grandparent caregivers. *Journal of Gerontological Social Work, 28*(1/2), 47–61.

Grunfeld, E. (2004). Family caregiver burden: Results from a longitudinal study of breast cancer patients and their principal caregivers. *Canadian Medical Association Journal, 170*(12), 1795–1801.

Hoagwood, K., & Johnson, J. (2003). School psychology: A public health framework I. From evidence-based practices to evidence-based policies. *Journal of School Psychology, 41*(1), 3–21.

Jackson, R., Howe, N., & Nakashima, K. (2010). *Global Aging Preparedness Index*. Washington DC: CSIS.

Kelley, S. J., Yorker, B. C., Whitley, D., & Sipe, T. (2001). A multimodal intervention for grandparents raising grandchildren: Results of an exploratory study. *Child Welfare, 80*(1), 27–50.

Kolomer, S. (2008). Grandparent caregivers. *Journal of Gerontological Social Work*, 50(Supp. #1), 321–344.

Lee, S. L., Colditz, G. A., Berkman, L. F., & Kawachi, I. (2003). Caregiving and risk of coronary heart disease in U.S. women: A prospective study. *American Journal of Preventive Medicine, 24*(2), 113–119.

Lorig, K., Sobel, D., Stewart, A., Brown, B., Bandura, A., Ritter, P., Gonzolez, V., Laurent, D., & Holman, H. (1999). Evidence suggesting that a chronic disease self-management program can improve health status while reducing hospitalization. *Medical Care, 37*, 5–14.

Lorig, K., Sobel, D., Stewart, A., Brown, B., Bandura, A., Ritter, P., Gonzolez, V., Laurent, D., & Holman, H. (2001a). Chronic disease self-management program: 2-year health status and health care utilization outcomes. *Medical Care, 39*, 1217–1223.

Lorig, K., Sobel, D., Ritter, P., Laurent, D., & Hobbs, M. (2001b). Effects of a self-management program on patients with chronic illness. *Effective Clinical Practice, 4*, 256–262.

Marks, N., Lambert, J. D., & Choi, H. (2002). Transitions to caregiving, gender, and psychological well-being: A prospective U.S. national study. *Journal of Marriage and Family, 64*, 657–667.

McCallion, P., Janicki, M. P., Grant-Griffin, L., & Kolomer, S. R. (2000). Grandparent Caregivers II: Service needs and service provision issues. *JGSW, 33*(3), 63–90.

McCallion, P., & Kolomer, S. R. (2003). Aging persons with developmental disabilities and their aging caregivers. In B. Berkman & L. Harootyan (Eds.). *Social work and health care in an aging world*. (pp. 201–225). New York: Springer.

McCallion, P., Janicki, M. P., & Kolomer, S. R. (2004). Controlled evaluation of support groups for grandparent caregivers of children with developmental disabilities and delays. *American Journal on Mental Retardation, 109*(4), 352–361.

Musel, C., Warner, C., Zauszniewski, J., Wykle, M., & Standing, T. (2009). Grandmother caregiving, family stress and strain and depressive symptoms. *Western Journal of Nursing Research, 31*(3), 389–408.

National Alliance for Caregiving & AARP (2004). *Caregiving in the U.S.* Washington, DC: Author.

National Alliance for Caregiving & Evercare (2006). *Evercare® Study of Caregivers in Decline: A Close-up Look at the Health Risks of Caring for a Loved One*. Bethesda, MD: National Alliance for Caregiving and Minnetonka, MN: Evercare.

Navaie-Waliser, M., Feldman, P. H., Gould, D. A., Levine, C. L., Kuerbis, A. N., & Donelan, K. (2002). When the caregiver needs care: The plight of vulnerable caregivers. *American Journal of Public Health, 92*(3), 409–413.

Pinquart, M., & Sorensen, S. (2003). Differences between caregivers and noncaregivers in psychological health and physical health: A meta-analysis. *Psychology and Aging, 18*(2), 250–267.

Robinson, M. M., Kropf, N. P., & Myers, L. (2000). Grandparents raising grandchildren in rural communities. *Journal of Aging and Mental Health, 6*, 353–365.

Smith, A. B., & Dannison, L. L. (2002). Educating educators: Programming to support grandparent-headed families. *Contemporary Education, 72*(2), 47–51.

Strozier, A. L., Elrod, B., Beiler, P., Smith, A., & Carter, K. (2004). Developing a network of support for relative caregivers. *Children and Youth Services Review, 26*, 641–656.

Toseland, R. W., Smith, G., & McCallion, P. (2001). Helping family caregivers. In A. Gitterman (Ed.). *Handbook of social work practice with vulnerable populations*. (pp. 548–581). New York: Columbia University Press.

Vitaliano, P. P., Echeverria, D., Yi, J., Phillips, P. E. M., Young, H., & Siegler, I. C. (2005). Psychophysiological mediators of caregiver stress and differential cognitive decline. *Psychology and Aging, 20*, 402–411.

Wilson, K. M., & Fridinger, F. (2008). Focusing on public health: A different look at translating research to practice. *Journal of Women's Health, 17*(2), 173–179.

14 Promoting Resilience

Counseling Grandparents to Raise Effective Grandchildren

Craig Zuckerman and Robert J. Maiden

Abstract

Counselors and clinicians are being presented with an explosion of grandparents who are parenting their grandchildren coming to their practices. The grandparents are often reluctant to take on the role of parenting their grandchildren, but are willing to do so to provide a safe haven for their neglected or abused grandchildren or to keep their grandchildren out of foster care (Minkler, 1994). These burdened families enter therapy with a plethora of challenging problems. Clinicians faced with these families require solutions that are multi-layered, complex, and challenging to help the grandchildren to thrive and to prosper. One such solution is to build on the naturally occurring resilience in the grandparents and to nurture it in the grandchildren. A family systems approach along with cognitive-behavioral model is employed to build resilience and to aid a multigenerational family to bounce back. This is presented in a case study on Josephine and her grandson, DeShaun.

Resilience is a word that has its roots in Latin and literally means to "bounce back" much like a tree bounces back after receiving a burst of wind. When resilience is applied to grandparents raising their grandchildren it has implications for the well-being of their grandchildren. Resilient grandparents can benefit their custodial grandchildren who often come to their homes experiencing the trauma of devastating change and overwhelming stressors. It is extremely difficult for grandchildren to arise from the ashes of a broken home and relationships, chaotic family circumstances, and impoverishment to develop into mentally healthy individuals. These grandchildren are frequently faced with adversity, tragedy, and significant sources of daily stressors within their families that few of us ever see on a consistent basis—often including the presence of alcohol or drug abuse, and verbal, physical, and sexual assault. Of course, not all multigenerational families experience such negative life events. Nevertheless, the majority we see in counseling do. However, partially due to the resilience of their grandparents (and perhaps partially due to their own resilience), these grandchildren can make positive gains in their self-development, though these gains in development are incremental, generally occur at a very slow pace, and take years or decades to accomplish.

When children feel abandoned by their natural parent or parents, their security is placed at risk. Children lose trust in the ability of significant people in their lives to protect or to provide support or comfort them. Although the parents may be dysfunctional and causing the children considerable unhappiness, the situation can, from the children's perspective, become worse when the parent is unavailable to raise them. The children experience a constant state of mistrust along with a myriad of other negative feelings including fear.

Biopsychosocial Model of the Child

Besides having social and psychological components, fear, mistrust, and perils also have a biological component. The children first experience this as a "flight or fight" internal response. But children can do neither. They cannot run nor can they fight. The children don't understand what's happening and feel like they have been dropped into the middle of a battle zone. This leads the children into a state of intense paralysis and feelings of powerlessness which intensifies their fear and anxiety.

If more stressors are added to the mix, which is the most common experience of children whose grandparents become their surrogate parents, they become depressed and when depression and fear become a chronic condition, the children's immune system can be compromised which damages brain cells that involve memory and emotions (Stix, 2011). Thus, the grandchildren often are caught up in a seemingly endless and nasty interactive spiral of biological, sociological, and psychological forces.

Fortunately, there is a pathway out of this cycle of deep suffering. Many grandchildren can rely on and gain strength through the resilience of their grandparents. The resilience of the grandparents helps their grandchildren overcome the harmful effects of being constantly bombarded by unpleasant physiological, sociological, and psychological stressors experienced as abandonment, financial deprivation, and emotional trauma which would otherwise place the grandchildren on a perilous pathway to long-term or even permanent behavior problems, cognitive difficulties, and emotional suffering.

The Power of Resilience

Grandparents who are more resilient can help their family heal in the face of these adversities, trauma, tragedy, physical, and emotional threats and other significant sources of stress frequently experienced in these families. While some aspects of resilience may be an innate part of the character of some grandparents, resilience can also be taught and nurtured. Thus, psychologists and counselors and other professional helpers can assist multigenerational families in developing strategies to promote or enhance resilience. In this vein, the American Psychological Association (2011) published a pamphlet that outlines a program for building resilience.

Twelve Ground Rules for Building Resilience

1. Make connections. Good relationships with close family members, friends, church, and community can help. Also assisting others helps.
2. Avoid seeing crises as an insurmountable problem. Reframe the situation or change your perspective. Look for the long haul down the road. Work on identifying the positives.
3. Accept that change is part of living. In adverse conditions, some things can't change. Accept them and move on to what you can change.
4. Move toward your goals. Every small step in the direction you want to go in is positive. Be realistic and plan your goals in small increments. Keep track of your goals and successes. Measure them. Reconsider and reflect on them, noting what you are achieving, and whether you are moving in the right direction.
5. Take decisive action. When possible, take decisive action. Rather than avoiding the problem, taking action is best. Wishing your problems would just go away won't work, taking action will. People feel better and more in control when they are actively challenging their problems.
6. Find positive ways to reduce stress and negative feeling. Sometimes taking a break from your problems is a good idea. Engaging in pleasant distracters such as reading a good novel or mystery, watching a movie or taking a long stroll can be restorative. Such activities allow you to renew your energy so you can refocus on your issues and challenge them with a fresh approach.
7. Look for opportunities for self-discovery. Getting in touch with your spirituality or looking for positive ways to engage in self-discovery nurtures a perspective in which you can see how you grow from wrestling in the mud with your issues and your losses. Many people who have experienced tragedy, or great loss, or faced overwhelming odds find that the experience of vulnerability strengthens them and heightens their appreciation of life, helping them to live more intensely and they are grateful for the blessings, if you will, that they have. They find life more meaningful.
8. Nurture a positive view of yourself. Learn to believe in yourself. Trust your instincts. Have confidence that you will prevail, that you have the ability to problem solve and can achieve your goals.
9. Take care of yourself. Recognize that at times you need to take care of your needs first. Make sure you eat well and get the rest or exercise that you need. Or just take that little extra time to get your personal tasks or duties done.
10. Where to look for help. Be aware of the community resources that are available through social service, foster care or the courts. Participate in self-help groups on the internet or within your community that focus on grandparents' needs. Be cognizant of your legal rights and the types of assistance you can get from the local school system.

11. Additional ways of strengthening resilience. Work as a team. Locate the many resources that are available such as case management, respite care, not-for-profits, social services, and counselors in school, at the county counseling centers, in private practice, or your spiritual leader. Share with these people on your team, describe your hardships, talk about the loss of a loved one, forge a common goal of developing the best strategies and discovering the most appropriate resources to receive the support and encouragement you need to break through the cycle of negativity, deprivation, and helplessness. You might get stuck at times, but your team can give you the comfort of knowing you are not alone.
12. Do it your way. Listen, but recognize that everyone's path to success is a little different. What works for one family may not work for you and vice versa. Be inventive. Constantly try new avenues when old ones fail. Engage in positive self-talk when things look bleak and daily life is very stressful. Recognize that you react in your social interaction differently with different people. Above all, be the little engine that could. Never give up hope.

These are the ground rules that we as astute therapists can use to right the ship of multigenerational families that are experiencing the perfect storm of turmoil and tragedy. Below, we systematically apply these cognitive-behavioral ground rules to build resilience in a case study on an individual called Josephine.

The Case of Josephine

Josephine is a 67-year-old grandmother who currently lives in a blended family. She and her husband raised three children, two of whom grew up and married, and have maintained a stable family and economic lifestyle. The middle daughter showed signs of oppositional defiant tendencies as a young child. Childhood problems included a history of doing poorly in school, gravitating towards other children who misbehaved, which resulted in frequent attempts at psychotherapy.

As a teenager, the daughter began abusing marijuana and alcohol. Legal intervention was not successful in stemming the tide of her dependencies. In a defiant act, she moved away from home at age 18, prior to completing high school. Continued involvement with drugs and alcohol led to multiple partners and criminal activity. She became pregnant and was incarcerated. Her infant son was born while she was incarcerated on charges of drug dealing as well as possession.

The grandparents filed for and were awarded custody. Visitation was to be at the grandparents' discretion. The daughter, angered by her parents' perceived interference in her life and after two failed legal attempts at regaining custody of her son, fled to California.

Sadly, four years later, her parents were informed of their daughter's death due to complications from HIV-AIDS infection. Twelve years later, the grandparents have struggled with their grandson's behavior and educational problems. He was diagnosed with Attention Deficit Hyperactivity Disorder, inattentive and hyperactive type, and borderline intellectual functioning.

Fetal Influences

Following an assessment by a geneticist, a medical diagnosis of fetal alcohol effect was made. Because of financial burdens associated with their grandchild's legal and medical situation, the couple was forced to sell their home and move to their hometown, to reclaim a family home that they inherited, which represented a less expensive residence recognizing that change is a part of life.

Initial Referral

Subsequently, Josephine's husband passed away, leaving her to struggle with feeling isolated and depressed. Josephine came to me (the first co-author) for counseling because of depression and a feeling of hopelessness regarding her circumstances, now raising a very defiant and difficult 12-year-old, named DeShaun. Josephine has since remarried and at the time of the initial appointment was struggling with the resentment of her new partner, as a result of the time and commitment that her grandchild required.

Assessment

We believe that counseling strategies are best developed when taking into account data gathered during an assessment process, leading to appropriate intervention from a variety of theoretical models. Assessment for treatment planning should take into consideration several factors: social history, mental status examination, and selection of psychological measures. Given that psychological stress can cause stress to grandparents who take on full-time parenting of grandchildren, (Burton, 1992), global measures of stress such as the Symptom Checklist 90 (SCL-90-R) Inventory (Derogatis, L.R. 1994), and the Parenting Stress Index (PSI), (Abidein, 1995) were administered.

Other specific measures of psychological functioning such as the Beck Depression Inventory-2 (Beck, Stern, & Brown, 2003) and the Beck Anxiety Scale (Beck, 1990) were considered as well. Both tests are composed of 21 items that provide a total score of assessing symptoms of depression and anxiety. Also, a social history and mental status exam was administered that assessed carefully for health-related difficulties, social support, family resources.

Careful attention to assessment from a family systems perspective required the combination of gaining an understanding of the dyadic relationships in Josephine's current household, followed by an evaluation of the structural issues and communication patterns and their subsequent effect on individual behavior targeted for change. It became clear from this evaluation that Josephine's individual difficulties with depression, coupled with a disconnection between herself and her husband, Jim, were contributing to a lack of effectiveness in addressing the grandson's emotional and behavior problems.

All three members of this family were seeking control and attention by dysfunctional means. For example, when Josephine became angry and frustrated, she resorted to the use of aversive behavior management strategies such as yelling, criticizing, and lecturing.

Jim reacted with more emotional and psychological distance, thus isolating himself from his wife and step-grandson, DeShaun. The grandson's defiant behavior became strengthened by the combined process of ineffective parenting from the grandmother, who received little backup from her husband.

A Multisytemic Evaluation Was Used

Finally, a multisystemic evaluation of the family was undertaken. The purpose of which was to assess how the family was interacting with systems, such as mental health, school, legal and social services, and how these systems connected to the family and how they connected to the grandson's life. This evaluation was completed by listening to the family as well as personnel from the child's school and other agencies, resulting in an understanding of this family's increased isolation from other family members, as well as potential positive support in the community. Involvement with legal, and social service agencies, for example, were perceived by Josephine and Jim as sources of stress. They were not accustomed to speaking to others about their problems, and felt inconvenienced by the time required to complete the same.

Outcomes and Evaluation

Josephine scored very high on all three global indices of distress—anxiety, depression, and demoralization, assessed by the Symptom Checklist-90-Revised. Further problems with stress were identified by a clinically significant elevation of 98% on measures of the parenting stress inventory as well as the Beck Depression Inventory.

In terms of family functioning, an evaluation resulted in a clear picture of a woman who is still grieving the loss of her first husband, as well as her daughter, and the independence that she sought at this stage of her life. Sources of stress included financial difficulties, a combination of retirement with the financial burden of raising grandchildren, and coping with her grandson's behavior problems and school concerns.

Treatment Interventions

The treatment implemented for these custodial grandparents was based on using a cognitive behavioral model to build resilience. Cognitive behavior therapy (CBT), as a treatment model, aims to improve mental health functioning using therapeutic strategies to assess and change unhelpful thoughts, beliefs, and assumptions, as well as specific ways of behaving and reacting. Specifically, regarding treatment of depression, common negative belief patterns called schema, generate unhelpful and negative self-evaluations, which in turn contribute to unhelpful behaviors. Effective change of belief patterns coupled with an increase of positive behavior change are the key components of CBT and contribute heavily to increasing resilience in these families.

Cognitive Therapy

Aaron Beck, a pioneer in the development of cognitive therapy, identified cognitive biases such as pessimism, over-generalization, over personalizing outcomes, dichotomous or "black-white thinking" that require challenge and change during the therapeutic process (Beck, 1975).

Another therapeutic treatment consideration of CBT is to increase behavioral activation of pleasant and rewarding activities in the patient's life, as well as to improve specific behaviors such as interpersonal skills directly relevant to enhancing resilience in these individuals.

Josephine's problems with depression could be traced to a combination of well-engrained faulty cognitions and thinking patterns. She reported feeling as if the sense of loss due to the death of both her first husband and her daughter were never completely grieved. As important, the sense of freedom she had hoped for as a retired individual did not materialize. Thoughts of hopelessness and pessimism about her situation were further exacerbated by Josephine's feelings of guilt that she failed as a parent and grandparent, as well as a spouse.

Josephine's guilt was further exacerbated by dwelling on what she "should" have done in her life, as well as her tendency to dwell on negative and punishing experiences such as financial distress, social isolation, quarreling with her current husband, struggles with her grandson's behavior at home, and dealing with the frequent calls from the school because of DeShaun's behavior and learning difficulties.

Additionally, Josephine lamented no longer having time to spend on her hobbies and interests.

The Therapeutic Agenda

Utilizing the cognitive behavior model, counseling was initiated by educating Josephine on the development of depression, followed by assisting Josephine in understanding how negative cognitions are triggered automatically by current and past events.

During individual counseling treatment sessions, the Socratic method was employed to help Josephine understand she could not, for example, predict her future, but that she could manage one day at a time. Thus, a "day by day" perspective on managing significant family problems helped Josephine from becoming overwhelmed with the long range view. In addition to triggering a more optimistic rather than pessimistic view, another goal of her therapy was to normalize the extent of her parenting challenges.

Rational Emotive Behavioral Therapy

Ellis (2001) used the terms "catastrophizing" and "awfulizing" to describe people's tendency to think in extreme and irrational ways. Josephine was taught to recognize and change her extreme thought patterns to recognizing that although things were bad, they were not signs of the end of the world and can be successfully resolved.

Helping Josephine recognize the link between her multiple loss experiences and automatic negative cognitions proved to be a beneficial therapeutic step as it encouraged her to avoid seeing her crisis as insurmountable, as well as to reinforce the sense that she could cope with her difficult situation. In addition, the fact that these relationship issues were addressed early in therapy served the purpose of providing emotional support for Josephine.

Ancillary Treatments

Facilitating a psychiatric consultation referral was also arranged to address medical management of depression, which she accepted.

Further Therapeutic Steps

Josephine found positive ways to reduce stress and negative feelings and to build resilience in developing a variety of social skills including relationship and stress management, assertiveness training, time management, and seeking a variety of support services designed to enhance her feeling of mastery of her life and to encourage increasing pleasant events in her life.

For example, Josephine found respite care for her grandson, so she and her husband could socialize with peers. They enjoyed reconnecting with friends to play cards or eat at a restaurant. Josephine also agreed to increase some time and effort spending small but important time re-engaged with favorite hobbies.

Stress Management Techniques

Typical for a stress management plan, Josephine prioritized the many issues that have become present in her life with the purpose of focusing on solving one problem at a time. After respite services were arranged for her grandson, and time socailizing with her Jim and friends was increased, she agreed it was time to concentrate on her grandson's situation at school to seek out better ways to improve his educational program. She agreed to meet with a local agency provider who provided advocacy services prior to seeking to alter DeShaun's educational plan.

Furthermore, Josephine was instructed in using effective stress management and resilience building techniques such as the use of guided imagery, and breathing exercises to divert Josephine's mental focus from her stressful situations. During her guided imagery, Josephine learned to concentrate on specific details of her favorite place in her backyard. She was coached to focus on creating in her "mind's eye," the sensory details of her image, such as sights, sounds, smells, and the temperature of the air.

Josephine was exposed to a relaxation technique using deep or diaphragmatic breathing. This was helpful as well. This strategy was practical and easy for Josphine to learn. After learning to recognize the contrast between shallow and deep breathing, Josephine was able to relax better by using this simple process of inhaling deeply through her nose, and exhaling slowly through the mouth. These relaxation techniques helped Josephine nurture a positive view of herself and to gain a sense of control over her life.

Further Therapeutic Interventions

Josephine was encouraged to invest in her spousal relationship, to not only serve the purpose of providing her with pleasant experiences with her fairly new partner, but also to resolve the domestic conflict that occurred between Josephine and Jim. They spent more quality time together. This resulted in Jim feeling less as an outsider in the family as well as someone "left out" of her life. He then expressed more willingness to join her effort to parent their difficult grandson, DeShaun. The ultimate goal of these efforts was to strengthen the partnership between her and Jim.

Multi-Dimensional Therapy

The above stated case highlights the multiple family dynamics that must be addressed as part of an effective treatment plan and to boost resilience. For example, during joint sessions with the grandparents, they were coached to discuss differing views on household rules and daily responsibilities for the grandson. The process of encouraging both to listen, and to validate each other's perspectives, facilitated a sense of compromise both felt was reasonable. These changes also allowed Jim to enjoy an emerging relationship with DeShaun.

Further Ancillary Referrals

Josephine was directed to where to look for additional help. Josephine appeared to benefit from a support group referral. Typical of curricula for therapeutic support groups, Josephine gained an opportunity to learn from others in a similar situation how to take better care of herself physically and emotionally. By engaging in mutual storytelling, as well as receiving psycho-educational intervention, Josephine appeared to gain insight from appropriate role models, and in-service training on various topics including mental health resources, health care, parent training, and legal issues (Dannison & Smith, 2003).

Drawing from Research

Similarly, results of a pilot study completed by Kelly, Yorker, Whipley, & Sipe (2001) suggests that Josephine and other grandparents might build resilience from a multi-modal intervention plan that includes a six session social support group coupled with individual in-home social work and problem solving sessions resulting in improvement of grandparents' mental health, confidence in parenting knowledge and ability to provide adequate care for their grandchildren. This type of approach is generally beyond the scope of the individual practitioner.

Augmenting Resilience

Assessment and treatment of Josephine's depression and stress related concerns, facilitated her resilience and her ability to better utilize social networks and family support, as well as school personnel, mental health therapists, and medical professionals. As a result, DeShaun emerged after treatment with improved behavior and competence at home and school.

He became more compliant with the basic rules of the household, including better adherence to expectations for helping with chores around the house, with much less verbal complaining and arguing. At school, the grandson became far less disruptive in the classroom, and was making and keeping friends. Challenges with academic achievement, especially in reading and math instruction were still present, but met with far less resistance on the child's part.

He was making positive social connections both informally by playing with peers around the neighborhood, but also formally by participating in one organized sport each season. The end result for the therapist was to facilitate helpful connections between grandparent and grandchild as well as between the family unit and service providers in school and other social service agencies (Edwards & Taub, 2009).

Following the successful implementation of the above treatment plan, DeShaun displayed considerable improvements in behavior and resilience, as family stressors were ameliorated and his emotional state began to return to normal levels. Management of Josephine's depression was a top therapeutic priority due to the clear link between caregiver depression and parenting difficulties (Minkler, Fuller-Thompson, Miller, & Driver, 1997). She made significant improvements with a combination of medication management and important changes in thinking about her life circumstances and in applying a cognitive behavioral model aimed at increasing resilience.

Josephine developed increased clarity about her parenting challenges and skills. She learned how to take a "day by day" approach to problem solving.

Specifically, more "rational" thinking patterns adopted by Josephine helped her feel more optimistic. Moreover, Josephine connected her grandson with professionals who could help her improve DeShaun's functioning.

The grandson's ADHD was also treated successfully with medication. As a sign of her growing resilience, Josephine obtained medical insurance coverage for medical and mental health care for him. Josephine moved toward obtaining case management services, which provided numerous benefits such as transportation to and from appointments. The case manager also assisted Josephine in her interactions with the school district.

Everything's Connected

Josephine's participation in meetings at the school resulted in the implementation of an Individual Educational Plan. The plan included provision of academic support and accommodations, counseling and a behavioral consultant to work with Josephine and the school staff. With his school behavior problems under much better control, DeShaun's educational competence also improved further enhancing his self-confidence and self-efficacy. He joined pro-social after school activities and made a few close friends.

As a result of her improvements in stress management and mood, Josephine was encouraged to set important behavioral goals for her grandson, and take advantage of training in parenting skills. As a result Josephine learned to improve her ability to use effective commands, and provide verbal praise. A weekly contract system was implemented to help the family to focus on concrete behavioral goals and to keep them current from week to week. While her grandson's behavior was far from angelic, Josephine began feeling as if she possessed a structure to cope and to react to her grandson's misbehaviors more effectively.

The Muscle of Resilience

Josephine's positive outlook helped her to develop greater reliance and to be less punitive to her grandson's behavioral challenges. The result was an improved balance of use of rewards and punishment. Josephine discovered that DrShaun's rate of compliance improved as her use of positive parenting techniques increased.

As a result, both she and her grandson were feeling less resentful toward each other. This change improved their emotional connection, as well as quality of life in the family contributing to their resilience. Furthermore, during joint sessions, Josephine and DeShaun were able to share positive memories about his mother. She was encouraged to build a scrapbook of photos and other mementos for her grandson. They grew closer. Together they agreed to a yearly family picnic as a ritual to honor the mother's memory.

These experiences helped Josephine's grandson immensely. He became more resilient. He learned important social skills such as shared decision making, appropriate expression of feelings, and willingness to co-operate with and please an adult parent figure.

Jim found it easier to emotionally accept the role of becoming another mentor for the grandson. His willingness to take DeShaun on garage sales and antique buying trips proved to be a mutually pleasing connection. The now resilient grandson learned to buy and sell his own garage sale items, and learn the responsibility of making money for himself.

With the above changes in place, DeShaun felt more connected to Jim. He began referring to them as "mom and dad." For his part, he took on more physical chores such as lawn mowing, and yard work, which were too physically demanding for his aging grandparents.

Conclusions and Implications for Helping Professionals

Counselors and clinicians are seeing an explosion of grandparents parenting their grandchildren being referred into their practices. The grandparents are often reluctant to take on the role of parenting, but are willing to do so to provide a safe haven for their neglected or abused grandchildren or to keep their grandchildren out of foster care (Minkler, 1994). These burdened families enter therapy with a plethora of challenging problems. For example, the children have ever changing educational needs.

The demands of a modern curriculum may put a strain on the grandparents' ability to help with homework. Grandchildren who have special education needs also are a contributing factor to further stress. Involvement in the legal system can also be daunting and overwhelming. Typical legal difficulties facing grandparents raising their grandchildren include clarifying custody. In the face of competing in courts with their own children, grandparents must work cooperatively with law guardians who represent their grandchildren, their own attorneys, and social workers that represent the Department of Social Services and other interested parties.

Interacting with the Department of Social Services and family courts can be time consuming, emotionally draining, and financially costly. The stressors grandparents face frequently cause many of them to feel defeated, depressed, and in poor health.

The clinician faced with these families requires solutions that are multilayered and complex. A family systems approach along with cognitive-behavioral model to build resilience in the grandparents is most productive in treating multigenerational families. Despite the trials and tribulations these grandparents are experiencing, they are proud to help their grandchildren and find their role meaningful and worthwhile.

As these families bounce back from a plethora of burdensome problems and difficulties, they manifest growing resilience. Building on the positive affect and love family members have for one another, the astute practitioner starts by developing rapport and trust in the family members, listens to their individual stories and perspectives, and makes changes gradually in small steps.

Generally, multigenerational therapy is long-termed and the therapist develops a strong relationship with his clients. The successful transaction and culmination of these cases is profoundly rewarding and meaningful to the clinician and family alike. Promoting the health and welfare of these families and watching the grandchildren grow and prosper has been extremely satisfying for us as clinicians and provides us with the energy and confidence to treat enthusiastically and to build resilience in newly referred grandparents who are parenting their grandchildren.

References

Abidin, R. R. (1995). *Parenting stress index.* Odessa, FL: Psychological Assessment Resources.

Beck, A. T. (1975). *Cognitive therapy and the emotional disorders.* International Universities Press, Inc.

Beck, A. T. (1990). *Beck anxiety inventory manual.* San Antonio TX: The Psychological Corp.

Beck, A. T., Steer, R. A., & Brown, G. K. (2003). *Beck depression inventorymanual* (2nd ed.) San Antonio, TX: The Psychological Corp.

Burton, L. M. (1992). Black grandparents rearing children of drug-addicted parents: Stressors, outcomes, and social services needs. *The Gerontologist, 32*(6), 744–751.

Dannison, L. L., & Smith, A. B. (2003). Custodial grandparents community support program: Lessons learned. *Children & Schools, 25*, 87–95.

Derogatis, L. R. (1994). *Symptom checklist-90-R.* Minneapolis, MN: Pearson Publishing Company.

Dimidjian, S. (2006). Randomized trial of behavioral activation, cognitive therapy, and antidepressant medication in acute treatment of adults with major depression. *Journal of Consulting and Clinical Psychology, 74*(4), 658–679.

Edwards, O., & Taub, G. (2009). A conceptual pathways model to promote positive youth development in children raised by their grandparents. *School Psychology Quarterly, 24*(1), 160–172.

Ellis, A. (2001). *Overcoming destructive beliefs, feelings, and behaviors: New directions for rational emotive behavior therapy.* New York: Prometheus Books.

Kelly, S. J., Whitley, D., Sipe, T. A., & Yorker, B. C. (2000). Psychological distress in grandmother kinship care providers: The role of resources, social support, and physical health. *Child Abuse & Neglect, 24*, 311–321.

Minkler, M. (1994). Grandparents as parents: The American experience. *Aging International, 21*, 24–28.

Minkler, M., Fuller-Thomson, E., Miller, D., & Driver, D. (1997). Depression in grandparents raising grandchildren: Results of a national longitudinal study. *Arch Fam Med, 6*, 445–452.

Stix, G. (2011, March). The neuroscience of true grit. *Scientific American*, 29–33.

15 Resiliency and Custodial Grandparents

Recognizing and Supporting Strengths

Andrea B. Smith, Linda L. Dannison, and Melodye James

Abstract

The diverse challenges associated with raising grandchildren are widely recognized as daunting. Custodial grandparents, however, frequently demonstrate commitment, creativity, and tenacity in their attitudes and their approaches to activities associated with their caregiving role. This chapter will highlight grandparents' readiness to learn and will illustrate effective service delivery practices for this population. Inherent strengths and a process for enhancing resiliency in grandparent caregivers will also be addressed.

Introduction

Parent education programs historically focused on providing services to first time parents in traditional families. This model of parent education has changed dramatically during the past generation. Parenting classes now serve varied populations, including parents whose children have been removed from their homes due to abuse and/or neglect, parents in the process of divorce, blended families, teen parents, single parents, incarcerated parents, military families, and grandparents who are raising grandchildren. Effective parent education programs need to recognize specific challenges and unique strengths common to the population being served. This chapter will highlight the development, implementation, and evaluation of a program designed to capitalize on the prior experiences, motivation, and capabilities of custodial grandparents. As shown within this chapter, there is no one "right" way to provide services to custodial grandparent family members. Effective services may look different in various communities but all share the common mission of assisting grandparents to acquire new skills and knowledge, establish vital relationships, and recognize and enhance their own personal resiliency.

Program Development: The Parent Topics Questionnaire

The Parent Topics Questionnaire is a standardized assessment measure developed to identify informational priorities of participants in diverse parent education programs (Smith & Dannison, 2003). Four "parent" groups—Teen, Grandparents, Single and Parent Education group participants—were surveyed. Results from this survey were shared with parent education group facilitators and provided information about needs, desires, and expectations of potential participants. More importantly, these results showed a high readiness for information among teen parent and custodial grandparent survey respondents (Gerard et al., 1996; Smith & Dannison, 2003). All participants were surveyed on perceived needs for information and strategies related to 11 topic areas: *Health and Safety, Social Issues, Family Relations, Guiding Behavior, Parenting Patterns, Parenting and Working, Pregnancy, Infancy, Early Childhood, Middle Childhood, and Adolescence.* On eight of these 11 scales, grandparents' desire for information was higher than any other parent group surveyed. (Dannison, 2011; Gerard et al., 1996; Smith & Dannison, 2010). Grandparent caregivers' recognition of their readiness and need for additional information to support their life circumstances was an initial indicator of the inherent resiliency common to many custodial grandparents, and lead to the development of the *Second Time Around* program (Dannison & Smith, 2010; Gerard et al., 1996; Smith & Dannison, 2010).

Programming for Custodial Grandparent Families

The *Second Time Around* program is a holistic program, initially developed in 1996 to provide services to caregiving grandparents, their young grandchildren and the professionals who work with these family members. Curricular materials were initially designed to facilitate group services for grandparents, and were soon expanded to include literacy-based playgroups for grandchildren and in-service education for community-based professionals. In 2006, the *Grandparent Resource Site* project was established with support from the WK Kellogg Foundation. This project was conceptualized as a multiyear initiative that capitalized on the unique strengths and needs inherent in each community. An RFP was published and 10 sites, in nine locations, were funded. In an effort to examine best practices across the country, locations that provided geographic and ethnic diversity were selected (see Figure 15.1). Sites operated under the guidance of a *Local Advisory Committee* (LAC) to insure that selected GRS services were relevant and appropriate for varying community needs.

The *Grandparent Resource Site* project provided basic financial assistance, curricular materials, staff training, programmatic evaluation, and ongoing support to all 10 locations. Several sites had already established some programming for custodial grandparents, although none were offering specific services to grandchildren. All sites received the same materials, training opportunities, and evaluation protocols. Site coordinators were able to communicate with each other and project directors via scheduled conference calls and email. A conscious decision was made to have project directors make multiple visits to each individual site to allow for regular training of program staff and observations

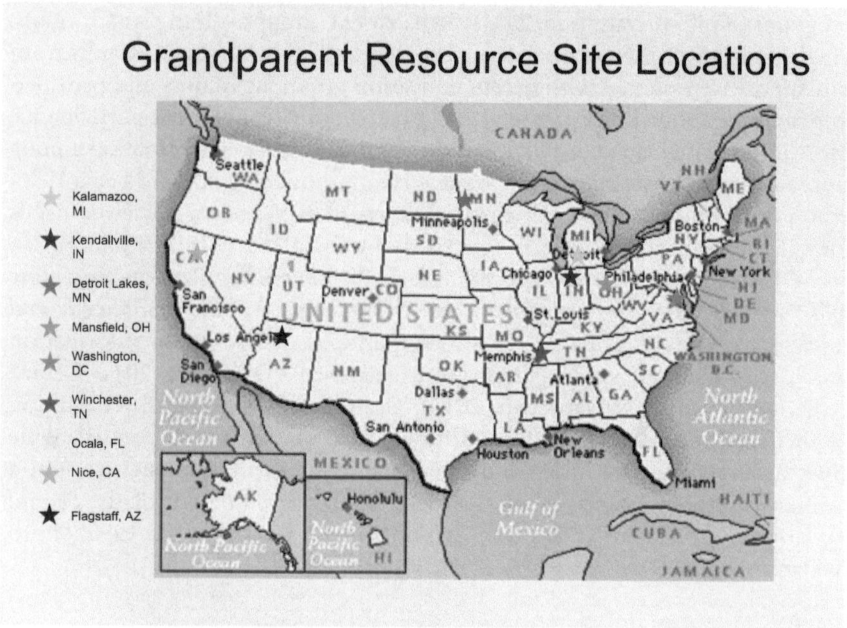

Figure 15.1 Map of Grandparent Resource Site locations

of services being provided. These visits were reciprocally beneficial, with sites receiving updated materials, training and support and project directors having opportunities to observe unique strengths inherent in the programs and delivery methods chosen by each site.

Common challenges faced by GRS Program Facilitators included recruiting grandparents, establishing group loyalty, learning to effectively manage group dynamics, and dealing with financial issues related to ongoing funding. Sites commonly experienced strong group cohesiveness and dedication after approximately three to four meetings. Facilitators in all sites highlighted grandparents' readiness to take on new challenges and to learn information and strategies to better equip them for their not-so-new parental role.

The program model (see Figure 15.2) identifies common services—Custodial Grandparent and Grandchildren's groups and Professional In-service Opportunities with their communities—for all sites during the first year of this project. During subsequent years, sites were encouraged to work with their Advisory Committees to determine which services (Continuation Groups, In-Home Services and Child Care Providers Trainings) were most appropriate. A listing of services selected by each GRS is provided in Figure 15.3. The varying services selected by each site allowed all sites to become more individually responsive to their particular clientele.

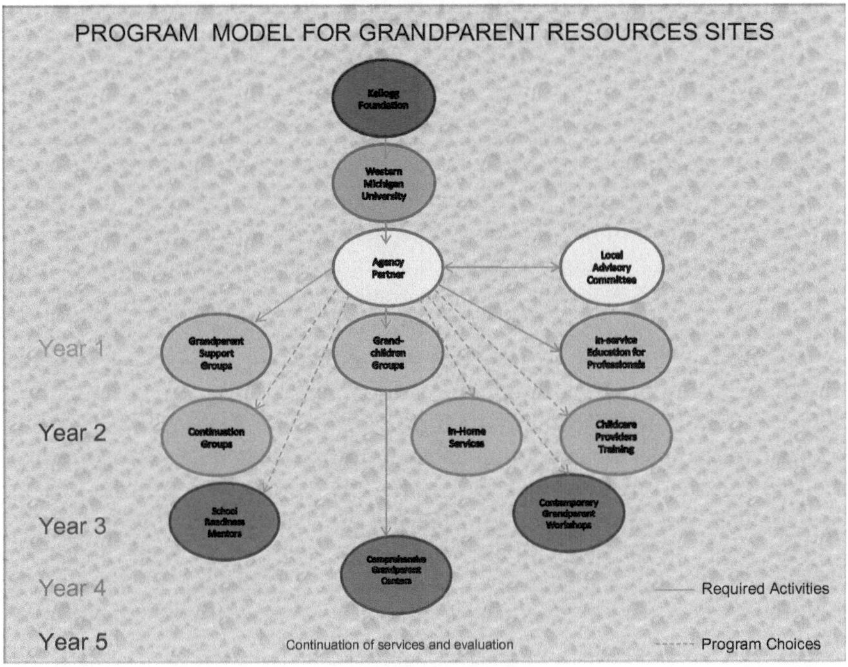

Figure 15.2 Grandparent Resource Site Program Model

Services Selected at 10 Sites

State	Grand-Parent Groups	Grand-Childrens Groups	Professional Outreach	Continuation	In-Home	Child Care
MI	X	X	X	X	X	
OH	X	X	X	X	X	
IN	X	X	X	X		
FL	X	X	X	X	X	X
FL	X	X	X	X	X	X
W-DC	X	X	X	X		
TN	X	X	X	X		X
CA	X	X	X	X	X	
MN	X	X	X	X	X	X
AR	X	X	X	X		X

Figure 15.3 Services Provided at GRS

Unique Aspects of Grandparent Resource Sites

Despite their similarities, some differences emerged when comparing the 10 Grandparent Resource Sites. One major difference related to the sites' prior experiences delivering services to grandparent-headed families. While some sites had an established history of service delivery to this specific population, other sites were "start-ups" and needed to begin with the basic tasks associated with any program. Some challenges for the newer sites included finding a convenient location, training facilitators, locating grandparents, and securing additional funding. Another difference for participating sites was related to their sponsoring organizations, which included Cooperative Extension, Human Services, Senior Services, Rehab Services, Faith-Based, School Districts, and a Native American Indian Reservation. Additional site-based challenges highlighted the cultural and community history of the grandparent families being served. For example, transportation issues in the Washington DC group revolved around utilizing public transportation services, while more rural sites, such as Tennessee and Minnesota, were challenged by finding funding to support grandparents and/or facilitators driving long distances to attend or provide group services. Additionally, each site developed a unique mission that supported and moved grandparent participants toward greater resiliency (Dannison & Smith, 2010; Smith & Dannison, 2010).

The Flagstaff, Arizona site is administered by the University of Arizona Cooperative Extension. Services were initially offered in two adjacent counties serving very diverse grandparent populations. Grandparents comprising one county's group were lower income and sessions often focused on identifying and utilizing local supports. In contrast, grandparents in the adjacent county were more affluent and their financial questions revolved around issues including long term financial security for their grandchildren. Grandparent group facilitators continued to receive training to enhance their knowledge and skills related to relationship building between group members. This resulted in building successful Continuation Group services, as grandparent participants remained eager about their group membership.

The Robinson Rancheria Grandparent Resource Site is located on a Native American Indian Reservation in Nice, CA. The reservation of Pomo Indians is supported in part by an on-site casino. Rurally located, this population has a long history of relatives providing care for children. One indicator of this is their high-quality local child care center, which is available to members of the reservation. Challenges for group members included financial struggles, geographic isolation, transportation issues, and community substance abuse. In addition to regular group services, this site effectively emphasized respite activities for all grandparent-headed family members.

The University of DC in the District of Columbia houses the largest urban Cooperative Extension Center in the United States. This location had no prior history working with grandparent-headed family members; staff worked hard to develop a program that was intimately connected to their members' needs.

Relationship building among participants was an identified area of emphasis, as was outreach and advocacy around issues common to custodial grandparents. Due to their location in the nation's capital, members of this site's groups were able to attend legislative rallies and meetings and developed ongoing relationships with members of a grandparent group from the Philadelphia, PA area.

Kids Central of Ocala is located in central Florida and incorporates a three-district Human Services Site. This GRS served the largest number of grandparent-headed family members and also initiated an annual state-wide Kinship Care Conference. This two-day event features nationally recognized speakers and is attended by both community-based professionals and kinship care providers. Some veteran grandparent group participants were eventually hired by Kids Central to serve as Grandparent Group Facilitators and office workers. Partnerships with existing community agencies allowed groups for grandparents and grandchildren to be offered through the local school districts and the community's public libraries.

A partnership between a local church and the community school district in rural Indiana resulted in the origination of the Northeast Indiana Grandparents Raising Grandchildren program. Religious leaders and school personnel had noticed increasing numbers of grandparents raising grandchildren in the local community and were concerned about effectively meeting these families' unique challenges. Within three months, this site identified and trained facilitators and began programming. Ties to other existing programs for custodial grandparents were established, allowing this site to continue to expand and eventually merge with a larger regional group. One of the facilitators, an ordained minister, has begun writing and speaking about responding to kinship care issues within faith-based organizations.

Michigan State University's Cooperative Extension program has a long history serving custodial grandparent families. Their involvement in the Grandparent Resource Site project lead to greater individualization of program services to more effectively meet existing community needs. Working with a dedicated Local Advisory Committee of professionals and grandparents, this site identified unique needs that were not being met by current resources. They provided leadership to translate programmatic materials into Spanish and were the first site to utilize in-home services for geographically isolated kinship care providers. Pro-bono legal services were secured to further support custodial grandparents.

Mahube Community Council is a non-profit Community Action Agency located in northwestern Minnesota. The agency serves three rural counties and had previous history working with grandparent-headed families. This site offered services to both grandparents and grandchildren in seven different locations, often necessitating that facilitators travel long distances to reach group meetings. In addition to regular program content, facilitators also addressed grandparents' challenges with geographic isolation and long winters. This site obtained additional grants to manage the higher costs of fuel, travel and food for both grandparent participants and facilitators.

The Mansfield, Ohio Grandparent Resource Site is located in a substance abuse rehabilitation center. This site offered strong integration with other community services providers and emphasized holistic programming to address the multiple challenges experienced by many of the site's grandparent group participants. Legal, vocational, medical, and educational professionals are now brought together in an Annual Grandparent Rally to raise awareness and support for kinship care family members.

The Campora Family Resource Center is a rural site housed in an adult education center in southern Tennessee. Grandparent group participants willingly drive long distances to attend meetings and other activities and maintain strong group loyalty. This large group (40–50 active members) is service oriented and coordinates and staffs a county-wide food pantry. Grandparents and their grandchildren come together monthly to sort, package, and deliver food boxes throughout their community. Funds raised through their efforts are directed to support college scholarships for grandchildren raised by grandparents.

Current Grandparent Resource Site Activities

Support to these sites through the *Grandparent Resource Site* project officially ended in June, 2009. Follow-up interviews were conducted with all nine site facilitators during the summer of 2011. These interviews focused on the evolution of the sites, current activities, and facilitators' perspectives related to grandparents' ability to cope with stress, grandparents' proficiency meeting their grandchildren's needs and grandparents' feelings of positivity and meaningfulness about raising their grandchildren.

Interview questions focusing on sites' evolution and current activities illustrate that, despite tight economic constraints, all former GRS agencies continue to respond to the needs of kinship care families in their communities. In all cases, funding issues are very challenging. Sites have moved beyond exclusively meeting grandparents' initial needs for information, socialization, and respite and are working to enhance and nurture grandparents' inherent resiliency in varying ways.

Services in several sites have been expanded and intentionally tailored for grandparent-headed family members in each community. These services reflect specific geographic and cultural differences. Examples include grand-family camp with the theme of "Finding Your Inner Playfulness," additional intergenerational recreation activities, expanded home visits in rural settings, meal deliveries, and increased access to Continuation Groups and Child Care Providers training opportunities. Several sites offer case management programming which support grandparents' efforts in securing legal, educational, and financial assistance. Services are being offered in more diverse settings, including public libraries, Head Start sites and recreational centers. Some sites are relying on technology for communication and networking. Partnerships with other organizations, including colleges and universities, the foster care system, the prison system, and other agencies serving kinship care families leads to the creation of unique services that recognize and work to enhance resiliency in kinship care family members.

Economic constraints are reflected in agencies' increased focus on more efficient service delivery models that continue to support grandfamilies. Collaboration with educational settings, including a local science center and utilizing college students from a local university to assist grandparent and grandchildren's groups have proven useful. Other sites have incorporated cost-effective strategies including writing a county-wide newsletter to reach greater numbers of grandparents at lower costs and increasing reliance on grandparents' leadership to keep groups going. One group prioritized and raised money to pay for child care costs of group members. Another site highlighted their efforts to use veteran grandparents to locate and recruit potential members for new group services. At one site, experienced grandparents have been hired to mentor other relative caregivers. Volunteer discussion group leaders are being trained in several counties to reduce costs associated with providing group services.

Experienced Grandparent Resource Sites have developed a more future-oriented focus. With immediate needs for information, support and respite provided, grandparents often gain the strength to look to the future. This is reflected in sites' current activities, which include taking high school-aged grandchildren to orientation at a local university, training grandparents to assist grandchildren with a science curriculum, and providing enhanced opportunities for respite and recreation. One group developed programming priorities that emphasized four areas of desired improvement: financial, physical, emotional, and spiritual. Other sites have become more active in speaking, writing, and educating within the mental health, educational, medical, legal, and religious professions. Regional and state-wide conferences have originated to raise awareness of kinship issues among professionals and to provide additional support and information to local custodial grandparents.

The Continuum of Resiliency

Professional work in the field with custodial grandparents, pilot-testing a comprehensive curriculum for grandparent caregivers, observations of multiple grandparent group facilitators, conversations with custodial grandparents both nationally and internationally, and interviews with grandparent-site coordinators and other professionals working with kinship care families lead to the development of a *Continuum of Resiliency in Custodial Grandparents* (Dannison, Smith, & James, 2011). This continuum highlights why some grandparent caregivers are more effective than others at fulfilling their parental roles, serves as a direction in which to "move" grandparent caregivers through support services, and provides a basis for capitalizing on inherent family strengths (see Figure 15.4).

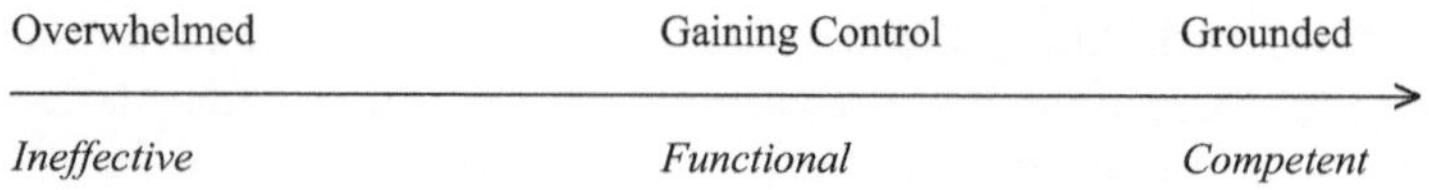

Figure 15.4 Continuum of Resiliency in Custodial Grandparents

Many custodial grandparents experience feelings of being overwhelmed for many reasons including a sudden change of life circumstances, isolation from friends and lack of family support. Over half of custodial grandparents are single parents (U.S. Bureau of the Census, 2009) and many are grappling with issues associated with living in poverty (U.S. Bureau of the Census, 2009). Grandchildren in the care of many of these grandparents experience emotional, cognitive, social and/or physical challenges (Dannison & Smith, 2004; Smith & Dannison, 2008; Smith & Dannison, 2003; Smith, Dannison, & Vacha-Haase, 1999).

Grandparents often struggle to meet their grandchildren's needs, while simultaneously meeting the needs of their own adult child and, in many cases, their own aging parents (Dannison, Smith, & Vacha-Haase, 1999; Smith & Dannison, 2008; Smith & Dannison, 2003). Grandparents' behaviors are often ineffective and inefficient at this stage and are focused on meeting the immediate needs of both grandparents and grandchildren. Questions such as "How do I discipline a ten year old?", "Can my grandchild qualify for Head Start?", "Where can I get a copy of his birth certificate?" and "Who can help me find a daycare provider that I can afford?" are common. Grandparents talk about feeling stressed, lonely, angry, and incapable of fulfilling their new role (Dannison, Smith, & James, 2011; Dannison & Smith, 2003; Grinwys, Smith, & Dannison, 2004; Smith & Dannison, 2003).

Grandparents move through this continuum, demonstrating increased control as they gain confidence and experience. Group services which offer information, support, and respite are very effective at this stage (Dannison & Smith, 2010; Vacha-Haase, Ness, Dannison, & Smith, 2000). Successful management of tasks associated with the custodial grandparent role often occur in small steps, with grandparents gaining confidence from their own successes and the acknowledgment and support of group members and facilitators. Friendships evolve between group members and often fill an important void in many grandparents' lives. Statements such as "These are my new friends," "I can say anything here," "My grandson's teacher told me that he's doing better," and "I'm not all alone" become more common. Grandparents' behaviors become more effective and efficient. They are better able to manage their multiple roles and show more confidence about seeking support and asking questions (Dannison, Smith, & James, 2011).

In time, many grandparents become grounded in their new parental roles. They display increased abilities to manage both familiar and new challenges and often use their own experiences as a basis for helping others. Leadership qualities may emerge as grandparents take pride in assisting those who are struggling with challenges they have overcome (Smith, Dannison, & Curtis, 2008). Grandparents acknowledge that they can't "do it all" and become more effective at prioritizing and making objective decisions. Behaviors are more effective and competent, with grandparents taking pride in their successes. Comments such as "I can sleep at night because I know my grandbaby is safe," "Her teacher and I are on the same page," "I'm bringing my friend to meet our group tonight," and "I called her up because I knew she was having a hard time with her daughter" are reflective of grandparents' movement into this stage of the continuum and toward greater resiliency.

Building Resiliency in Custodial Grandparents

Interviews with Grandparent Resource Site coordinators highlighted five themes that appeared to reoccur among custodial grandparents who were effective in their roles. These grandparents' behaviors consistently showed attributes of resiliency and can be conceptualized as the following "5 P's of Resilient Grandparent Caregivers": *Proud, Positive, Persistent, Protective and Problem-Solvers* (Dannison, Smith, & James, 2011).

Proud custodial grandparents are loyal to their grandchildren. They're proud of the role they are playing in grandchildren's lives and learn to accept the challenges of their not-so-new roles. Grandparents' pride is displayed in their empathy toward other grandparent caregivers and their willingness to share information and support. Deb, a 52-year-old grandmother of three grandsons, personifies this pride. She is unfailingly loyal to her grandchildren and accepts their behavioral and physical challenges related to prenatal drug exposure. Following juvenile court's ruling that she could not be considered as her grandchildren's legal guardian without entering a drug treatment program, she willingly began a program , submitted to daily mouth swabs for over a year, obtained individual counseling and completed a care plan with Children's Services. Deb also attended the *Second Time Around* support group for custodial grandparents in her community, where she built supportive relationships with other group members and the facilitator. Determined that she would not fail her grandchildren as she had her daughter, her mantra became "Whatever it takes." Today, Deb is proudly caring for her three grandsons and continuing to do what it takes.

Resilient custodial grandparents display *positivity* about their daily lives. They are open to working hard to meet their changed circumstances and adhere to a "glass half full" philosophy. These grandparents can see humor in small things and take delight in living with their grandchildren. Positive grandparents recognize that they care deeply for their grandchildren and are able to put grandchildren's needs ahead of their own. Many grandparents express a conviction that "family comes first" and that caring for grandchildren is what they should be doing at this time in their lives. Dianne, age 69, effectively portrays this sense of positivity as she cares for her 12-year-old grandson. She believes that God has given her the role of caring for this child, who was diagnosed with Attention-Deficit Hyperactivity Disorder (ADHD) and Autistic Spectrum Disorder (ASD). Diane has self-educated herself about these disabilities and has become her group's resident expert on children with special needs. She has secured the services of a young male mentor for her grandson, and advocates for his mental health and educational needs. Diane has embraced her role as a caregiving grandparent and feels positive about the successes she can observe in her grandson's life.

Persistence is another attribute demonstrated by resilient grandparents. These caregivers model strength on a daily basis as they juggle multiple demands to find the time and energy necessary to meet their changed family circumstances. Custodial grandparents bravely navigate unfamiliar systems in the legal, medical, educational and/or social service arenas, often returning multiple times before getting the answers and/or services they feel are essential. Many work extremely hard to fill the role of caring for multiple generations—their grandchildren, their own children, and often their aging relatives—within their own families. These grandparents are strongly motivated to learn and do what is needed to better care for their grandchildren. Barb, an 82-year-old great-grandmother raising two girls, ages five and seven years, exemplifies this persistence. Denied access to education during her own youth, Barb is determined that her great-granddaughters will have access to opportunities and advantages that were unavailable to her. She negotiated unfamiliar territory of her community's school voucher system so that her grandchildren could attend a private Catholic school. Barb sought out scholarships for ballet lessons and enrolled herself in a math tutoring program so that she could better assist with homework. She sets firm boundaries and appropriate limits for the girls but remains kind and tender in her interactions with them. Barb is not afraid to knock on any doors and consistently and persistently advocates for her grandchildren's needs.

Resilient custodial grandparents are *protective*. They are unfailingly loyal and assume the caregiving role because "this is family." Many care for grandchildren with special needs and/or challenges and who may need significant amounts of time and attention from their grandparent caregiver (deToledo & Brown, 1995; Sawyer & Dubowitz, 1994; Smith & Dannison, 2008). The continuation and establishment of family rituals and traditions, loving nicknames, and a fierce dedication to the children in their care are all characteristics of this protective attribute. Betty is 75 years old and is raising her 14-year-old granddaughter. Betty was raised in a close and supportive family and is determined to pass these values and unconditional love onto her granddaughter. Betty became aware of her grandchild's concern about Betty's age and what would happen if Betty was not able to raise her to adulthood. Betty engaged in some long and often difficult conversations with extended family members. She secured commitments from selected persons about what their roles would be in her granddaughter's life if Betty is unable to continue to care for her. Betty communicated this plan to her grandchild, who feels more secure in the knowledge that, no matter what, she will continue to stay with family members.

Family always comes first for Betty, and she protects those she cares about in many different ways.

The final attribute demonstrated by resilient custodial grandparents relates to *problem solving*. These grandparents make sure that they are knowledgeable about the information and/or support that will benefit their grandchildren. If they don't have an answer, they develop creative strategies. They are able to effectively put aspects of their own lives on hold and demonstrate the ability to prioritize tasks and goals. Custodial grandparents frequently have unique insight and knowledge related to family history. This personalized knowledge fills a void in the lives of children in kinship care families (Smith & Dannison, 2008). Above all, resilient grandparents are action-oriented. They evaluate situations, set goals, determine plans and then make things happen. Barb, age 40, displays these problem solving abilities. Raising a four-year-old child who is not biologically related to her, Barb faced state and county policies and regulations that were not inclusive of fictive kin providers. She was unable to secure mental health counseling for her child and get him enrolled in school. Unwilling to accept no for an answer, Barb has been seeking help from the very agencies who initially refused to help. As a result of her problem solving approach to this situation, a meeting has been scheduled with the superintendent of her school district, the county is working with an attorney to address the issue of non-relative representation, and a local attorney is assisting Barb to complete pertinent paperwork. In addition, Barb has volunteered to attend a state-wide kinship care coalition to better understand these issues and to share her own experiences with decision makers. On a more personal level, Barb has taken classes to become foster care certified and volunteers to provide respite for other kinship caregivers.

Conclusion

The keys to building resiliency in grandparents raising children are clearer after becoming familiar with the life circumstances of the kinship care providers. Specifics of their situations may vary but many commonalities exist (Dannison, Smith, & James, 2011; Dannison, 2010; Dannison & Smith, 2003; Whitley, Smith, & Goyer, 2011). It is essential to recognize that many grandparents feel overwhelmed as they assume their new roles and that the process of gaining control and becoming more grounded takes time. Resiliency is enhanced when grandparents are assisted in recognizing that *knowledge is power*. Services aimed at assisting kinship care providers to refine parenting skills and locate and utilize existing resources are especially beneficial. Secondly, resiliency will be enhanced when grandparents are encouraged to *find support*. Building relationships with others sharing similar circumstances is an important step toward reducing the isolation, depression, and helplessness initially felt by many custodial grandparents. Finally, grandparents should be encouraged to *seek respite*. Taking good care of one's own self is an essential aspect of being able to effectively care for others.

References

Dannison, L., Smith, A., & James, M. (2011, October). Resiliency in kinship care families: Capitalizing on family strengths. *4th Annual Kinship Care Conference and Grandfamily reunion*. Detroit, MI.

Dannison, L. (2011, April). Building and sustaining support groups for relative caregivers. *Relatives as Parents Program Annual Conference*, Denver, CO.

Dannison, L. & Smith, A. (2010, November). Enhancing personal competency: Lessons learnred. *Gerontological Society of America Annual Conference*, San Francisco, CA.

Dannison, L. & Smith, A. (2004). Understanding emotional issues in your grandchildren's lives. Minneapolis, MN: *Family Information Services.*

deToledo, S. & Brown, D., (1995). *Grandparents as parents: A survival guide for raising a second family*. New York: The Guilford Press.

Gerard, N., Smith, A., & Dannison, L. (1996, November). Assessing information needs of parents: Evolution of an instrument. 58th Annual Conference of the National Council on Family Relations, Kansas City, MO.

Grinwys, B., Smith, A., & Dannison, L. (2004). Custodial grandparent families and health care: Steps for developing responsive services. *Michigan Family Review, 9*, 37–44.

Sawyer, R. & Dubowitz, H. (1994). School performance of children in kinship care. *Child Abuse and Neglect, 18*, 587–597.

Smith, A. & Dannison, L. (2010, November). My glass is half-full: Positive grandparent caregivers. *Gerontological Society of America Annual Conference*, San Francisco, CA.

Smith, A. & Dannison, L. (2008). Preschool children and caregiving grandparents: Enhancing family strengths. In Hayslip, B., & Kaminski, T. (Eds), *Parenting the custodial grandchild: Implications for practice*. New York, Springer, 237–250.

Smith, A. & Dannison, L. (2003). Grandparent-headed families in the United States: Programming to meet unique needs. *Intergenerational Programming Quarterly, 1*(3), 35–47.

Smith, A., Dannison, L., & Curtis, T. (2009, July). Findings from the Grandparent Resource Site project. *15th Generations United International Conference*, Washington DC.

Smith, A. Dannison, L., & Vacha-Haase, T. (1999). When "Grandma" is "Mom": What today's teachers need to know. *Childhood Education, 75*, 12–16.

U.S. Bureau of the Census (2009). United States Census Bureau's 2005–2009 American Community Survey. Washington DC: *US Government Publication.*

Vacha-Haase, T., Ness, C., Dannison, L., & Smith, A. (2000). Grandparents raising grandchildren: A psychoeducational group approach. *Journal for Specialists in Group Work, 25*(1), 67–78.

Whitley, D., Smith, A., & Goyer, A. (2011, April). Grandparents raising grandchildren: Preliminary results of a national survey on research and practice. *American Society on Aging*, San Francisco, CA.

16 Promoting Family Empowerment Among African American Grandmothers Raising Grandchildren

Deborah M. Whitley, Susan J. Kelley, and Peter E. Campos

Abstract

Empowerment is often a focal outcome of community-based support services designed to enhance the well-being of grandparent-headed families. The authors in the present study conducted a correlational analysis to determine possible links between perceptions of empowerment, using the Family Empowerment Scale, perceived family support, and community resources. Using a convenience sample of 311 custodial grandparents participating in a comprehensive, multi-disciplinary program, pre/post test findings suggest the custodial grandparents experienced an enhanced perception of empowerment across all dimensions and subscale ($p \leq .001$), except competence. However, weak correlations were found between empowerment and perceptions of family support and community resources, suggesting using independent measures of perceived community resources and family support may not serve as surrogates for a specific empowerment measure. In addition, qualitative statements from six grandparents supported the quantitative findings, providing further insight on the program's effect on perceived empowerment.

Introduction

In the U.S., there are 2.4 million grandparents serving as primary caregivers for their grandchildren (Simmons & Dye, 2003). Parental substance abuse, psychiatric disorders, incarceration, homicide, HIV-AIDS are the primary reasons grandparents are raising their grandchildren (Dowdell, 1995; Kelley, Whitley, & Sipe, 2007; Poindexter & Linsk, 1999; Vega, et al., 1993). Clearly, many custodial grandparents are raising grandchildren under very difficult circumstances. The myriad of challenges faced by custodial grandparents is defined in the literature, including limited financial resources, emotional distress, social isolation, inability to access necessary community-based private/public support services (Landry-Meyer, Gerard, & Guzell, 2005; Waldrop & Weber, 2001). In addition, as older custodial grandparents experience the effects of aging, many become anxious about parenting grandchildren as their physical/mental capacity declines, further exacerbating any perceived lack of competence to fully meet the demands of parenting (Fuller-Thomson & Minkler, 2000). The literature also provides descriptions of various service delivery initiatives that offer a range of support services for grandparents. Case management, respite care, health services, support groups, parent education classes, legal assistance, and material aid are notable services targeted to custodial grandparents (Cox, 2002; Dannison & Smith, 2003; Kelley, Whitley, & Campos, 2010; McCallion, Janicki, Grant-Griffin, & Kolomer, 2000). Program descriptions often suggest empowerment is a desired outcome for program participants. There is the expectation that through specialized intervention services, grandparents' will feel empowered to manage their parenting responsibilities with competence, to acquire a positive perspective about their support networks, and to master advocacy skills to benefit their families. However, past studies have based conclusions about empowered participants largely on small sample sizes and anecdotal statements. In response to this limitation, this chapter extends a previously published study on empowerment of African-American grandmothers that describes an intervention service for custodial grandparents in parent-absent households, with the specific goal of empowering its participants (Whitley, Kelley, & Campos, 2011). The described program accentuates the strengths of grandparents through a comprehensive, interdisciplinary service structure, and facilitates the development of appropriate problem-solving skills to address family needs. The current study presents a portion of the data results from the previous work, but also tests grandparents' perceptions of family support networks and community resources to ascertain how they might be associated with perceptions of empowerment. In addition, qualitative statements from former program participants further elucidate program effects.

Background

Previous literature reviews describe the concept of empowerment and empowerment practice (Chadiha, Adams, Biegel, Auslander, & Gutierrez, 2004; Cox & Parsons, 1996; Dunst, Trivette, & Deal, 1988; Freir, 1983; Gutierrez, 1995; Kieffer, 1984; Parsons, 1991; Rappaport, 1987). There is a consensus that empowerment involves individuals gaining control over life situations and motivating others for positive change. Solomon (1976) conceptualized empowerment as a process where individuals acknowledge and utilize their personal strengths and attributes to bring about positive change. According to Dunst, Trivette, and Deal (1988), being empowered increases feelings of control that promote competence and positive action. Lee (2001) makes the point that empowerment is something that is inherent in an individual; it is not something "given" to another. However, perceptions of empowerment can become dormant when one is oppressed, discriminated against, or experiences social stigma. Kieffer (1984) notes when individuals believe they are *disempowered*, they may experience feelings of hopelessness and lack trust. To revitalize a sense of power, Gutierrez and Lewis (1999) suggest a "psychological transformation" for interpreting life events is required (p. 6). What is critical in the transformation process, according to the authors, is the full participation of individuals to recognize needs and their sources, to develop a sense of confidence in solving problems, and to share experiences within a supportive social network.

Hodges, Burwell and Ortega (1998) expounded on empowerment perspectives within a family context. They state, "Collaborative relationships, capacity building and connections to extended family networks are central themes of family empowerment" (p. 149). The authors suggest family-based collective action allows all members to use their talents and assets to address barriers to family well-being. A role of empowerment practitioners is to help families recognize and use their varied sources of strength, to target their inner "powers" for positive change.

Clarifying how African-American custodial grandparents are empowered is notable because social and economic disparities exacerbate their sense of lost power as many of them struggle to manage multiple and difficult life challenges, with restricted resources. Social oppression, economic marginality, and discrimination among caregivers of color are important contexts that enhance feelings of lost power, which practitioners cannot ignore. Although, many African-American grandparents may experience feeling disempowered, most assume their parenting responsibilities with considerable hope and optimism.

Published studies on empowerment practices with custodial grandparents are limited. Several authors suggest grandparent caregivers were empowered when they recognized their own inner strengths, took an active role in the decision making process for setting priorities, and collaborated with service providers as partners to resolve issues (Cox, 2008; Graves & Shelton, 2007; Joslin, 2009). Their findings are based on descriptive studies, with small sample sizes (less than 30 participants), using group service models singularly, and qualitative outcome measures (Okazawa-Rey, 1998; Cox, 2002; Joslin, 2009).

For the purposes of this study, empowerment is a positive, collaborative process between grandparents and service providers. Grandparents view service providers as partners, rather than adversaries; grandparents are seen as "experts" and have influence and authority over service decisions. Specific empowerment-focused outcomes are *self-efficacy, knowledge building, and advocacy engagement. Self-efficacy* is feeling one has the capacity to control/modify their environment for one's own benefit, or the benefit of others; *knowledge building* is receiving shared information about new or existing services/benefits, including how to access and use them effectively; finally, *advocacy engagement* is the individual or collective action to promote institutional response to meet expressed needs.

Perceived social support and community resources are frequently studied in grandparent studies (Butler & Zakari, 2005; Gerard & Roe, 2006; Gladstone & Fitzgerald, 2009; Sands & Goldberg-Glen, 2000). Some studies have recognized the importance of perceived social support and community resources as it relates to psychological well-being (Kelley, Whitley, Sipe, & Yorker, 2000). They provide information on separate expressions of family functioning, and draw conclusions just short of stating the participants are "empowered" if they experienced enhanced perceptions of social support and community resources following an intervention. The present study will conduct a correlation analysis exploring if there is a possible link between perceptions of empowerment with perceived family support and community resources with a sample of African-American grandparents.

Program Description

Project Healthy Grandparents (PHG) is an intervention model for custodial grandparents raising grandchildren in parent-absent households in the Atlanta metropolitan area. The program draws upon the resiliency model of family stress, adjustment, and adaptation (McCubbin, Thompson, & McCubbin, 1996) to conceptualize the influence of stressors on family systems. A stated goal of the program is to *empower* grandparents by increasing their personal attributes to manage individual and family circumstances. Specific objectives were to help grandparents to: (1) gain a sense of control over difficult life challenges; (2) work collaboratively with service providers to obtain needed resources; and (3) advocate for necessary individual and community-based support services to address family needs. The core service design included social work/nursing case management, monthly support groups, parent education classes, and referrals to legal services. A full description of program services is available in previous publications (See Whitley, White, Kelley, & Yorker, 1999). In brief, the case management service was a collaborative process between the social workers/nurses and grandparents to determine appropriate service referrals, and facilitate problem resolution and action plans. Both nurses and social workers used a strengths-based perspective to identify needs, provide individualized support, introduce new and existing community-based services, and help link grandparents to necessary social, legal and medical resources (Saleeby, 1997). Social workers completed a minimum of two home visits per month, while nurses completed a minimum of one home visit per month. Grandparents received case management services for 12 months; families needing extended case management services following their 12-month participation in PHG received a referral to another service provider.

Participants were offered monthly support group meetings and parent education sessions. Facilitated by a social worker, the support groups and parent education sessions served as primary resources for information sharing, knowledge building, parenting skill development, peer support, and socialization. During the group meetings, grandparents had the opportunity to share their personal stories, which helped to affirm their collective identity and enhanced group cohesion. Grandparents were able to attend any group meeting without any time restrictions. Transportation to group meeting sites was available through the program.

Partnering with other community-based agencies and organizations, additional services provided to families included legal referrals, early child development screenings and evaluations, and material aid distribution (e.g., food, clothing, furniture, toys). There were opportunities for grandparents to participate in community-wide advocacy initiatives. Over the course of the program's operation, grandparents met with county administrators, state legislators, and participated in national advocacy activities sponsored by AARP and Generations United.

Participant Description

Custodial grandparents were eligible for participation in PHG if they were raising one or more grandchildren, aged birth to 16 years, in parent-absent households. Only grandmothers and great-grandmothers participating in the project were included in the current study (generally referred to as grandmothers); grandfathers were eligible to receive program services, but their numbers were too small for comparative statistical analysis. Race was not an inclusion criterion for the study; however, the program's service boundaries were limited to participants residing in one of two counties in the Atlanta area. The racial makeup in those counties was predominately African-American. A variety of community agencies, including health care clinics, child care centers, schools, churches, and child welfare agencies referred families to PHG. All families entered the program voluntarily; formal or informal custodial grandparents were eligible for participation. An institutional review board approved the research protocol; all participants signed letters of informed consent agreeing to participate in case management services, at a minimum.

Data Collection Procedures

Data collection occurred at two time points: *project entry* before the receipt of any services, and *project exit* after 12 months of service participation. Using computer-assisted data collection procedures, trained research assistants collected data in the grandparents' homes; they read all questions to grandparents because the average educational attainment was less than high school. Data collectors downloaded the final datasets into SPSS for later descriptive and comparative statistical analysis.

Measures

Grandparents' perceptions of empowerment, family support, and community resources were measured using standardized scales.

The Family Empowerment Scale (FES) is a 34-item rating scale designed to measure levels of perceived empowerment in parents of children with disabilities (Koren, DeChillo, & Friesen, 1992). The FES is comprised of three dimensions (family, service, and community/political systems) within four subscales (advocacy, knowledge, competence, and self-efficacy). The scale's original item wordings reflected its focus on parents as caregivers; the word "grandparents" and "grandchild(ren)" were substituted for "parents" and "child(ren)" to reflect the sample group. Responses were rated on a 5-point Likert-type scale (1 = *not true at all*, 5 = *very true*), higher scores indicating greater perceived empowerment. Scores range from 12–60 for the family and service dimensions; 10–50 for the community/political dimension. Psychometric analyses indicated the FES has good test-retest reliability. Internal consistency coefficients ranged from .87 to .88; test-retest scores ranged from .77 to .85 (Koren et al., 1992; Singh & Curtis, 1995). Kappa coefficients were computed from independent ratings of scale items made on the basis of defined dimensions; results were .83, .70, and .77 for the family, service system, and community/political categories, respectively, the overall coefficient was .77 (Koren et al., 1992).

The Family Resource Scale (FRS) (Dunst & Leet, 1987; Dunst, Trivette, & Deal, 1988) measures caregivers' perceptions regarding the adequacy of family resources. The FRS is a 31-item, self-report Likert-type scale and is derived from a conceptual framework that predicts that an inadequacy of resources will negatively impact personal well-being and parental commitment. Items refer to specific resources and are rated on a 5-point scale from 1 (*does not apply*) to 5 (*almost always adequate*). The total score is obtained by adding the score for each item, with higher scores indicating more resources. A total score is obtained by adding the scores for the items. The FRS has been used by numerous researchers examining the resources available to low-income, African-American families with children. The measure has good internal consistency (.92) and test-retest reliability (.52).

The Family Support Scale (FSS) (Dunst & Trivette, 1989) measures the helpfulness of sources of support to families raising children. The FSS includes 18 items that are rated on a 5-point scale from 1 (*not at all helpful*) to 5 (*extremely helpful*). A total score is obtained by adding the score for each item. Higher scores are indicative of increased social support. The measure has strong validity and reliability. The FSS has been used by numerous researchers examining social support in low-income, African-American families with children.

Demographic Form (DF). Background information on grandparents, including educational attainment, employment status, reasons for parenting, as well as information on the grandchildren (e.g., number of grandchildren in household, ages of grandchildren) was obtained on each participant.

Analysis

A sample of 311 grandmothers receiving intervention services from Project Healthy Grandparents completed the Family Empowerment, Family Resource, and Family Support scales. Demographic data indicate participants were African-American grandmothers (95.5%), or great-grandmothers (4.5%). The grandmothers ranged in age from 36 to 83 years, with a mean of 56.8 years. Only 13.5% of the grandmothers reported to be married at the time of the study. Nearly 45% of the participants did not have a high school diploma, and 29.6% worked outside the home. Collectively, the grandmothers were raising

Table 16.1 Paired Samples *t*-Test for FES Dimensions ($n = 311$, $df = 310$)

	Pre-intervention Mean (SD)	*Post-intervention Mean (SD)*	t-*test*
Family	53.1 (5.9)	54.3 (5.7)	3.5*
Service System	52.9 (6.5)	54.5 (5.9)	4.1*
Community/Political	33.7 (8.8)	38.4 (7.7)	9.5*

Note: *$p < .001$

Table 16.2 Paired Sample *t*-Test for FES Subscales ($n = 311$, $df = 310$)

FES Subscales	*Pre-intervention Mean (SD)*	*Post-intervention Mean (SD)*	t-*test*
FES—Advocacy	23.3 (7.3)	26.4 (6.5)	7.8*
FES—Knowledge	32.9 (7.7)	36.3 (6.8)	7.8*
FES—Competence	28.8 (3.5)	29.0 (3.5)	1.0
FES—Self-efficacy	20.8 (3.3)	21.5 (2.9)	3.3*

Note: *$p > .001$

721 grandchildren, ranging in age 1–8 years. On average, the grandmothers were caring for 2.3 children per family. The primary reasons for raising their grandchildren include all forms of parental child maltreatment (74%), parental substance abuse (63%), and neglect (61%). In many cases, the grandmothers reported multiple reasons they were raising their grandchildren.

Table 16.1 presents the descriptive results on the three independent dimensions of the Family Empowerment Scale. Based on the measured responses, participants' experienced comparable increases in the dimensions of family management, service systems, and community/political involvement, ($p \leq .01$).

Statistical results for the four FES subscales are shown in Table 16.2. The findings suggest the participants' sense of advocacy ($p < .00$), knowledge ($p < .00$), and self-efficacy ($p < .00$) increased significantly. Only their sense of competence did not improve following their participation in the program.

Table 16.3 shows the comparisons on the family support and family resource measures. Data results suggest grandparents experienced enhanced perceptions of family resources and social support following their participation in the program ($p \leq .01$). Finally, to determine if there was a relationship among the studied variables, a correlation analysis of family empowerment with family support (.21) and family resource (.21) showed a relatively weak, but statistically significant correlation ($p < .01$).

Table 16.3 Univariate Statistics for Family Scales ($n = 311$, $df = 1{,}310$)

	Pre-test	*Post-test*	t-*test*	p
Family Resources				
M	99.44	104.96	7.0	.000
SD	18.43	17.83		
Family Social Support				
M	24.26	28.68	5.6	.000
SD	9.97	10.94		

Qualitative Responses

To continue to demonstrate how PHG impacted grandparents, a focus group of six current/former participants shared their viewpoints on the empowering aspects of participating in the program. Facilitated by a third party, questions were framed around experiences with project staff and peers, reactions to service units, and changes in personal and family circumstances attributed to the program's services. All focus group participants were grandmothers, ranging in age from 45–70 years. The grandmothers were raising an average of two grandchildren, ranging in age 6–17 years at the time of the focus group meeting. Each participant signed a consent form and received $20.00 for their time. The program provided transportation to the focus group site.

In speaking with the grandmothers in the focus group, one immediately realizes the absolute commitment and dedication the grandmothers have toward their grandchildren. One grandparent remarked how taking in her grandchildren affected her marriage:

> I have six kids, plus I have three daughters of my own at home . . . he doesn't want to be a part of the girls' lives . . . So he left and I said goodbye. So I lost a marriage, but I wasn't even concerned about it. I was concerned about my grandkids.

Yet in spite of the challenges, the grandmothers spoke about specific empowering effects on their lives and the lives of their grandchildren that occurred because of their participation in the program. Major themes that emerged from the focus group discussion included the concepts of self-efficacy, knowledge building/skill development, and engagement/advocacy,

Self-Efficacy

The grandmothers had many positive comments about the program, including the staff and the service units. They spoke about the positive life changes that occurred because of their participation in the program. Gaining control of their lives is an essential outcome that many participants try to achieve. While the grandmothers understood the importance of gaining control of their personal and family challenges, they did not always have the appropriate information or had an awareness of the urgency to control certain aspects of their lives for the sake of their grandchildren. One grandmother spoke about her health and the support from program nurses to manage her chronic illness. She stated:

> I am a diabetic. The nurse comes to my house and she taught me how I was not eating right. I knew that I was not doing right, but with the stress, I just did not care. But she helped me to understand that if I do not take care of myself, who was going to take care of my grandchildren. So she told me things like I was not drinking enough water. I told her I did not like water. She said it was not a matter of liking it but what I needed to do for my grandchildren, so I started drinking more water. They also told me how to cook and what to eat to keep my diabetes under control. I used to be on high blood pressure medicine, but I am not on it anymore. My doctor says I am doing well so I do not have to be on it anymore. That was because of [the program].

Another grandmother spoke about how participating in the program helped to keep her focused on her parenting responsibilities. She stated:

> [the program] has helped me not only with self-esteem but with . . . keeping me focused on [my grandson] as far as making sure that I take care of [him] . . . Because they say things and tell me things as far as making sure I stay focused, making sure I take care of myself. And it's all about I have to make sure I take care of myself because, like I said, that's it. Who is going to be there to take care of them? So I have to take care of myself, as well as them. I'm just looking out for them.

Knowledge-Building/Skill Development

Knowledge and skill building are essential elements of the empowerment process. Grandmothers spoke about what they learned from individual meetings with project staff and during group meetings. One grandmother spoke about the support group meetings:

> The meetings were most helpful, so much to educate us, help us. We received information on financial aid to teach us how to budget, get credit, how to save, how to purchase a home, how to maintain good credit, save money.

Another grandmother who is raising a teenage grandson, stated:

> I had problems with my older grandson; his attitude was a problem; he did not want to listen to me; his grades went down. But I learned how to talk to him, to be firm with love, discipline with love. I talked to him

> about where would he be without me. After our talking, his attitude changed, his grades improved. He graduated from high school and got a band scholarship. So he is doing much better.

Finally, another grandmother spoke about how the program informed her about other services and programs in the broader community. She stated:

> They let me know there is information out there that I can get instead of just saying I can handle things better on my own. There are places out there that you can go and try out different things. It's truly helped me.

Engagement and Advocacy

Several grandmothers spoke about how they became advocates for themselves, their grandchildren, and for the program. One grandmother stated:

> I tell other grandparents about the program. I brought in 3 new grandparents to the program; identified two other grandparents for the program also . . . I also enjoy meeting with other grandparents. I had other grandparents come to my home to visit and I visited them at their homes. I talk on the telephone with other grandparents about once or twice per month.

Another grandmother spoke about the process that helped her to become self-reliant and independent:

> Since I was in [the program], I learned how to ask questions. In the first year in the program, they do not leave you alone. The social workers and the nurses come to your home and help you with anything you need. They provide transportation and everything, until you become an adult, until you can stand alone. They put a great foundation in me so that I can do great things on my own . . .

One grandmother spoke passionately about the need to take individual responsibility and actively used any information provided by program staff. Her statements characterized the concept of empowerment:

> I have two grandchildren that are with me and to me I have got a lot out of the program. They have a lot of interesting people that come in and tell you [things]. The thing about it is you've got to make these things happen. They are not going to happen on their own. So when you get the information that they have to offer, you've got to put it to use. You've got to make it happen, it's got to come. The only way that the program can be successful is that the information you have, whatever information it is, you've got to make it happen.

Discussion

The findings from the present study suggest custodial grandparents experienced an enhanced perception of empowerment following their participation in a comprehensive, interdisciplinary program. According to statements from focus group members, grandparents valued PHG services because it helped them to acquire new knowledge, attain a level of self-efficacy, and learn how to advocate for themselves and their grandchildren. Prior to participating in the PHG, grandparents spoke about their being so overwhelmed with focusing on the immediate needs of their grandchildren that they often neglected their own needs, and failed to recognize their innate strengths. Yet in spite of their challenges, grandparents viewed having their grandchildren living with them as positive; they did not see their grandchildren as a source of strain. They expressed a total commitment to their grandchildren, and were willing to make any necessary sacrifices to support them. Any acknowledged strains were the results of weakened relationships with other family members, or associated with a lack of access to needed services or resources.

According to early theorists, knowledge building, self-efficacy, and engagement in advocacy are recognized features of the empowerment process (Cox & Parsons, 1996; Ozer & Bandura, 1990). PHG incorporates these attributes within program services. Early in the case management process and during monthly group meetings, grandparents acquired new knowledge about community-based services previously unknown to them, or viewed as inconsequential (e.g., mutual support from a neighbor, material aid from a local church). Acknowledging and drawing upon newly recognized resources to address needs is a starting point toward empowerment. In addition, grandparents received individualized "coaching" from their assigned nurses and social workers, as well as coaching from their peers during group sessions. Program staff helped grandparents to recognize and use their positive assets to address challenges, to develop/refine problem-solving skills that may benefit them over the long term. Grandparents, during group sessions, often instructed peers about accessing community services, becoming skilled in asking service providers questions, learning how to manage difficult family situations, or navigating service delivery systems.

The FES self-efficacy subscale scores increased between pre and posttest. Interestingly, the differences on the subscales over time were not dramatic, possibly suggesting participants had an unrecognized level of control over their family situations. Grandparents sometimes remarked that they often were not aware of how they compared with other families until they interacted with them during the monthly group meetings. During that time there was often the realization that their situations were not as severe as previously believed. It is possible that gaining a perspective about their family situation, when compared to others, validated their actions. Statements from the focus group session illustrated the subscale results. The grandparents spoke eloquently about how they gained control over specific elements of their lives. Various statements noted how they gained control of personal health problems, emotional stresses, and grandchild behaviors.

Lorraine Gutierrez (1995) defined empowerment as "the process of increasing personal, interpersonal, or political power so that individuals, families, and communities can take action to improve their situations" (p. 229). Taking direct action to improve one's situation or influence the institutions they depend upon is the heart of the advocacy attribute of empowerment. Based on the FES subscale, significant increases from pretest to posttest were evident. Statements from the focus groups provided some insight into how participants exhibited advocacy skills. Grandparents spoke about engaging other grandparents to enroll in the program, self-advocating with service providers, and taking an active role in using acquired information to bring about positive change. This is an area requiring more in-depth description and analysis with a broader representation of program participants.

The one FES subscale that did not show statistical significance is competency. There are several possible explanations for this result. First, program staff worked with grandparents to enhance skills to promote family well-being. Grandparents might have practiced various skills in their home setting or within the safe environment of the group setting. However, they may not have had adequate opportunities to execute their new skills in real situations. Secondly, in some complex situations involving various service institutions, professional intervention was required to bring about positive change, disallowing grandparents to demonstrate their skills independently. Finally, it is likely participants needed additional time to master certain skills. Since the full service intervention was in effect for 12 months, participants may need to experience additional opportunities to "practice" their skills with successful outcomes before a sense of competency is obtained.

The results from the Family Resource and Family Support scales suggest the grandparents did experience enhanced perceptions of support and community resources, a knowledge building benefit. However, the weak correlations with the Family Empowerment scale suggests to use measures of perceived community resources and family support are not adequate as surrogates for an empowerment measure. Clearly, the concept of empowerment is more complex than simply enhancing one's perceptions about family support and community resources. As noted by Vanderslice (1994), the empowerment process requires active participation. It is not enough to have participants passively receive information from service providers, even when such information addresses immediate needs.

Future Directions for Research and Practice

The present study provided a perspective of empowerment that extends earlier works on empowerment research and practice. Our findings suggest a multidisciplinary program with home-based services appears to have a positive effect on perceptions of empowerment. But there are additional inquiries needed. The population of grandparents in the current study was a homogeneous group. A more diverse group of grandparent caregivers will provide insight on how the program promotes empowerment among participants varying on income, race, residential locality, and various dimensions of grandparent caregiving (e.g., raising grandchildren with special needs, raising grandchildren while caring for elderly parents, comparisons between oldest grandparents vs. young grandparents).

Varying the program design also provides an area of future study. Must grandparents participate in all aspects of the service intervention to acquire a sense of empowerment? Are support groups adequate to help grandparents enhance their sense of empowerment? Is there a difference in the process of empowerment if a grandparent only participates in case management vs. group support? For which grandparents is the full complement of services necessary to become empowered? Answers to these types of questions require further study, preferably using a mixed-methods design.

Social and familial factors that predict family empowerment is another line of future study. Previous studies suggest parental stress, employment, and family functioning are associated with empowerment among families raising children with emotional needs (Scheel & Reickmann, 1998). In addition, future study designs that include randomization and control/comparison groups, as well as extended qualitative methods, will only strengthen the initial positive results presented in this study.

The findings in this study provide some thoughts for practitioners working with grandparent-headed families. Program services that include individualized case management were positively acknowledged by focus group participants; similarly support groups also had a positive response. Both of these services acknowledge and/or utilize personal and familial strengths to address life challenges. Practitioners should consider if providing one or both of these services is feasible and beneficial for custodial grandparents in their communities. Providing home-based programs would service the needs of isolated families unable to travel to office locations; similarly offering transportation to grandparents with limited travel accommodations to attend group meetings broadens the potential outreach to families who may attend support groups. Giving grandparents new knowledge about existing community resources is another important feature of the described program that potentially enhanced perceptions of grandparent empowerment. Service delivery systems are constantly changing benefit levels, eligibility requirements, service hours and locations, making it difficult for families to know when or how to access systems of care. Practitioners may create innovative communication strategies (e.g., newsletters, peer exchanges, face book pages) that support information sharing and dissemination. Finally, it is essential practitioners provide opportunities for grandparents to acquire and use empowerment skill sets (asking questions of providers, comparing alternative services, creating a collective voice with peers) to be effective self-advocates. In every community, practitioners can collaborate with child welfare or aging services to help custodial grandparents find their collective voice to address community-wide issues.

While the described service program focused on empowering the dyadic relationship between the grandmother and the grandchild, practitioners also need to acknowledge the whole family system. In fact, the grandmothers in the focus group spoke very little about their relationships with other family members, what support they received from them, if their relationship changed in any way since raising their grandchildren. The empowerment process may be hampered if there is tremendous stress and conflict between grandparent couples, or other family members, as a result of raising grandchildren in the household. Practitioners may need to explore familial relationships when working with grandparents, to learn how both grandparents, step-grandparents, or other family members define/redefine their roles and relationships when assuming the care of grandchildren. Practitioners may have to help family members, especially marital couples, transition into their new roles, and determine what the new roles mean for their relationship with spouses, other grandchildren not living in the household, or other family members. Reducing potential areas of family stress and conflict promotes a family environment that is supportive, nurturing and potentially enhances empowerment among all family members.

Conclusion

It is encouraging to know that grandparents who are raising grandchildren under very difficult circumstances view their responsibilities with a positive sense of commitment to their grandchildren, and a great deal of optimism for themselves, their families, and the community of grandparent caregivers. Interdisciplinary interventions incorporating varied service strategies, within a collaborative context, provide a means to empower grandparent caregivers, to help them reach their inner power to transform their families, as well as others. As noted by one grandparent "People can change from support; . . . if I can help one [person], then my living won't be in vain."

References

Butler, F. R., & Zakari, N. (2005). Grandparents parenting grandchildren: Assessing health status, parental stress and social supports. *Journal of Gerontological Nursing, 3*(3), 43–54.

Chadiha, L. A., Adams, P., Biegel, D., Auslaner, W., & Gutierrez, L. (2004). Empowering African American women informal caregivers: A literature synthesis and practice strategies. *Social Work, 49*(1), 97–108.

Cox, C. (2002). Empowering African American custodial grandparents. *Social Work, 47*(1), 45–54.

Cox, C. (2008). Empowerment as an intervention with grandparent caregivers. *Journal of Intergenerational Relationships, 6*(4), 465–477.

Cox, E., & Parsons, R. (1996). Empowerment-oriented social work practice: Impact on late life relationships of women. *Journal of Women & Aging, 8*, 3–4.

Dannison, L. L., & Smith, A. B. (2003). Custodial grandparents community support program: Lessons learned. *Children and Schools, 25*(2), 87–95.

Dowdell, E. B. (1995). Caregiver burden: Grandmothers raising their high risk grandchildren. *Journal of Psychosocial Nursing, 33*, 27–30.
Dunst, C. J., & Leet, H. E. (1987). Measuring the adequacy of resources in households with young children. *Child Care, Health, and Development, 13*, 111–125.
Dunst, C. J., & Trivette, C. M. (1989). Toward experimental evaluation of the family, infant, and pre-school program. In H. Weiss & F. Jacobs (Eds.), *Evaluating family programs* (pp. 315–346). New York: Aldine Publishing.
Dunst, C. J., Trivette, C. M., & Deal, A. G. (1988). *Enabling and empowering families: Principles and guidelines for practice.* Cambridge, MA: Brookline Books.
Freire, P. (1983). *Pedagogy of the oppressed.* New York: Seabury Press.
Fuller-Thomson, E. & Minkler, M. (2000). The mental and physical health of grandmothers who are raising their grandchildren. *Journal of Mental Health and Aging, 6*, 311–323.
Gerard, J. M., & Roe, J. G. (2006). Grandparents raising grandchildren: the role of social support in coping with caregiving challenges. *International Journal of Aging and Human Development, 62*(4), 359–383.
Gladstone, J., & Fitzgerald, K. (2009). Grandparents raising their grandchildren: Tensions, service needs and involvement with child welfare agencies. *International Journal of Aging and Human Development, 68*(1), 55–78.
Graves, K. N., & Shelton, T. L. (2007). Family empowerment as a mediator between family-centered systems of care and changes in child functioning: Identifying an important mechanism of change. *Journal of Child and Family Studies, 16*, 556–566.
Gutierrez L. M. (1995). Understanding the empowerment process: Does consciousness make a difference? *Social Work Research, 19*, 229–237.
Gutierrez, L. M., & Lewis, E. A. (1999). *Empowering women of color.* New York, NY: Columbia University Press.
Hodges, V. G., Burwell, Y., & Ortega, D. (1998). Empowering families. In L. Gutierrez, R. Parsons & E. Cox (Eds.), *Empowerment in social work practice: A sourcebook* (pp. 146–162). California: Brooks/Cole Publishing Company.
Joslin, D. (2009). Custodial grandparent empowerment: Models of practice. *Families in Society, 90*(2), 196–204.
Kelley, S. J., Whitley, D. M., & Campos, P. E. (2010). Grandmothers raising grandchildren: Results of an intervention to improve health outcomes. *Journal of Nursing Scholarship, 42*(4), 379–386.
Kelley, S. J., Whitley, D. M., & Sipe, T. A. (2007). Results of an interdisciplinary intervention to improve the psychosocial well-being and physical functioning of African American grandmothers raising grandchildren. *Journal of Intergenerational Relationships, 5*, 45–64.
Kelley, S. J., Whitley, D., Sipe, T. A., & Yorker, B. C. (2000). Psychological distress in grandmother kinship care providers: The role of resources, social support, and physical health. *Child Abuse and Neglect: The International Journal, 24*, 311–321.
Kieffer, C. H. (1984). Citizen empowerment: A developmental perspective. *Prevention in Human Services, 3*, 9–36.
Koren, P. E., DeChillo, N., & Friesen, B. J. (1992). Measuring empowerment in families whose children have emotional disabilities: A brief questionnaire. *Rehabilitation Psychology, 37*, 305–321.
Landry-Meyer, L., Gerard, J. M., & Guzell, J. R. (2005). Caregiver stress among grandparents raising grandchildren: The functional role of social support. *Marriage & Family Review, 37*(1/2), 171–190.

Lee, J. (2001). *The empowerment approach to social work practice: Building the beloved community*. New York: Columbia University Press.

McCallion, P., Janicki, M., Grant-Griffin, L., & Kolomer, S. (2000). Grandparent carers II: Service needs and service provision issues. *Journal of Gerontological Social Work, 33*, 57–85.

McCubbin, H. I., Thompson, A. E., & McCubbin, M. A. (1996). Resiliency in families: A conceptual model of family adjustment and adaptation in response to stress and crisis. In *Family assessment: Resiliency, coping, and adaptation*. Madison, WI: University of Wisconsin Publishers.

Okazawa, Rey, M. (1998). Empowering poor communities of color: A self-help model. In L. Gutierrez, R. Parsons, & E. Cox (Eds.), *Empowerment in social work practice: A sourcebook* (pp. 52–64). California: Brooks/Cole Publishing Company.

Ozer, E., & Bandura, A. (1990). Mechanisms governing empowerment effects: A self-efficacy analysis. *Journal of Personality and Social Psychology, 58*(3), 472–486.

Parsons, R. (1991). Empowerment: Purpose and practice principle in social work. *Social Work with Groups, 14*(2), 7–21.

Poindexter, C. C., & Linsk, N. (1999). HIV-related stigma in a sample of HIV-affected older female African American caregivers. *Social Work, 44*(1), 46–61.

Rappaport, J. (1987). Terms of empowerment/exemplars of prevention: Toward a theory for community psychology. *American Journal of Community Psychology, 15*(2), 121–149.

Sands, R., & Goldberg-Glen, R. (2000). Factors associated with stress among grandparents raising their grandchildren. *Family Relations, 49*(1), 97–105.

Saleeby, D. (Ed.) (1997). *The strengths perspective in social work practice* (2nd ed.). New York: Longman Publishers.

Scheel, M. J., & Rieckmann, T. (1998). An empirically derived description of self-efficacy and empowerment for parents of children identified as psychologically disordered. *American Journal of Family Therapy, 26*, 15–27.

Simmons, T., & Dye, J. L. (2003). Grandparents living with grandchildren: *2000* (Census 2000 Brief No. C2KBR-31). Retrieved from Census Bureau website: http://www.census.gov/prod/2003pubs/c2kbr-31.pdf.

Singh, N., & Curtis. W. (1995). Psychometric analysis of the family empowerment scale. *Journal of Emotional & Behavioral Disorders, 3*(2), 85–92.

Solomon, B. B. (1976). *Black empowerment: social work in oppressed communities*. New York: Columbia University Press.

Vanderslice, V. (1984). Empowerment: A definition in progress. *Human Ecology Forum, 14*(1), 2–3.

Vega, W., Noble, A., Kolody, B., Perter, P., Hwang, J., & Bole, A. (1993). Prevalence and magnitude of prenatal substance exposures in California. *New England Journal of Medicine, 329*, 850–954.

Waldrop, D., & Weber, J. (2001). From grandparent to caregiver: The stress and satisfaction of raising grandchildren. *Families in Society, 82*, 461–472.

Whitley, D. M., Kelley, S. J., & Campos, P. E. (2011). Perception of family empowerment in African American custodial grandmothers raising grandchildren: Thoughts for research and Practice. *Families in Society, 92*(4), 110–119. doi: 10.1606/1044-3894.4148.

Whitley, D., Kelley, S., & Sipe. (2001) Grandmothers raising children: Are they at increased risk of health problems? *Health and Social Work, 26*(2), 105–114.

Whitley, D. M., White, K. R., Kelley, S. J., & Yorker, B. (March/April, 1999). Strengths-based case management: The application to grandparents raising grandchildren. *Families in Society, 80*(2), 110–119.

Epilogue

Bert Hayslip Jr. and Gregory C. Smith

Resilience and Grandparent Caregivers: Assuming the Positive

The study of resilience began over three decades ago when developmental researchers began to notice positive adaptation among subgroups of children who were considered "at risk" for developing later psychopathology. Indeed, it could be argued that interest in resilience among adults and older persons has been driven by the Positive Psychology movement (Seligman & Csikszentmihalyi, 2000). Specific examples of the application of resilience to later life are found in discussions of strength-based approaches to counseling and therapy (Arean & Huh, 2006; Ronch & Goldfield, 2003), grief and bereavement (Moore & Stratton, 2002; Stroebe, Hansson, Schut, & Stroebe, 2008), dying (Nakashima & Canda, 2005), and the notion of cognitive reserve capacity (Staudinger, Marsiske, & Baltes, 1993).

Given the above shift in our orientation toward the study of adults and older persons, we argue that an awareness of resilience's potential contribution to the study of grandfamilies is *necessary* to (1) better understand grandparent caregivers and the grandchildren they are raising and to 2) improving the quality of their lives (Hayslip, Davis, Neumann, Goodman, Smith, Maiden, & Carr, this volume). Likewise, acknowledging resilience's potential in this respect not only has implications for the development of prevention and intervention efforts designed for grandfamilies, but it may also influence public policy and social programs whose goal is to improve psychosocial and health-related outcomes for grandparent caregivers and their grandchildren.

How Should We Understand Resilience in Grandparent Caregivers?

In this volume, we have attempted to understand resilience as a *personal characteristic* as well as in terms of *relationships with others*, and *resources available* in the broader environment. In addition, we have presented numerous examples of interventions designed to foster resilience in grandparent caregivers. In doing so, we acknowledge that grandparent caregiver resilience is complex, and recognize that such resilience needs to be understood in terms of the risks and adversities of caregiving, protective factors that are at once personal and social in nature that buffer grandparents in the face of the difficulties they may face in raising their grandchildren, and the positive outcomes that are associated with resilience. Thus, resilience may lead to better caregiver functioning and adjustment, or result from it. Likewise, it may be that focusing on the behaviors that persons display in coping with caregiving is as important in understanding resilience as is viewing it as an individual attribute that grandparents possess in varying degrees.

Irrespective of age, resilience has typically been defined as a pattern of positive (or the avoidance of negative) adaptation in the context of past or present adversity or risk that poses a substantial threat to healthy adjustment (Rutter, 2007). As there are many paths to resilience and grandparent caregivers are indeed quite different from one another in many ways (Hayslip & Patrick, 2006), it is not surprising that Zuckerman and Maiden (this volume) stress the importance of "doing it your way" in becoming more resilient. This idiosyncratic path to resilience is reflected in the multiple themes underlying the development of resilience identified by Bailey, Letiecq, Erikson, and Koltz (this volume), e.g., positive appraisal/acceptance of the new family, being a survivor/never giving up, having healthy boundaries, being connected to others, adapting new routines, commitment to the grandchild.

Many chapters in this volume approach resilience as reflected a variety of individual attributes in the study and assessment of resilience. These include predispositional characteristics or personality trait(s) (Hayslip, Davis, Neumann, Goodman, Smith, Maiden, & Carr; Goodman, Scorzo, Ernandes, & Alvarez-Nunez), as well as related constructs such as resourcefulness (Zauszniewski & Musil), empowerment (Whitley, Kelley, & Campos) and benefit finding (Castillo, Henderson, & North; Conway & Consedine). Other chapters take a more dynamic approach, stressing that resilience is a *process* involving a grandparent's interactions with the environment, i.e., other grandparent caregivers, service providers, their grandchildren, their adult children (Smith & Dolbin-MacNab; Kolomer, Himmelheber, & Murray; Dolbin-MacNab, Roberto, & Finney; Fruhauf & Bundy-Fazioli). On the basis of each of these chapters' contributions, we conclude that resilience is best understood as an individual attribute *and* as an adaptive process growing out of one's interactions with the environment and others in one's life.

While Smith and Dolbin-MacNab and Bailey, Letiecq, Erickson and Koltz each stress the importance of the process of positive appraisal of one's life circumstances, other authors (James & Ferranti; Whitley, Kelley, & Campos) focus on empowerment via one's interactions with others in the family and in the community. Other examples of adaptive resilient processes are learning to ask for help from others, attending to one's health and making good decisions regarding one's health/illness, being active, making good lifestyle choices, becoming one's own advocate, developing positive, proactive coping skills, being able to seek both emotional and instrumental support from others that is timely and effective, self-care, boundary-setting, flexibility in the face of change, and the provision of support to others (James & Ferranti; Fruhauf &

Bundy-Fazioli; McCallion, Ferretti, & Kim; Dolbin-MacNab, Roberto, & Finney; Goodman, Scorzo, Ernandes, & Alarez-Nunez; Kolomer, Himmelheber, & Murray; Zauszniewski & Musil; Castillo, Henderson, & North; Bailey, Letiecq, Erickson, & Koltz).

Reflecting resilience as an ongoing process that evolves over time within persons, wherein different persons may be at different points in the development of resilience, Smith, Dannison, and James discuss the *continuum* of resilience, which varies from being overwhelmed to gaining control to being grounded, producing adaptive processes and related outcomes that are described in terms of being ineffective, being functional, and being competent, respectively. Consistent with this emphasis on the evolution of resilience is the importance of seeing the process of caregiving itself as giving rise to resilience, greater well being, and greater role satisfaction (Goodman, Scorzo, Ernandes, & Alvarez-Nunez; Kolomer, Himmelheber, & Murray; Yancura & Greenwood).

Regardless of which approach one takes to understanding resilience (possessing greater internal resilience or developing and utilizing coping skills, reflecting the operation of resilient processes), being resilient or behaving in a resilient manner each enhances the chances of a grandparent's ability to respond productively to the physical, emotional, and psychosocial challenges accompanying caregiving. Indeed, possessing greater resilience or developing resilient processes may enable one to *grow* and *prosper* in the face of adversity. In this light, it is not surprising that many of the chapters in this volume reflect themes of strength, virtue, honor, responsibility, hope, faith, a never give up attitude, flexibility, and proactivity.

The Ecology of Grandfamily Resilience

Ungar (2010) has noted that "a social ecological understanding of resilience is congruent with systemic approaches to intervention that emphasize the need to change social interactions, environmental structures, and the availability of health resources (like access to health care, safety, education, and social support) rather than just changing individuals to adapt to the threats posed to them" (p. 423). Many chapters in this volume reflect the attention necessary to understanding the ecology of resilience among grandparent caregivers, as it is reflected in an emphasis on cultural values and rituals (Yancura & Greenwood), the dynamics of the interaction between grandparent and grandchild (Goodman, Scorzo, Ernandes, & Alvarez-Nunez), or interactions with service providers (Dolbin-MacNab, Roberto, & Finney).

As is true for resilience in general (see Smith & Hayslip, 2012, pp. 3–28), grandparent caregiver resilience encompasses personal resources that interact with environmental support and constraints in producing outcomes that benefit both grandparent and grandchild. Thus, in both understanding and promoting resilience, we might consider resilience as (1) an adaptive dispositional *attribute* possessed in varying degrees by different grandparent caregivers, (2) in the context of relationships with others, to include the family as a whole, wherein families as such may be more or less resilient, (3) as a dynamic and fluid *process* stressing continual adaptation to/coping with change (Bailey, Letiecq, Erickson, & Koltz, this volume) as well as with adverse experiences per se (see Leipold & Greve, 2009), and as (4) an *outcome, derived from* one's experience in dealing with stress and adversity, i.e., "What does not kill me makes me stronger" (Nietzsche, 1888). This complex approach to grandparent caregiver resilience is reflected in the distinctions made by Zauszneiwski and Musil (this volume) between personal and social resourcefulness. It also reflects the fact that grandparents may be resilient in some respects (e.g. in dealing with the loss of a relationship with an adult child) and not others (e.g. in dealing with threats to their physical health).

How Can We Best Foster Resilience in Grandparent Caregivers?

The key elements of the resilience process are *risk/adversity; protective factors; and positive outcomes* (Smith & Hayslip, 2012, pp. 3–28). Indeed, the complexity of resilience in terms of the interaction of risk and protective factors is consistent with the conclusion that there are *many* ways to foster resilience in grandfamilies. In this respect, Hildon et al. (2010) has recommended a dual approach to practice and policy that consists of finding effective ways to minimize adversity and its impact where possible; and promoting systems and services that can deliver support when necessary. Thus, as much attention should be directed to altering the environmental context in which grandparent caregivers function as might be given to helping such persons increase resilient behaviors. This way of understanding helping efforts with grandparents is consistent with the notion of levels of intervention (Danish, 1981) and person-environment fits (Lawton & Nahemow, 1973), where our goal might be, for example, to intervene *simultaneously* with grandparents (e.g., in learning better methods of coping or in changing attitudes), service providers (e.g., in educating them about how to productively interact with the grandparents they serve), and the programs serving grandparent caregivers (e.g., in increasing access to services, removing red tape hindering the determination of one's eligibility for services). Even educating the public about the strengths grandparents bring to raising their grandchildren is a form of intervention, even though it does not directly target grandparent caregivers themselves. Many of the chapters in this volume reflect this multi-leveled perspective on fostering resilience and resilient behavior processes, and this view of intervention is underscored by the importance of the therapist's understanding and promoting a "resilience narrative" in grandparent caregivers who are at risk for adverse outcomes (Bailey, Letiecq, Erickson, & Koltz). Indeed, Dolbin-MacNab, Roberto, and Finney suggest that interventions be aimed at both the individual/proximal environmental level (altering grandparents and beliefs) and a distal environmental level (improving program accessibility and educating/training program staff).

According to Rutter (2010), the best way to minimize the impact of adversity is by developing resistance coping strategies as well as psychological and physical defense mechanisms. Along these lines, many chapters here stress the importance of key coping skills that act as protective factors to buffer grandparents in the face of adversity, and in this respect, such skills can be seen as key to either developing resilience or as enhancing factors that otherwise protect one from the negative effects of caregiving. Examples of these skills are positive appraisal (Smith & Dolbin-MacNab; Bailey, Letiecq, Erikson, & Koltz), benefit finding (Castillo, Henderson, & North; Conway & Consedine), reframing (Zuckerman & Maiden), both physical and emotional self-care (Fruhauf & Bundy-Fazioli; McCallion, Ferretti, & Kim), positive coping/stress reduction (Zauszniewski & Musil; Zuckerman & Maiden), or asking for help and support from others (Kolomer; Himmelheber & Murray; Dolbin-MacNab, Roberto, & Finney).

The development of these skills can insulate the grandparent from the negative effects of adversity, or modulate/buffer such effects in reducing their severity. These skills are all in varying degrees solution or resource-based (Smith & Dolbin-MacNab), and are consistent with the fact that resilience mediates or links the experience of stress and a variety of emotional, interpersonal, or behavioral outcomes (see Hayslip, Davis, Neumann, Goodman, Smith, Maiden, & Carr, this volume; Wallace, Bisconti, & Bergeman, 2001). Likewise, enlisting the support of others (Kolomer; Himmelheber & Murray; Dolbin-MacNab, Roberto, & Finney) can be conceived as a protective factor in minimizing adversity (see Fuller-Iglesias, Sellars, & Antonucci, 2008).

In drawing attention to the larger context in which efforts to help grandfamilies should be understood, Conway and Consedine advocate for a shift in the research agenda adopted by those who seek to understand grandfamilies as well as for a change in public policy that reflects an orientation away from a needs perspective to one emphasizing supportiveness. At a more individual level of understanding, Conway and Consedine suggest that acknowledging that one is facing adversity and that sacrifice is necessary are key to understanding resilience among grandparent caregivers.

Reflecting this "assumption of the positive" orientation to intervention is the *Skip Generation* program discussed by James and Ferrante that emphasizes self-advocacy, the benefits of mentorship to other grandparent caregivers, and finding one's inner strengths. McCallion, Ferretti, and Kim also reflect this proactive approach in describing a health education program stressing health and illness management and health promotion that is both remedial and preventative in nature. Whitley, Kelley, and Campos in describing *Project Healthy Grandparents*, take an empowerment approach that is multi-leveled in educating grandparent caregivers about how to self advocate and enhance their awareness of community resources, leading to greater self efficacy. Zuckerman and Maiden, who adapt a multigenerational family system approach to treating grandfamilies, describe a multi-layered approach that builds upon the intrinsic resilience of the grandparent in benefiting the grandchild, emphasizing such acquired skills as: reframing crises as amenable to being coped with, goal-setting, self care, self-discovery, developing positive ways of coping with stress, and learning to ask for help. Smith, Dannison, and James, in discussing the nationally organized multi-site *Grandparent Resource Site* program, stress a number of characteristics underlying the resiliency found among program participants, i.e., pride, being positive, persistence, being protective of the family, and being a good problem-solver.

Attending to Differences Among Grandparent Caregivers

As there are differences between grandparent caregivers in the extent to which they possess resilient characteristics, engage in resilient behavior processes, and interact with environments that are in varying degrees, supportive of their efforts to see life in terms of the "glass is half full", interventions to promote resilience should be carried out with these differences in mind, regardless of the level at which they are designed to be effective. In this way, not only will we be better able to understand grandparent caregivers by adopting a positive focus on their strengths, but we can more effectively work with grandfamilies to nurture hope, optimism, and growth.

References

Arean, P., & Huh, T. (2006). Problem solving therapy with older adults. In S. Qualls & B. Knight (Eds.), *Psychotherapy for depression in older adults* (pp. 133–151). New York: Wiley.

Danish, S. (1981). Life-span development and intervention: A necessary link. *Counseling Psychologist, 9*, 40–43.

Fuller-Iglesias, Sellars, B., & Antonucci, T. (2008). Resilience in old age: Social relations as a protective factor. *Research in Human Development, 5*, 181–193.

Hayslip, B., & Hicks-Patrick, J. (2006). *Custodial grandparents: Individual, cultural, and ethnic diversity*. New York: Springer.

Hildon, Z., Montgomery, S. M., Blane, D., Wiggins, R. D., & Netuveli, G. (2010). Examining resilience of quality of life in the face of health-related and psychosocial adversity at older ages: What is "right" about the way we age?. *The Gerontologist, 50*, 36–47.

Lawton, M. P., & Nahemow, L. (1973). Ecology and the aging process. In C. Eisdorfer & M. P. Lawton (Eds.), *The psychology of adult development and aging* (pp. 619–674). Washington, DC: American Psychological Association.

Leipold, B., & Greve, W. (2009). Resilience: A conceptual bridge between coping and development. *European Psychologist, 14*, 40–50.

Moore, A., & Stratton, D. (2002). *Resilient widowers: Older men speak for themselves*. New York: Springer.

Nakashima, M., & Canda, E. (2005). Positive dying and resiliency in later life: A qualitative study. *Journal of Aging Studies, 19*, 109–125.

Nietzsche, F. (1888). *Twilight of the idols*.

Ronch, J., & Goldfield, J. (2003). *Mental wellness in aging: Strength-based approaches.* Baltimore: Health Professions Press.

Rutter, M. (2007). Resilience, competence, and coping. *Child Abuse & Neglect, 31,* 205–209.

Rutter, M. (August, 2010). *From individual differences to resilience: From traits to processes.* Presented at the 118th Convention of the American Psychological Association. San Diego, CA.

Seligman, M. E. P., & Csikszentmihalyi, M. (2000). Positive psychology: An introduction. *American Psychologist, 55,* 5–14.

Smith, G., & Hayslip, B. (In Press). Resilience in adulthood and later life: What is it and why arewe going? In B. Hayslip & G. Smith (Eds.), *Annual review of gerontology and geriatrics: Emerging perspectives on resilience in adulthood and later life.* New York: Springer.

Staudinger, U. M., Marsiske, M., & Baltes, P. B. (1993). Resilience and reserve capacity in later adulthood: potentials and limits of development across the lifespan. In D. Cicchetti & D. J. Cohen (Eds.), *Developmental psychopathology (Vol. 2: Risk, Disorder, and Adaptation)* (pp. 801–847). New York: Wiley.

Stroebe, M., Hansson, R., Schut, H., & Stroebe, W. (2008). Bereavement research: 21st century prospects. In M. Stroebe, R. Hansson, R. H. Schut, & W. Stroebe (Eds.), *Handbook of bereavement research and practice* (pp. 577–605). Washington, DC: American Psychological Association.

Ungar, M. (2010). Families as navigators and negotiators: Facilitating culturally and contextually specific expressions of resilience. *Family Process, 49,* 421–435.

Wallace, K., Bisconti, T., & Bergeman, C. (2001). The meditational effect of hardiness on social support and optimal outcomes in later life. *Basic and Applied Social Psychology, 23,* 267–279.

Index